THE ADOLESCENT IN FAMILY THERAPY

THE GUILFORD FAMILY THERAPY SERIES
Michael P. Nichols, Series Editor

RECENT VOLUMES

The Adolescent in Family Therapy, Second Edition:
Harnessing the Power of Relationships
Joseph A. Micucci

Essential Skills in Family Therapy, Second Edition:
From the First Interview to Termination
*JoEllen Patterson, Lee Williams, Todd M. Edwards, Larry Chamow,
and Claudia Grauf-Grounds*

Doing Couple Therapy: Craft and Creativity
in Work with Intimate Partners
Robert Taibbi

Doing Family Therapy, Second Edition:
Craft and Creativity in Clinical Practice
Robert Taibbi

Collaborative Therapy with Multi-Stressed Families,
Second Edition
William C. Madsen

Working with Families of the Poor, Second Edition
Patricia Minuchin, Jorge Colapinto, and Salvador Minuchin

Couple Therapy with Gay Men
David E. Greenan and Gil Tunnell

Beyond Technique in Solution-Focused Therapy:
Working with Emotions and the Therapeutic Relationship
Eve Lipchik

Emotionally Focused Couple Therapy with Trauma Survivors:
Strengthening Attachment Bonds
Susan M. Johnson

Narrative Means to Sober Ends:
Treating Addiction and Its Aftermath
Jonathan Diamond

Couple Therapy for Infertility
Ronny Diamond, David Kezur, Mimi Meyers, Constance N. Scharf, and Margot Weinshel

Short-Term Couple Therapy
James M. Donovan, Editor

THE ADOLESCENT IN FAMILY THERAPY

Harnessing the Power of Relationships

SECOND EDITION

JOSEPH A. MICUCCI

THE GUILFORD PRESS
New York   London

© 2009 The Guilford Press
A Division of Guilford Publications, Inc.
72 Spring Street, New York, NY 10012
www.guilford.com

Printed in the United States of America

This book is printed on acid-free paper.

Last digit is print number: 9   8   7   6   5   4   3

Library of Congress Cataloging-in-Publication Data

Micucci, Joseph A.
  The adolescent in family therapy : harnessing the power of relationships /
Joseph A. Micucci. — 2nd ed.
      p. cm. — (The Guilford family therapy series)
  Includes bibliographical references and index.
  ISBN 978-1-60623-330-6 (hardcover : alk. paper)
  1. Adolescent psychotherapy.   2. Family psychotherapy.   3. Family—
Psychological aspects.   4. Parent and teenager.   I. Title.
  RJ503.M495 2009
  616.89′140835—dc22

                                                                    2009014593

To
Dominick Micucci
(1920–1981)
for pointing me in the right direction

About the Author

Joseph A. Micucci, PhD, ABPP, received his AB in Psychology from Cornell University and his PhD in Clinical Psychology from the University of Minnesota. In 1984, he joined the staff of the Philadelphia Child Guidance Center, where he served as Director of the Adolescent Unit from 1987 to 1993 and as Chief Psychologist from 1991 to 1993. Currently, Dr. Micucci is Professor of Psychology and Chair of the Division of Psychology at Chestnut Hill College in Philadelphia, Pennsylvania. He is Director of the PsyD Program in Clinical Psychology and has taught courses in psychological assessment, adolescent development, and family therapy. Dr. Micucci is a member of the American Psychological Association and the American Family Therapy Academy, and is an Approved Supervisor for the American Association for Marriage and Family Therapy. He holds specialty board certification in Clinical Psychology from the American Board of Professional Psychology. Dr. Micucci has a private practice in Bryn Mawr, Pennsylvania.

Preface

In the decade since the first edition of *The Adolescent in Family Therapy* was published, my approach to working with adolescents and their families has continued to evolve. As in the first edition, I continue to stress the importance of family relationships in promoting optimal developmental outcomes for adolescents. While adolescents are certainly growing more independent of their families, they continue to need the affection, attention, support, and guidance of their parents in order to negotiate successfully the challenges of the second decade of life. Problems may arise when family relationships have not adapted to the adolescent's changing needs, or when parents have withdrawn their attention and support in ways that leave the adolescent feeling abandoned or isolated.

In the first edition of this book I also emphasized that clinicians who work with adolescents and their families must be familiar with the trends and themes of normal adolescent development. A developmental perspective is essential so that normal and typical behavior can be differentiated from atypical or abnormal behavior. Families sometimes overreact to behavior that is typical of adolescents in our culture, and in overreacting run the risk of exacerbating problems. On the other hand, widespread myths about "storm and stress" during adolescence can lead to reduced expectations and failure to provide the necessary guidance to an adolescent who is off track.

My work continues to be guided by the fundamental ideas of family systems theory. Symptoms tend to arise, evolve, and persist because of particular interactional patterns that become attached to the symptoms. Over time, the symptoms and the interactional patterns become inextricably linked, such that they tend to elicit and reinforce one another. I have termed this interrelationship between symptoms and patterns of interpersonal interaction the *symptomatic cycle*. Effective intervention requires an understanding of the particular form that the symptomatic cycle takes in a family and a mastery of a variety of techniques that can help replace these ineffective interactional patterns with more adaptive and flexible patterns.

Questions and comments from readers of the first edition, my students, supervisees, and attendees at workshops have guided me in writing this revised, second edition. The format of this edition follows that of the first edition. After summarizing essential points about normal adolescent development, I present my basic framework for understanding how problems arise and evolve in families. In the subsequent chapters, I apply this framework to a variety of common presenting problems. All of the chapters have been revised or expanded, some more than others. Some of the features of this revised, second edition include:

- Addition of an entirely new chapter on anxiety (Chapter 7).
- Expanded treatment of attachment issues and how they can be incorporated into family treatment.
- Expanded discussion of the development of lesbian, gay, and bisexual adolescents in Chapter 2.
- Addition of a section on racial and ethnic identity to the chapter on adolescent development (Chapter 2).
- Expanded discussion of techniques of intervention. Chapter 2 ("The Process of Therapy") from the first edition has been expanded into two chapters, one that reviews theoretical concepts, and one that describes specific techniques of intervention.
- Addition of over 200 new and updated references.
- Addition of new case examples.

A word about the case examples in this book. My intention in presenting case examples is not to offer empirical evidence for the efficacy of the principles and techniques I am advocating, but rather to provide a concrete demonstration of how these principles and techniques might be applied in situations commonly encountered by clinicians. The cases in this book are not "case studies" in the strictest sense of the term. In order to protect confidentiality, all of the cases have been extensively disguised and altered in important ways. Whenever I report dialogue from clinical sessions, the words of the family members have been paraphrased to protect their privacy and anonymity. Some of the cases are generic cases. Many of the cases are composite cases, created from clinical situations cobbled together from several cases. A few of the cases discussed in this book were not actual clinical families at all, but rather "simulated families." The latter refers to a procedure developed by my colleague Scott Browning for the purposes of training students in family therapy

(Browning, Collins, & Nelson, 2005). An experienced family therapist trains actors to portray a family and to interact as if they are actual members of a family coming for treatment. The therapist meets this "family" for the first time when they are in character, and then proceeds to conduct one or more sessions of family therapy with them as if they are an actual family. Throughout this process, the coach continues to guide the actors to remain in character and interact in ways typical of actual families in treatment. When I have been the therapist in these situations, I have found that my subjective experience is virtually identical to what I typically experience when treating families in actual clinical settings. I am grateful to Dr. Browning for his assistance in helping to create the simulated families, and I am also grateful to the actors for the time and energy they contributed to this project.

My editor at The Guilford Press, Jim Nageotte, has been a helpful presence throughout this revision project. I am also grateful to Series Editor Michael P. Nichols for his insightful comments on early drafts of some of the chapters. Mike was intensively involved in critiquing drafts of the chapters for the first edition of this book, and his influence continues to permeate this revised edition.

The ideas in this book germinated during my years at the Philadelphia Child Guidance Center (PCGC) in the 1980s and early 1990s. I am especially grateful to John Brendler and Michael Silver for all that they taught me during my tenure at PCGC. The spirit of other colleagues who contributed to the first edition continues to be present in this revised edition: Molly Hindman, Steve Simms, John Sargent, Guy Diamond, and the late Peggy Spiegel.

I am grateful to President Carol Jean Vale, SSJ, PhD, William T. Walker, PhD, and the Board of Directors of Chestnut Hill College for granting me sabbatical leave in 2005 to work on an article that evolved into the ideas presented in Chapter 8 of this revised edition. My parents and family provided me with a "secure base" that allowed me to become all that I am today.

Finally, and most important, the companionship, devotion, and encouragement of Jim Davis continue to nurture me and remind me that our close relationships form the foundation for all that we are and all that we achieve.

Contents

1 Introduction   1
My Orientation and Influences   3
Diagnosis and Labeling   4
Biology, Medications, and Systems   5
The Paradox of Control   6
Harnessing the Power of Relationships   7
The ARCH   8
Adolescents Need Nurturance   9
The Plan of This Book   11

2 Adolescent Development   12
Developmental Issues of Adolescence: An Overview   13
Early Adolescence   16
Middle Adolescence   29
Late Adolescence   45
Summary   56

3 Basic Concepts   59
A Core Assumption   59
Family Systems and Family Therapy   60
The Symptomatic Cycle   62
Consequences of the Symptomatic Cycle   64
Common Patterns in Symptomatic Families   68
The Pattern Is the Problem   71
Summary and What's Next   71

4 How to Assess and Treat Problems   73
General Principles Guiding Effective Intervention   74
How to Build an Alliance with the Family   80
How to Identify Symptomatic Cycles   82
Setting the Course for Treatment   87
Techniques for Changing Patterns   89

When to Conduct Individual Sessions   101
Benefits and Risks of Consultations   105
Summary   106

5   Eating Disorders   108
Perspectives on Eating Disorders   110
Principles of Treatment   115
Step 1: Negotiating a Treatment Contract   121
Step 2: Encouraging Parental Collaboration   125
Step 3: Addressing Unresolved Conflicts   127
Step 4: Handling Relapses   132
Step 5: Supporting Individual Development   136
Step 6: Supporting the Transformation   139
Pitfalls and Complications   141
Summary   145

6   Depression and Suicide   146
The Role of Gender in Adolescent Depression   147
Assessment of Adolescent Depression   150
Treatments for Depression   151
The Role of Family Dynamics in Adolescent Depression   153
Common Family Patterns Associated with Adolescent Depression   154
Helping Suicidal Adolescents   162
Case Example: The Crying Father   172
Summary   183

7   Anxiety   185
Anxiety and the Family   186
Cognitive Factors in Adolescent Anxiety   189
Anxiety and Abandonment   191
Freeing the Family from the Grip of Anxiety:
   A Detailed Case Example   198
Summary   216

8   Defiant and Disruptive Behavior   217
How Common Is Problem Behavior during Adolescence?   220
Developmental Perspectives   221
Factors Related to Adolescent Defiance   222
Assessing the Severity of the Problem   225
Interventions When the Problem Is Mild   228
Interventions for Moderately Severe Defiance   232
Interventions for Severe Defiance   238
Summary   253

9   Psychosis   255
Theoretical Perspectives   255
Psychosis and Isolation   258

Reducing Isolation in Psychotic Systems 261
Summary 267

**10 Underachievement and Other   269
School-Related Problems**
Factors Contributing to Adolescent Underachievement 271
Strategies for Intervention 279
Identifying and Avoiding Triangulation 291
Summary 293

11 Leaving Home   295
Perspectives on Leaving Home 297
Assessment 299
Intervention 302
Summary 304

12 Families with Multiple Problems   306
*Principles for Working with Overwhelmed,
   Low-Income Families 310*
Case Example: Two Tokens 318
Summary 321

Epilogue: The ARCH   323

References   329

Index   359

1

Introduction

Louis (age 16) is locked in a bitter battle with his father. Every discussion turns into an argument. Meanwhile, Louis's grades continue to slip and the relationship between his parents is becoming tenser.

Caleb (age 13) can't go to bed until he performs an elaborate ritual that is taking more and more time each night. His parents are afraid to stop him because he becomes terrifyingly agitated if his ritual is interrupted.

Tina (age 16) has lost over 20 pounds in the past 6 months because she won't eat. Her divorced parents, Bill and Rose, seem more interested in fighting with one another than in finding a way to help their daughter.

Jenny (age 15) ingested a handful of acetaminophen tablets minutes after what both she and her mother described as a pleasant conversation over dinner.

Keith (age 15) is staying out all night and using drugs. He threatens his parents with violence if they try to impose any restrictions or consequences. As a result, his terrified parents shrink from confronting him.

This book is about adolescents like Louis, Caleb, Tina, Jenny, and Keith. Along the way, we will meet other young people like them: Bart (age 16), whose intractable abdominal pain allowed him to say "no" to his overbearing father; Tyrone (age 17), on the verge of leaving for college, who can't seem to follow his mother's simple rules about curfew; and Tammy (age 14), whose sexual promiscuity terrified her parents. If you are a therapist who works with adolescents, the stories I tell will have a familiar ring. If you are a therapist who is looking for a compass to orient you through the sometimes frustrating journey of working with teenagers and their families, I hope to provide one in this book.

In one sense, working with adolescents is no different than working with any person who comes to us for help. The basic principles of family systems thinking that guide my work can be applied to problems that arise at any point in the human life cycle. On the other hand, work with adolescents poses particular challenges because of the developmental processes that are occurring during this period of life. For this reason, I believe that therapists who work with adolescents must be familiar with the typical developmental changes that are occurring during adolescence. In Chapter 2, I review the basics of normal adolescent development and provide guidance on how to differentiate normal adolescent behavior from atypical or problematic behavior. One of the major trends that is at the forefront during this phase of life is the push–pull between dependency and independency. How the parents and the adolescent negotiate this balance is a critical factor to determining how successful their passage through adolescence will be.

I discuss and illustrate many techniques that are useful in work with adolescents and their families. However, techniques must be embedded in a clear map for what the therapist hopes to accomplish. Techniques are like tools: The more you have, the more options for getting a job done— but you have to know what you are building first. Familiarity with a variety of techniques can give a therapist security in versatility, but relying on techniques without a formulation can lead to haphazard and reactive treatment that frustrates both the therapist and the family.

Many therapists find theories too abstract and therefore not particularly relevant to what they are trying to accomplish in their work with families. Seeing the merits in a number of different schools of therapy, many therapists consider themselves "eclectic," which usually means that they have refrained from committing themselves to a particular model. Unfortunately, eclecticism can breed hopeless confusion, leaving the practitioner a "jack of all trades, master of none," with no guidance on how to weave together ideas from a variety of theories into a coherent whole.

I hope to address this dilemma in this book by striking a balance between theory and technique. What I hope to offer are pragmatic solutions for common clinical problems. I have tried to spell out my rationale for my suggestions, and illustrate their use in clinical case examples. Sometimes, I recommend a step-by-step approach. I trust that readers will realize that steps and phases are rarely discrete or invariably sequential in all cases, and so will exercise sound clinical judgment in applying these ideas.

MY ORIENTATION AND INFLUENCES

The fundamental guiding beacon for my work is family systems theory. Thus, my focus is not on the individual alone, but on the network of relationships in which individuals participate. A basic premise of the family systems perspective is the idea that problems and symptoms occur in an interpersonal context. These problems are not internal to any single person, but rather arise and are maintained by particular, repetitive patterns of interactions among those who are in close contact with the person who exhibits the symptom or problem. I elucidate on these ideas in Chapter 3, when I discuss the concept of the *symptomatic cycle,* and in Chapter 4, when I describe a number of techniques derived from a family systems perspective.

There have been a number of important theoretical influences in my work and my thinking about adolescents and families. From structural family therapy (Minuchin, 1974, 1984; Minuchin & Fishman, 1981; Minuchin, Nichols, & Lee, 2007), I borrow many of the concepts that describe how a family is organized: subsystems, boundaries, hierarchy, and alignments. I also borrow from structural family therapy many techniques associated with this model, including joining, enactment, using complementarity, and unbalancing. I discuss these techniques in more detail in Chapter 4.

From Jay Haley (1987), I borrow the basic framework for conducting an initial session. From models of therapy termed "strategic" I borrow the idea that people get caught up in cycles that keep a problem alive, and that their efforts to solve the problem often make the problem worse (Fisch, Weakland, & Segal, 1982). From narrative therapy, I borrow the insight that language shapes our experience of reality, and the value of talking about problems as if they were external forces influencing all family members rather than defects or deficiencies within individuals (White & Epston, 1990).

My work has also been influenced by ideas that were originally developed within the context of psychodynamic theory. In particular, I find value in the work that has explored the importance of emotional attachments during the lifespan (Ainsworth, 1989; Bowlby, 1988). In particular, I believe that the emphasis on promoting adolescents' independence from parents has paid insufficient attention to the ways in which adolescents continue to need parental support and nurturance (Mackey, 1996). In this vein, I appropriate some of the ideas and methods from emotionally focused therapy (Johnson, 2004), particularly the emphasis on uncovering and emphasizing the "softer" emotions such as hurt and sadness that are often obscured behind angry interactions (see also Micucci, 2006). Also relevant in this context is the importance placed by contextual family therapy on mutual accountability and loyalties within families (Boszormenyi-Nagy & Spark, 1973).

In addition, I believe that a number of techniques that are traditionally associated with individual models of therapy could also be helpful in work with families. Many parents can benefit from training in parenting skills based on behavioral methods. There is much evidence that cognitive-behavioral techniques can be helpful in modifying symptoms of depression and anxiety (Cartwright-Hatton, Roberts, Chitsabesan, Fothergill, & Harrington, 2004; Lewinsohn, Clarke, Hops, & Andrews, 1990). Recently, attention has been given to supplementing cognitive-behavioral techniques with mindfulness and acceptance of negative feeling states (Segal, Williams, & Teasdale, 2002). These methods are not incompatible with a family systems perspective, and, in fact, integrating a family-based component with cognitive-behavioral treatments has been found to be effective in treating children and adolescents (Bogels & Siqueland, 2006; Kendall, Hudson, Gosch, Flannery-Schroeder, & Suvey, 2008).

DIAGNOSIS AND LABELING

The use of diagnostic labels from the fourth edition of the *Diagnostic and Statistical Manual of Mental Disorders* (DSM-IV-TR; American Psychiatric Association, 2000) can have value if used appropriately. Diagnostic labels can facilitate communication among therapists and help to alert therapists to aspects of a problem that might not be readily apparent from the presenting complaint. Labels such as these become problematic only when they are used to pathologize individuals and imply that the problem is "owned" by a single person rather than by the whole family. They are also problematic when they are viewed as the most important or defining characteristic of the individual, as, for example, when a parent says, "My son *is* ADD." For this reason, extreme care should be exercised when sharing diagnostic labels with families.

The same argument can be applied to the use of the term *dysfunctional* in reference to families. This term has been used to describe certain families who repeatedly engage in problematic interactions and in which a family member is symptomatic or functioning inadequately. Used in this way, the term is purely descriptive and can be innocuous. Unfortunately, the term can also be used to label or pathologize families in the same way that individual diagnostic labels can pathologize patients. For this reason, I prefer not to use the term *dysfunctional* as applied to a family. Instead, I think the term is more aptly used to describe interactional patterns that are unproductive in that they promote or sustain symptoms.

In contrast, *functional* interactions are those that promote conflict resolution, stimulate growth, or strengthen the connection among the family members. If the term is used in this way, it is clear that families engage in a mixture of functional and dysfunctional interactions. One of the ways to help families change dysfunctional patterns is to help them utilize their functional interactions more creatively.

BIOLOGY, MEDICATIONS, AND SYSTEMS

There is evidence that some emotional and behavioral symptoms are linked to brain physiology and neurochemistry. The subjective suffering associated with some of these syndromes can be reduced through the use of medications. Knowing how to recognize these patterns and syndromes when they occur can help nonmedical practitioners make a reasoned assessment of the need for a consultation from a medical practitioner. It does not mean that the therapist abandons a systemic perspective, but rather recognizes that biological factors can play a role in influencing emotions and behavior. It will enable the therapist to guide the family toward changing what they are able to change rather than expending energy trying to change something that is likely to be more resistant to change because of biological influences.

Even in cases where a strong biological influence is assumed, such as schizophrenia and severe mood disorders, family interactions influence the severity of the symptoms and the probability of relapse (Hooley, 2007; Rice, Harold, Shelton, & Thapar, 2006). Thus, in those cases where treatment with medications seems warranted, work on family interactions will help to reduce symptom severity and promote better functioning in the long run. For example, in the case discussed in Chapter 9, medications helped to relieve a girl's subjective suffering as a result of psychosis. The therapy, however, was focused on the intense conflict between the mother and grandmother that created stress for the girl and inhibited the adults from helping the girl to function to her full potential.

On the other hand, the use of medications has a downside, not the least of which is the presence of side effects, the unknown long-term effects of taking medications for many years, and the potential dangers of failing to comply with the prescribed dosage. Families can become overly reliant on medication and less motivated to do the hard work involved in changing the ways they interact with one another. Therapists can become overly focused on assessing symptoms and identifying disorders, rather than listening to people and trying to understand them. If the therapist is not the prescriber, conflicts between the therapist and psychiatrist can arise and undermine both the family therapy and the pharmacology.

To avoid these pitfalls, it is important to maintain a holistic perspective that views all potential influences on a problem as interacting with one another. This perspective advocates a *both/and* rather than *either/or* approach. Thus, while biological factors might play a role in the problem, they are not privileged as the sole or primary "cause" of the problem. The same can be said for a traumatic life experience, environmental deprivation, cultural prejudice, or family interactions. No single factor can be isolated as causative, but rather all factors work together. A systemic perspective calls attention to the ways in which multiple influences on a particular problem interact and mediate one another. So, by focusing on family interactions in this book, I do not intend to imply that these are the main "cause" of the problems of adolescents. However, I hope to show that viewing problems from a family systems perspective can provide a very useful lens, one that opens up options for promoting change and growth that go beyond what other models provide.

THE PARADOX OF CONTROL

Efforts to control other people are often at the core of the problems that are brought to the attention of therapists. Families come to therapy because someone in the family is behaving in an undesirable way. Other members of the family try to convince this person to change, using a variety of methods, such as reasoning, arguing, begging, bribing, criticizing, threatening, or punishing. These methods have not been effective in producing the desired change, hence the visit to the therapist, who is presumed to have special expertise in changing people.

One problem with this approach is that people are less likely to change when they feel they are being controlled or manipulated against their will. These efforts at control contribute to disconnection, estrangement, and resentment. Rather than feeling motivated to change in order to please another person whose feelings matter to them, people who feel controlled try to escape the feeling of being controlled and/or assert their autonomy by resisting the efforts to change them. In effect, they are placed in a bind: If they change in response to the efforts made by others to change them, they are giving up a part of themselves and acknowledging that their acceptance in the family is conditional on their changing.

As a further complication, the more the other family members direct their attention to changing or controlling the behavior of the symptomatic member, the more their behaviors are governed by the symptom. Unsuccessful attempts to eliminate the symptom breed more (unsuccessful) attempts, and the range of interactions in the family constrict to those that are organized around the symptom. The more this happens, the more the relationships in the family suffer. The more the family members concentrate on changing someone else, the less they concentrate on changing themselves. The more they focus attention on the symptom, the less they attend to important qualities of their relationships with each other and with the person who is showing the symptom. As I elucidate in Chapter 3, this process is called the *symptomatic cycle* and constitutes the basic dilemma faced by families who come to treatment.

HARNESSING THE POWER OF RELATIONSHIPS

In my view, the most powerful resource for helping a person change is the relationships in which he or she participates. It's about as close as we get to an axiom in therapy that the quality of the therapeutic relationship is a key determinant of the success or failure of therapy. Certainly, our relationships with clients are critically important. But I'm talking here not only about the therapeutic relationship, but about the healing potential of the natural relationships in a person's life.

As I discuss in Chapter 3, families who come to therapy are often experiencing profound isolation and disconnection in their relationships with one another. Perhaps they have become so focused on solving the problem that brought them to therapy that they have lost sight of other aspects of their relationships. Perhaps they have followed a policy of conflict avoidance for so long that they have concealed parts of themselves from one another, only to realize one day that they no longer feel connected to one another.

The relationships in these families are no longer sustaining. The family members see each other as obstacles rather than resources. They have settled into patterns of interaction that inhibit growth. Sometimes, relationships outside the family can compensate for unfulfilling family relationships. But all relationships are poisoned to some degree by the absence of a "secure base" in the family (Bowlby, 1988).

One of the features that differentiates individual therapy from family therapy is the relative emphasis placed on the relationship with the therapist versus the relationships with people in one's life. Family therapists view the therapeutic relationship as a means to an end rather than as an end in itself. The purpose of the therapeutic relationship is to help family members change their relationships with one another, from relationships that inhibit growth to relationships that promote growth. Family therapists see beyond the problematic patterns in the family to the potential healing power of family relationships.

It is in the context of a relationship with the therapist that family members experience aspects of themselves that had been suppressed in family interactions. For example, when a father and his teenage son are locked in conflict, I use my relationship with the father to encourage more tenderness from him, and my relationship with the son to encourage more restraint. In this way, both father and son will experience underutilized aspects of themselves that can provide the seed around which new relationship patterns can crystallize.

In my view, the purpose of therapy is to enable individuals to experience sustaining and growth-enhancing relationships with the real people in their lives. In the case of troubled adolescents who are still living with their families of origin, my goal is to help the family members become better resources to the youngster and to one another. If an adolescent is not living with his or her family, and instead resides in a group home or residential facility, my goal is to help him or her make better use of the available relationships in his or her life. If an individual client is disconnected and isolated from other people, I cultivate a relationship with the client that will inspire him or her to seek out sustaining relationships with others.

I consider therapy successful when the family members (or individual clients) have discovered ways to get what they need from their relationships with the people in their lives, so that their relationship with me is no longer necessary to sustain them. Like a chemical catalyst that facilitates a reaction between two other substances, the therapeutic relationship catalyzes the transformation of relationships in the lives of clients. But the real healing takes place not in the therapeutic relationship but in the client's relationships with significant others.

THE ARCH

I suggest that therapists pay particular attention to cultivating relationships with each member of the family and to use these relationships as springboards for facilitating change. Minuchin (1974) has called this process *joining*. But joining is not simply a technique. It requires an experiential change on the part of the therapist and is achieved by making a conscious and deliberate effort to engage each family member in a relationship. To join effectively, therapists must listen carefully to each family member, try to see the problem from each family member's unique point of view, and find something about the person that they like. Then, the relationship is maintained just like any other relationship that is important to the therapist, by communicating what I like to call the ARCH of therapy: Acceptance, Respect, Curiosity, and Honesty.

• *Acceptance* means appreciating the family's struggles and understanding that they are all affected by the problem and suffering as a result of their problematic interactions. Acceptance does *not* mean communicating that it is "OK" for people to be verbally or physically abusive to one another. It means refraining from judging people and reducing them to only one particular facet of their complex selves.

• *Respect* means treating everyone in the family as a unique individual with his or her own opinions, needs, and feelings. Finding something about each family member that we generally like or admire can help promote respect. The therapist makes a commitment to the relationship, and by holding the relationship in high esteem conveys to the other person the expectation that he or she also will hold the relationship with the therapist in high esteem. This is particularly important with adolescents, who often feel as if adults don't respect them and don't care what they think.

• *Curiosity* means maintaining an open mind and expressing genuine interest in understanding people and why they do what they do. Curiosity means avoiding rigid attachment to a particular hypothesis and instead always remaining open to new information. It also means that therapists feel free to ask whatever questions will help them understand the family members better.

• *Honesty* applies both to oneself and to others. Being honest with oneself means acknowledging and dealing with feelings that could interfere with our ability to help the family. Being honest with others means (respectfully) communicating to them information about how they are coming across.

ADOLESCENTS NEED NURTURANCE

This brings me to another point, and one that has been a major goal of mine in writing this book: the importance of strengthening the adolescent's relationship with the parents and other family members. Some writings on treating adolescents stress the importance of promoting greater individuation and encourage the therapist to serve as midwife to the separation of the adolescent from the family. Parents may be encouraged to "back off" and give adolescents space to define themselves as separate and autonomous individuals. However, by emphasizing adolescent autonomy and independence, too little attention can be paid to the adolescent's ongoing need for nurturance, guidance, and support from the parents.

Susan Mackey (1996) is one of the few authors who have addressed the importance of strengthening the quality of the relationship between parents and the adolescent as an essential component of treatment:

I believe that a secure attachment to parents may lessen the influence of peers and consequently increase the likelihood that the adolescent will respond to parental limits. Similarly, I believe that secure attachment allows the parents to feel safer about the normal acting-out behavior which is characteristic of adolescents and thus less prone to overreactions. Because they feel that their children are attached, they have greater trust that the children will contact them when they find themselves in situations they cannot handle. Therefore, it may be a mistake to guide parents who may already be feeling insecure in their attachment to the adolescent to "back off" without first addressing the relationship issues to increase security within the attachment. (pp. 497–498)

Other authors have also emphasized the importance of attachment and its role in adolescent development (Allen & Land, 1999). Feminist scholarship has noted that the equation of maturity and separation does not apply to women, who strive to maintain continuity in relationships even as they develop a clearer conception of a personal identity (Gilligan, Lyons, & Hanmer, 1990; Jordan, Kaplan, Miller, Stiver, & Surrey, 1991; Josselson, 1987). The emphasis on independence and invulnerability has been cited as contributing to difficulties in the psychological development of boys as well (Bergman, 1995; Pollack, 1998). Olga Silverstein and Beth Rashbaum (1994) have pointed out that parents, especially mothers, are wrongly encouraged to pull away from their teenage sons to avoid stifling their masculinity. They write:

Often, of course, in the teenage years just as in the earlier phases of our sons' lives, we don't recognize that it is we who are doing the withdrawing. There's a reciprocity to this dance of withdrawal that has been going on for so long, and there's our firmly held and culturally mandated belief that it is the inexorable destiny of the adolescent male to move away from his parents. If for some reason he doesn't—if he's not ready yet to make that move, or if he is comfortable and happy enough within his family circle not to see the necessity of making it—we become very alarmed. And then we are likely to force the issue, with results ranging from disappointing to disturbing to disastrous. (pp. 123–124)

In order to be appropriately nurturing—neither smothering nor overestimating the adolescent—the parents must be able to *empathize* with the adolescent. The "good-enough" parents for an adolescent will be attuned to the adolescent's needs and respond accordingly. It is for this reason that "how to" books on parenting adolescents can offer no more than general guidelines. Like a good therapeutic relationship, the essence of good parenting is a connection; one grounded in empathy and resting on the ARCH—Acceptance, Respect, Curiosity, and Honesty.

THE PLAN OF THIS BOOK

In the next chapter, I present a brief overview of current knowledge about normal adolescent development. I believe that familiarity with the literature on adolescent development is essential for any therapist who is working with this population. Therapists must be familiar with what is typical or atypical in adolescence in order to assess the severity of a presenting problem and to provide proper guidance to parents.

In Chapters 3 and 4, I present in more detail my framework for helping families. In Chapter 3, I present the foundations of the model, which rests on the concept of the *symptomatic cycle*. In Chapter 4, I outline a general framework for assessing and treating families that is based on this model. In Chapters 5 through 11, I apply these principles to problems that families with adolescents commonly present to therapists: eating disorders, depression and suicide, anxiety, defiant and disruptive behavior, psychosis, school-related problems, and problems associated with "leaving home." In Chapter 12, I discuss common pitfalls encountered in work with families with limited financial resources and multiple problems, and suggest ways to avoid these pitfalls. Along the way, I present case examples, some detailed and some brief, which highlight the challenges and delights of working with adolescents and their families.

2

Adolescent Development

Many adults, including many mental health professionals, continue to hold the view that adolescent turmoil is a universal phenomenon (Offer, Ostrov, & Howard, 1981). They are wrong. Developmental psychologists long ago abandoned the idea that adolescence is inevitably characterized by emotional turmoil and upheaval. This "storm-and-stress" view of adolescence was first proposed by G. Stanley Hall (1904) and reinforced by early psychoanalytic thinking (Blos, 1962; Freud, 1958). However, these early notions were formulated from clinical experiences with a biased sample of adolescents who were in treatment. Studies that have been based upon more representative, random samples of adolescents have failed to find support for widespread turmoil (see Offer & Schonert-Reichl, 1992).

On the other hand, while emotional turmoil is by no means universal during adolescence, there is considerable evidence that storm and stress is more common during adolescence than at other ages (Arnett, 1999). Adolescents are prone to greater extremes of mood and more frequent changes in mood than younger or older individuals. Conflicts with parents increase in frequency and intensity during adolescence, as do rates of risk behaviors, such as drinking, smoking, and sexual activity. For these reasons, most developmental psychologists today endorse a "modified" storm-and-stress view of adolescence (Arnett, 1999). Although adolescent turmoil is not universal, it is true that adolescence is a period of increased risk for the development of psychosocial difficulties that could have serious implications for the young person's future.

Clinicians who work with adolescents must be familiar with the typical developmental processes that occur during this phase of life. A basic understanding of normal adolescent development can help avoid the following errors:

12

1. *Ignoring serious problems.* Families and therapists can under-estimate the severity of disturbance in an adolescent who presents for treatment by misinterpreting problematic behavior as developmentally normal. If parents believe that it is typical for an adolescent to be moody, irritable, and sullen, they can aggravate the problem by ignoring it.

2. *Overreacting.* Families and therapists might overreact by assuming that a behavior signals pathology, when in fact it is typical for many adolescents. Biased and inaccurate perceptions of adolescents can create self-fulfilling prophecies (Rosenthal & Jacobson, 1968). If parents interpret innocuous and typical adolescent behavior as evidence of pathology, they could respond in an excessively punitive way that could push the adolescent to exhibit more such behavior in an effort to assert autonomy.

3. *Inhibiting growth by restricting freedom.* Widespread belief that adolescents are by nature out of control can lead institutions to develop restrictive policies that limit the civil rights of adolescents and deprive them of opportunities for growth through exploration (Quadrel, Fischhoff, & Davis, 1993). Stereotypes about adolescents as wild, rebellious, and disdainful of authority can lead parents to overreact when their child challenges them. Believing that teenagers aren't interested in a relationship with them, many parents back off too quickly, which deprives youngsters of the nurturance and guidance they continue to need (Mackey, 1996). In doing so, parents fail to provide the optimal context for growth during this stage of life. Adolescents need parents who allow them ample room to experience the consequences of their own decisions, but who also provide reasonable limits that mirror those the adolescent is likely to encounter in the adult world.

The purpose of this chapter is to review the literature on normal adolescent development in order to provide a context for the discussion of problems of adolescents and their families in the subsequent chapters. I shall not attempt to cover all of the voluminous literature on adolescent development, but rather highlight information that is most relevant to the practicing clinician. Readers who are interested in a more detailed discussion of normal adolescent development can consult one of the many fine textbooks in the field (e.g., Adams & Berzonsky, 2003; Feldman & Elliott, 1990; Lerner & Steinberg, 2004).

DEVELOPMENTAL ISSUES OF ADOLESCENCE: AN OVERVIEW

We can divide the second decade of life into three general phases, during each of which a particular set of developmental challenges is at the forefront. These phases and the accompanying issues are as follows:

Early adolescence (ages 11–13)

- Adjusting to pubertal changes
- Learning to use new cognitive capacities
- Finding a place among peers
- Dealing with gender-related expectations

Middle adolescence (ages 14–16)

- Handling sexuality
- Making moral decisions
- Balancing autonomy and accountability
- Developing new relationships with peers

Late adolescence (ages 17–19)

- Consolidating an identity
- Experiencing new levels of intimacy
- Leaving home

Although the unfolding of these developmental challenges describes the typical pattern for adolescents in our culture, it is also important to keep in mind four important considerations:

1. *Context and the definition of normality.* Any discussion of "normality" poses a paradox: How can we describe what is normal without being so inclusive that the description is meaningless, or so restrictive that any deviations from the norm are considered pathological? Needless to say, our ideas of what is normative are influenced by cultural expectations. Adolescents are often considered troubled when they exhibit behavior that violates the norms of a particular setting, such as home, school, or community. But labeling an individual "troubled" assumes that the problem exists *inside the person* rather than *in the context*. Efforts are then directed to treating the troubled individual rather than trying to understand why his or her behavior does not fit the context. A mismatch between the kid and the context does not necessarily signal a problem with either, but it does suggest that a change in context might be considered instead of or in addition to a change in the youth.

2. *Asynchronicity in development.* Consider the case of the 6-foot, 200-pound quarterback who was an "early bloomer" and at age 14 has essentially completed his physical growth. Now consider his classmate, who at 5 feet 5 inches and 140 pounds has hardly begun developing. The divergent physical appearances of these boys can elicit different expec-

tations from adults. Will not the quarterback be expected to act more mature, while less mature behavior will be tolerated from his classmate? Will not adults assume that the quarterback is capable of handling more privileges than his late-blooming classmate? The course of development is not necessarily linear or coordinated in all areas. An adolescent almost always develops at different rates in different areas. The youngster whose body has not yet physically matured could be capable of sophisticated reasoning, while the adolescent whose body appears similar to an adult's might be unable to appreciate the perspective of another person. The error of assuming that development proceeds at the same pace in all areas can lead parents to expect too much of a youngster. Just because an adolescent is mature in one area doesn't mean that he or she is mature in other areas as well.

3. *Individual differences.* When group developmental trends are discussed, there is the implication that all adolescents follow (or should follow) the same developmental trajectory. Abnormality or even psychopathology might be assumed if a particular adolescent does not follow the group developmental trends that are considered to be "normal." While knowledge of general trends and themes regarding adolescent development is essential for working with teens, it is important to keep in mind that group trends do not necessarily apply to all individuals. It is only relatively recently that developmental psychologists have begun to study how individual differences, such as gender, ethnicity, culture, socioeconomic status, geographical residence, and sexual orientation, influence the general trends and themes of adolescent development. These factors must be considered before concluding that an adolescent who appears off track according to typical developmental sequences is abnormal rather than simply different.

4. *Interaction between adolescent and parental developmental issues.* Psychological development continues throughout the lifespan. While our focus will be on adolescent development, we should also keep in mind that parents are facing developmental challenges as well. In some cases, it is the adolescent's struggle that triggers the complementary struggle in the parent (see Steinberg & Steinberg, 1994). For example, a mother who is experiencing menopause might feel threatened by her daughter's nascent sexuality, and so responds by attempting to restrict the girl, who reacts by hiding her sexual experimentation from her mother. In other cases, the adolescent is progressing normally, but it is the parent who is struggling with his or her complementary developmental challenge and projecting this struggle onto the adolescent. A father who is going through a "midlife crisis" of regret over his own achievement might exert pressure on his son to get higher grades in school. The boy responds to

his father's pressure by prematurely asserting his decision to forgo college and become a construction worker.

Try to keep in mind these considerations as we examine in more detail the developmental events that occur during the three phases of adolescence.

EARLY ADOLESCENCE

Adjusting to Pubertal Changes

Timing and Sequence of Pubertal Changes

The most public signs of adolescence are the physical changes associated with puberty. While the development of secondary sexual characteristics, such as breasts in girls and facial hair in boys, is the most obvious, the biological changes that initiate puberty start long before evidence of these changes becomes visible (Buchanan, Eccles, & Becker, 1992). Menarche, for example, occurs midway through the process of pubertal development for girls. For boys, first ejaculation, usually experienced between ages 11 and 14 during masturbation or nocturnal emission (Stein & Reiser, 1994), occurs only after several less obvious physical changes have occurred.

The adolescent "growth spurt" is a well-known phenomenon, as is the observation that girls, on the average, experience their growth spurt about 2 years earlier than boys (Marshall, 1978). The gangly appearance of many adolescents is associated with the fact that different parts of the body grow at different rates (Tanner, 1972). It is also well documented that puberty is occurring at an earlier age than in previous centuries. For example, the average age of first menstruation in 1990 was 13, while it was 15 in 1900. This phenomenon has been attributed to improved environmental conditions such as wider availability of good nutrition and better healthcare (Eveleth & Tanner, 1976).

The physical changes of adolescence generally follow a predictable sequence for both boys and girls, although there can be some variability, especially for girls. While the sequence of pubertal changes is more or less predictable, there is far more variability in the timing of these changes. Early-developing girls, for example, can experience first menstruation at age 10, while late-developing girls might not menstruate until age 16. For boys, testicular growth might start as early as age 10 or as late as age 13. There is also individual variability in the length of time an adolescent takes to complete the pubertal changes. The interval can range from 1 to

6 years in girls and from 2 to 5 years in boys. There does not appear to be a relationship between the age at which puberty begins and the rate at which it proceeds (Tanner, 1972).

Raging Hormones?

Although frustrated adults frequently cite "hormones" as the explanation for erratic adolescent behavior, the research literature does not support a strong link between mood or behavior and the hormonal changes associated with puberty. Adolescents do experience frequent, rapid, and intense mood shifts, and hormonal factors might play a small role in influencing these changes (Rosenblum & Lewis, 2003). However, hormonal effects tend to be small (Brooks-Gunn, Graber, & Paikoff, 1994; Buchanan et al., 1992) and are overshadowed and mediated by other factors in the adolescent's environment. For example, Booth, Johnson, Granger, Crouter, and McHale (2003) found that testosterone levels in boys were related to risk behavior and conflicts with parents. However, the quality of the parent–child relationship moderated the link between testosterone and behavior: When the parent–child relationship was strong, the link between testosterone and risk behavior was weaker. In a sample of girls, negative life events mediated the association between hormonal levels and aggression (Graber, Brooks-Gunn, & Warren, 2006). The association between hormonal levels and aggression was stronger for girls who had experienced negative life events compared to girls who had not experienced negative life events. Thus, hormonal influences on mood and behavior appear to be far less important than environmental and psychosocial factors.

Other Biological Changes during Adolescence

Aside from hormonal changes, there are other biological changes associated with puberty that might play a role in adolescent moodiness and risk taking. Many adolescents suffer from chronic sleep deprivation because they experience a "phase shift" in their sleep patterns such that the onset of sleepiness is later (Carpenter, 2001). As a result, they don't get enough sleep because they fall asleep later but nevertheless must wake up very early in the morning because of the early start time for high school classes. They might attempt to compensate for this sleep debt on weekends, but the disruption in their weekday pattern is likely to make it even more difficult for them to adjust their "biological clocks" to their school schedules.

It was once believed that brain development was essentially completed by the time a person reached adolescence, but recent research findings have shown that this is not the case (Casey, Getz, & Galvan, 2008). The brain is not fully developed until the early 20s. The part of the brain that is still undergoing considerable development during adolescence is the prefrontal cortex, the functions of which include impulse control, planning, and decision making. While adults have the capacity to reflect on their "gut" reactions, put situations into context, and consider their options before responding, these capacities are still developing during adolescence. Because brain regions that assist in the regulation of emotion and prediction of the consequences of actions are not yet fully developed, adolescents are apt to react quickly from their "gut" and insufficiently consider the impact of their response on others. Adults who find this behavior frustrating or annoying might then respond in ways that increase the intensity of the interaction and make it even more likely that the adolescent will respond in an impulsive manner. In contrast, adults who remain calm in their interactions with adolescents not only model appropriate mature behavior, but also keep the level of affect within a range that the adolescent's maturing brain can manage.

Psychological Impact of Pubertal Changes

The physical changes associated with puberty, in themselves, have little negative impact on the adolescent's self-image, except in one instance: when adolescents are going through puberty around the same time they are experiencing other changes in life, such as changing schools (Simmons, Burgeson, Carlton-Ford, & Blyth, 1987). Far more important than the physical changes themselves is the reaction of the social context to the adolescent's physical changes (Brooks-Gunn & Reiter, 1990). For example, girls are at risk for developing eating disorders because of the societal emphasis on thinness (Attie & Brooks-Gunn, 1989).

Boys who mature early are accorded respect and status among their peers, but not so for girls. Early-maturing girls are often the target of lewd remarks by adolescent boys—an experience that is devastating to many girls (Pipher, 1994). Early maturation has been associated with problem behavior among girls (Archibald, Graber, & Brooks-Gunn, 2003), especially among girls who exhibited behavioral problems prior to puberty. According to a study by Caspi and Moffitt (1991), early-maturing girls who did not exhibit behavioral problems prior to puberty were at only slightly higher risk for postpubertal behavior problems than girls who matured on time or late. In contrast, among girls who exhibited behavioral problems prior to puberty, early-maturing girls were more likely to display problem behavior in adolescence than girls who matured on time or late.

Impact of Puberty on Family Relations

At the onset of puberty, it is common for adolescents and their parents to experience increased distance in their relationship (Steinberg, 1987). Adolescents seem to become allergic to parental curiosity. Locked doors and hushed phone conversations serve only to make their parents more curious.

This change in family relationships seems to occur regardless of the age at which the adolescent enters puberty, suggesting that it is puberty itself that correlates with increased distance from parents, not simply age. It is likely that a process of mutual withdrawal is taking place. The adolescent prefers more privacy and the parents back off, either in deference to the adolescent's privacy or simply to avoid conflict.

Parents who are threatened by the pubertal adolescent's increased desire for privacy might elicit a backlash from the adolescent, who withdraws even more to avoid parental scrutiny. Parents who have relied on the child to meet their needs might feel personally rejected, and respond by becoming depressed or by rejecting the adolescent in retaliation. In other cases, the parental relationship comes into sharp relief when adolescents remove themselves from the picture. The triangulated child who begins to spend more time away from home puts the parents squarely in contact with one another and forces them to confront their own unresolved marital issues.

Learning to Use New Cognitive Capacities

The Shift to Formal Operational Thought

Adolescents begin to develop more sophisticated modes of thought that include increased ability to think about future possibilities, increased awareness of alternatives, abstract reasoning, and relative thinking. They also become aware that it is possible to think about thinking itself (metacognition). Jean Piaget has identified these cognitive abilities as *formal operational thinking* (Inhelder & Piaget, 1958).

It might come as a surprise to many adults that thinking becomes more sophisticated during adolescence. To them, adolescents appear rigid, unyielding, unable to foresee alternatives, and incapable of reflecting on themselves. If anything, it seems more difficult to reason with an adolescent than with a younger child.

It is possible to reconcile these apparently contradictory views. On the one hand, adolescents become capable of more sophisticated modes of thought. On the other hand, they are not yet experienced in the use of these new capabilities. Therefore, they are in transition from the more concrete modes of reasoning characteristic of children to the more sophisticated modes of reasoning associated with adulthood. Furthermore, because they are relatively unskilled in the use of these modes of thought, adolescents are prone to make certain types of cognitive errors.

Adolescent Egocentricism

David Elkind (1967) described the phenomenon of *adolescent egocentricism*, a tendency in younger adolescents to become extremely self-absorbed. According to Elkind, there are two aspects to adolescent egocentricism: the *imaginary audience* and the *personal fable*. The former refers to the tendency for many young adolescents to imagine that they are continually "on stage," that their behavior is the focus of everyone else's attention. The adolescent who agonizes over any flaw in his or her physical appearance or attire exemplifies this tendency. The personal fable refers to the belief that one's own experiences are unique and therefore impossible for another person to understand.

One manifestation of the personal fable is the belief that one is "invulnerable" to the dangerous consequences of risk-taking behavior. The youngster who claims to know that it can be dangerous to ride his or her bike along a dark road at night but nevertheless assures his or her parents that no harm will come from doing so exemplifies the personal fable. In support of the notion of the personal fable, Alberts, Elkind, and Ginsberg (2007) reported a positive association between endorsement of the personal fable and risk-taking behavior in early adolescence.

Although there is some controversy regarding whether these characteristics are typical of all adolescents, or whether they describe only a minority of adolescents (see Quadrel et al., 1993), these concepts can provide parents and clinicians with a helpful framework for understanding the seemingly irrational behavior of some adolescents. Many adults, for example, find it difficult to understand why teenagers place so strong an emphasis on the evaluation of their peers.

Some adults might conclude that a young adolescent's strong identification with the peer group reflects poor self-esteem and low self-reliance. However, the concept of the imaginary audience tells us that it is typical for young teenagers to worry almost obsessively about what their peers might be thinking about them. Ironically, what does not occur to the adolescent is that his or her peers are equally concerned about what he or she is thinking about *them*. Moreover, because adolescents at this age are not developmentally ready to infer accurately what others are thinking, they are likely to assume that others are thinking what they themselves are thinking. What seems to the youngster to be the real opinions of the peer group are actually their own projections and manifestations of the imaginary audience.

Adults who point out this irony and attempt to help the teenager gain insight into the workings of the imaginary audience are likely to fail, because they run into the wall of the other manifestation of adolescent egocentricism: the personal fable. The more adults try to convince adolescents that their way of thinking is erroneous, the more kids feel misunderstood and compelled to defend their own position more strongly.

The concept of adolescent egocentricism also explains the apparently greater tendency of teenagers to take what adults consider foolhardy risks. Studies of risk taking have shown that the process of weighing benefits over possible losses is very similar in adolescents and adults (Quadrel et al., 1993). However, for youngsters under the gaze of the imaginary audience, the risk of being ridiculed or ostracized by the peer group is far more threatening than many adults can comprehend. Furthermore, as noted above, because their prefrontal cortexes are not yet fully developed, adolescents are still developing the capacities to plan behavior effectively and anticipate consequences.

Add to these observations four other factors and we can understand why conflicts between teens and adults are so common. First, adolescents become more facile at arguing, which makes them more formidable opponents for adults than are younger children, whose concrete reasoning doesn't stand a chance against an adult's more sophisticated and abstract formal operational thinking (Steinberg, 1996). Second, adolescents have less idealized views of their parents than do younger children and are therefore more likely to question parental perceptions (Steinberg & Silverberg, 1986). The father who was idolized by his 9-year-old daughter experiences an understandable blow to his ego when his daughter, now 14, blithely points out all his faults, most of which he secretly acknowledges but tries to hide. Third, parents and teenagers define issues very differently; in a sense, they live in "separate realities" (Larson & Richards, 1994; Smetana, 1989). Parents tend to define issues as matters of values and personal accountability while adolescents define the same issues as matters of autonomy or differences in personal taste. A parent might challenge an adolescent's choice of clothing on the grounds that "People just don't dress like that to go to school," while the teenager argues that all of his or her friends dress that way. Fourth, early adolescents are not yet fully capable of adopting the point of view of another person, particularly one whose reasoning seems alien to their own. Robert Selman (1980) has proposed an interesting theory that encompasses this latter tendency.

Taking the Perspective of Another Person

Selman posits that the capacity to take the perspective of another person progresses through a number of stages. Younger teens are just entering the stage when they can imagine what the point of view of another person might be, and so are not adept at recognizing when others experience a situation differently than they do. A girl who is surprised by a friend's strong reaction to a comment about her appearance is a case in point. She is surprised by her friend's response to her remark because she does not yet fully appreciate that other people might experience a situation very differently than she does.

During early adolescence, young people are just beginning to adopt what Selman calls the "third-person perspective," which allows them to analyze a conflict between themselves and another person from a more objective and less personalized point of view. It is only later in adolescence (and for some, not until adulthood) that the young person can accurately infer the perspective of another person and also consider how an impartial third party might view the situation. Two years later, at age 17, an adolescent could think, "I have to be careful what I say to Tracey about her hair because she is very sensitive about it," or, "Tracey and I often get into arguments because we're both so stubborn."

Selman's model provides a framework for understanding how adolescents reason about social situations. It would be futile to expect kids in their early teens to appreciate the merits of points of view different from their own. They realize that the same situation could be viewed differently by different people, but they still remain invested in their own points of view and are likely to designate the others as "wrong."

It is only later that teenagers can recognize that there are elements of right and wrong in all perspectives, and that compromise is the most prudent course. Parents who engage head-to-head with teenagers in a futile battle over whose point of view will prevail can lose sight of the importance of achieving a workable compromise that takes into account the adolescent's perception of the situation and the fact that the youngster is likely to have radically different needs and tastes (Larson & Richards, 1994).

Selman, Brion-Meisels, and Wilkins (1996) have applied this model to an understanding of interpersonal conflicts involving adolescents. These authors posited a relationship between the ability to negotiate interpersonal problems and the capacity to coordinate social perspectives. Adolescents at the earliest stage of development view fighting or fleeing as the solution to conflicts. The next developmental step involves the use of verbal means (e.g., arguing) rather than physical means to prevail in a conflict. At the next stage, adolescents are capable of appreciating the other person's perspective, and so might offer trades or exchanges to get what they want. Finally, at the most mature level of the developmental sequence, adolescents recognize that there is validity to both parties' points of view, and so collaboration or compromise is the preferred solution to conflict. According to Selman et al. (1996), adolescents at the first three levels prefer "other-transforming" strategies to resolve conflicts while adolescents at the most mature level manifest "self-transforming" strategies. In the former, adolescents attempt to change the other person's behavior or point of view, while in the latter, adolescents acknowledge the importance of changing one's own viewpoint or behavior.

This model provides a useful framework for setting realistic goals for adolescents who have difficulty with interpersonal conflict resolution. Since effective and mature conflict resolution lies at the end point of a developmental sequence, it is approached only by moving through the earlier stages of the sequence. Thus, it is not realistic to expect that an adolescent who uses physical threats or intimidation will abandon this strategy in favor of collaboration or compromise. Rather, it is more realistic to work first on helping the adolescent learn to argue more effectively (without physical violence). After this skill is mastered, the next step entails helping the adolescent to barter behavioral changes with his or her "opponent." Finally, and only much later, would it be realistic to work on collaboration or compromise as conflict-resolution strategies.

Finding a Place among Peers

The Importance of Peers

Early adolescence marks a dramatic shift in the importance of the peer group. The young child still puts the approval and attention of adults before peer approval. After puberty, this balance shifts. Children in their early teens appear to throw themselves into the peer group, to the point that many parents feel that they are fighting a losing battle with peers for the adolescent's time and attention. Sometimes the parents, adolescent, and peers become locked in a triangular struggle: The child uses the peer group as a way of challenging parental authority; the parents blame the peer group for the child's "bad" behavior, and the adolescent bonds with peers through shared contempt of parents.

Despite the attendant frustrations to parents, the peer group nevertheless serves important developmental functions. First, the peer group is a context where young people learn the skills that are the foundation for adult friendships and intimacy. Second, the peer group provides adolescents with a temporary reference point for their emerging sense of identity (Brown, 1990). Through identification with peers, adolescents begin the process of defining who they are and how they differ from their parents. Third, the peer group serves as a "transitional object" that mid-wives the process of individuation from the family of origin. It becomes a surrogate family that provides a secure context in which the adolescent can begin to experiment with independence. Thus, acceptance by a peer group becomes almost a matter of psychological survival for a young teenager. However, the adolescent believes that acceptance requires con-formity. Thus, it is during early adolescence that peer conformity is at its height, declining steadily after age 14 (Berndt, 1979).

Peer Pressure?

Parents often blame "peer pressure" when their adolescent misbehaves, but peer cliques simply do not operate in this fashion. An adolescent does not passively respond to peer pressure; peers are actively exerting pressure on *each other*. According to *peer cluster theory* (Oetting & Beauvais, 1987), peer cliques develop their membership and norms through a pro-cess of mutual influence. Kids who share values, attitudes, and beliefs are attracted to one another, forming highly homogeneous "peer clus-ters." Then, each member of the cluster participates in actively shaping the norms and behaviors of that cluster. In other words, both *selection* (choosing a friend who is similar to oneself) and *socialization* (becoming more similar to one's friends) are equally important in the formation and maintenance of adolescent peer groups (Kandel, 1978).

While association with so-called "deviant" peers is strongly linked to problem behaviors among adolescents (Ary, Duncan, Duncan, & Hops, 1999; Aseltine, 1995; Dishion & Loeber, 1985; Heinze, Toro, & Urberg, 2004), the quality of the relationship with parents moderates the ado-lescent's susceptibility to peer influence. Adolescents who associate with deviant peers are less likely to engage in deviant behavior themselves if their parents effectively monitor them (Farrell & White, 1998; Galambos, Barker, & Almeida, 2003; Vitaro, Brendgen, & Tremblay, 2000; Wood, Read, Mitchell, & Brand, 2004). Moreover, strong attachment to par-ents is negatively correlated with attachment to deviant peers (Brown, Mounts, Lamborn, & Steinberg, 1993; Freeman & Brown, 2001) and also attenuates the link between association with deviant peers and prob-lem behavior among adolescents (Dorius, Bahr, Hoffman, & Harmon, 2004; Farrell & White, 1998; Vitaro et al., 2000; Wood et al., 2004).

What appears to promote a strong bond with parents is the oppor-tunity to be involved in decision making. Fuligni and Eccles (1993) found that adolescents who viewed their parents as asserting their power over them, restricting them, and giving them few opportunities to be involved in decision making were most strongly oriented toward peers. The more parents employ power-oriented techniques to "rein in" or control an "unruly" adolescent, the more alienated the adolescent feels and the more susceptible the adolescent will be to the influence of peers who are engaging in similar patterns of disruptive behavior.

Dealing with Gender-Related Expectations

Gender-Role Intensification

Around age 11, both boys and girls tend to adopt more rigid conceptualizations of gender roles, that is, what constitutes appropriate behavior for a boy or a girl (Basow & Rubin, 1999). This process has been termed *gender-role intensification* (Hill & Lynch, 1983). Messages from parents, peers, schools, and the media encourage boys to be strong, assertive, and self-reliant, and girls to be attractive, charming, and compliant. The extent to which the adolescent is successful in conforming to these expectations has a significant impact on his or her self-image. Masculine girls and effeminate boys are likely to be ostracized by peers and consequently experience a blow to their self-image, which can be even more intense if the adolescent is also coming to terms with sexual feelings for people of the same gender.

Androgyny

Earlier conceptions of masculinity and femininity as bipolar opposites have been supplanted by the realization that they are separate dimensions. Many individuals exhibit an equal mix of traditionally masculine and traditionally feminine traits, a characteristic that has been termed *androgyny* (Bem, 1975). While there is some evidence to support the idea that androgynous adults are better adjusted than those who are very masculine or very feminine, this does not appear to be the case for adolescents. Among teenagers, it is the masculine component of androgyny that seems to be associated with better adjustment (Markstrom-Adams, 1989). While androgynous girls show higher levels of both peer acceptance and self-acceptance than do very feminine or very masculine girls, very masculine boys show higher levels of peer acceptance and self-acceptance than do androgynous boys (Lau, 1989; Massad, 1981). For boys, "masculinity" is seen as incompatible with behaving in ways that are considered traditionally feminine (Pollack, 1998). Boys are actively encouraged to relinquish feminine traits. For girls, femininity is encouraged, but so are traditional masculine traits such as independence and self-reliance. The absence of masculine traits in girls is actually a disadvantage, both in terms of self-image and peer acceptance.

Gender-Role Pressures on Girls

At first glance, it might seem that the greater tolerance for masculinity in girls places girls at an advantage relative to boys, who are actively discouraged from exhibiting feminine qualities. However, what appears to be social tolerance is often experienced by girls as a bind that takes a toll on their self-concept. Many girls become consumed with worries about not being attractive or popular, characteristics that they assume are hallmarks of success as a woman. At the same time, girls become aware that the feminine traits they are being encouraged to develop are not those that society values most highly. It is not surprising, then, that girls score lower than boys on measures of self-esteem, particularly during the early adolescent years, when they have not yet developed the cognitive sophistication to recognize and challenge these mixed messages about gender (Simmons & Rosenberg, 1975). Some experts have argued that these conflicting cultural messages contribute to the higher incidence of depression among adolescent and adult females as compared to adolescent and adult males (Petersen et al., 1993).

Girls also experience other pressures related to gender-socialization messages. In *Reviving Ophelia*, Mary Pipher (1994) argued that adolescent girls experience intense conflict when socialization pressures come into conflict with their sense of self. Girls experience pressure to deny parts of themselves in order to fit in or to maintain relationships that are important to them. Girls are in a bind: They value relationships and put much energy into them, but at the same time the preservation of these relationships might require them to deny important aspects of themselves. As a result, adolescent girls experience a *loss of voice* (Jack, 1991, 1999). They silence themselves in order to preserve relationships or to avoid hurting people who are close to them. For some girls, this process creates intense stress as they face the impossible dilemma of denying who they are or finding themselves abandoned or rejected.

Here are some important points to keep in mind when working with adolescent girls:

• Help girls to find their voices, and to listen to all of their internal voices without feeling compelled to silence any of them. There is an example of how this principle is applied in Chapter 5. Each of Tina's voices was given a name, and Tina was encouraged to give each its due attention rather than feeling she had to align herself with one of them or silence some of them in order to feel more in control of herself.

• Respect a girl's relationships and the importance of these relationships to her. Help her to articulate what she wants from her relationships and evaluate whether she is getting what she wants from them. Don't discourage her from talking about her relationships or the people who are important to her, as when she is doing so she is often expressing important information about herself.

• Encourage parents to understand and value the importance of relationships in their daughter's life. Some parents communicate disapproval of what they believe is their daughter's excessive "dependency" on her friends. Usually, what these parents mean is that their daughter seems to give more value to the opinions of her friends than to the wishes of the parents. The more the parents challenge a girl's loyalty to her friends, the more the girl feels compelled to defend her friends out of loyalty to them. Rather than pitting themselves in opposition to the girl's friendships, the parents should engage their daughter in discussions about ways in which they could help strengthen their daughter's attachment to them and to the family.

• Help girls to identify and articulate feelings of anger and outrage, and validate these feelings when they are expressed. Many girls have difficulty with these feelings because they believe that expressing them will threaten relationships that they value. Some girls resolve this dilemma by engaging in indirect, passive–aggressive ways of expressing anger. Others internalize their anger and become depressed. Often, girls will express anger with tears rather than with words. Help girls to recognize when they are angry and provide a safe context for them to express anger. It is especially important for therapists to permit and encourage girls to express when they feel angry at *them*, as doing so provides an opportunity for girls to experience anger openly without risking the loss of an important relationship.

• Encourage parents to use relationship-based methods of influencing their children rather than methods based in power and authority. These ideas are emphasized throughout this book, particularly in Chapter 8. While this principle applies to all adolescents, it is especially important with girls. When a girl is engaging in risky behavior, rather than relying entirely on rules to control their daughter's behavior, parents should express how worried and frightened their daughter's behavior is making them feel, and try to elicit their daughter's cooperation based on her concern for their feelings and loyalty to her attachment to the parents. However, doing so will be effective only if the parents are also willing to listen respectfully to their daughter's feelings and take them seriously.

Gender-Role Pressures on Boys: The Boy Code

More recently, attention has also been paid to the ways in which gender-role socialization is stressful for boys and young men. In *Real Boys,*

William Pollack (1998) claimed that boys are pressured to conform to an unwritten set of rules that define how a "real boy" must act in our society. Among the elements of this "Boy Code," Pollack claimed, are the injunctions to be stoic and independent, to never show weakness, to act as if everything is under control even if it isn't, and to avoid showing any feelings other than anger. If a boy breaks the code, for example, by openly displaying feelings of sadness or fear, he risks being shamed and humiliated, often by adult males who see it as their job to teach the boy "how to be a man."

Pollack argued that male gender roles are particularly inflexible when compared with female gender roles, even though white males still enjoy many benefits in our culture. People tend to react more negatively to boys who possess female-typed traits than to girls who possess male-typed traits. In our culture, "masculinity" is not an inherent quality a person has because he is male, but rather a status that must be earned and repeatedly proven. Pollack writes, "Becoming masculine is defined as avoiding the feminine. *Being a boy becomes defined in the negative: not being a girl*" (p. 28, emphasis in original).

Parents are under pressure too: "Many fathers fear that if they don't follow the old Boy Code by acting 'tough' around their sons—and by pushing their boys as early as possible to act strong and independent—their sons will become outcast sissies rather than 'real boys' destined for success in the mainstream ... *maybe if I don't do something, Alex is going to turn out to be effeminate*" (Pollack, 1998, pp. 128–129, emphasis in original). Mothers back off from their sons, out of fear of making them "mama's boys." Olga Silverstein and Beth Rashbaum (1994) discussed at length the dilemma faced by mothers of boys in *The Courage to Raise Good Men*. They claimed that mothers, in honoring society's prescriptions for raising men in our culture, back off from their sons, lest they be considered bad mothers who are smothering their boys. However, this not only deprives the mother of her relationship with her son but also works against the boy, who still longs for closeness with his mother and feels rejected when she backs away, yet fears being perceived as "unmanly" if he complains about it.

Pollack makes several recommendations for ways that parents and other adults can counteract the destructive power of the Boy Code. Some of his recommendations include:

• Establish a safe environment to talk about the Boy Code. Create opportunities to talk openly with boys about the ways in which they experience and deal with cultural prescriptions for acceptable masculine behavior.

• Recognize that many boys become uncomfortable if their parents insist that they talk about feelings. Rather, parents can foster connections with their sons by participating in mutually enjoyable activities, or by engaging in conversations with their sons while they are playing or working together.

• Avoid shaming language when talking with a boy. The weapon of the Boy Code is shame—if you transgress, you are supposed to feel ashamed of yourself. Rather than asking, "How could you do that?" Pollack advises parents to ask questions to draw their son out: "What happened? Has something happened between you two guys? What can we do to help?"

• Do not confuse action with violence. Help the boy find healthy and constructive ways to let off steam. Anger is the one emotion that is acceptable for males in our culture to express. So if a boy becomes angry easily, it is important to look beneath the surface to try to find other feelings that the boy might not be able to articulate.

Basically, the theme behind these recommendations is to recognize that a boy might be behaving in accordance with the Boy Code when he is silent or sullen or angry. Respect that this behavior might be the only way he has learned to express himself. Gradually, through interactions with him, create a more inclusive view of masculinity by modeling and patiently encouraging a greater range of behavior and feelings.

Table 2.1 summarizes the developmental issues, and typical and atypical behaviors of early adolescence.

MIDDLE ADOLESCENCE

Handling Sexuality

Whether adults choose to acknowledge it or not, adolescents engage in sexual activity. By 12th grade, about two-thirds of students admit to having experienced sexual intercourse (Crockett, Rafaelli, & Moilanen, 2003). While accurate statistics are not available, it is reasonable to assume that even higher percentages of adolescents have engaged in other forms of sexual activity that stop short of intercourse.

The good news is that adolescent sexual activity in itself is not associated with later negative outcomes. Bingham and Crockett (1996) reported that there were no net negative developmental outcomes that could be attributed directly to sexual activity, once the effect of prior problem behavior was statistically controlled. Thus, adolescents who are

TABLE 2.1. Early Adolescence (Ages 11–13)

Major developmental issues

- Adjusting to pubertal changes
- Learning to use new cognitive capacities
- Finding a place among peers
- Dealing with gender-related expectations

Typical behaviors

- Increased attention to physical appearance
- Concern about whether their body is developing normally
- Increased ability to reason in abstract ways
- A temporary period of extreme self-consciousness ("Adolescent egocentricism")
- Adolescent invulnerability—apparent disregard for rules of safety ("I know it's not safe, but it won't happen to me.")
- The personal fable—self-dramatization and belief that their experiences are so unique that no one (especially adults) could possibly understand them
- Increased argumentativeness, accompanied by what may seem to be rigid thinking, because they cannot objectively weigh the merits of their own point of view against that of the person with whom they are arguing
- Intense involvement with the peer group, perhaps even to the extent of neglecting other responsibilities
- Increased conformity to peers and concern about acceptance
- Increased attention to differences between "masculine" and "feminine" gender roles and discomfort with gender-atypical behavior in others

Signs of problems

- Appears unusually and consistently secretive about activities, particularly those that involve peers
- Consistently fails to practice personal hygiene, for example, refuses to bathe or groom
- Has no friends or doesn't seem interested in having any friends
- Gets along well with adults but doesn't relate well to peers

sexually active but who have no history of prior behavioral problems are no more likely to suffer negative psychological consequences in later life than those who refrain from sexual activity.

Adolescent sexual values are influenced by parental values, but are far more influenced by the prevailing peer norms (Crockett et al., 2003; Moore, Peterson, & Furstenberg, 1986; Newcomer & Udry, 1984; Treboux & Busch-Rossnagel, 1990). The availability of sexual partners in the peer group and the manner in which the peer group accords status to sexual activity are more influential than prohibitions issued by adults. Nevertheless, there is evidence that close relationships with parents are associated with postponement of intercourse, less frequent intercourse, and fewer sexual partners (Crockett et al., 2003). Among adolescents who are already sexually active, parental monitoring and supervision reduce the likelihood that these teens will engage in high-risk sexual behaviors, such as unprotected sex (Li, Stanton, & Feigelman, 2000; Rodgers, 1999).

Gay, Lesbian, and Bisexual Adolescents

During adolescence, some boys and girls gradually become aware that their sexual and emotional attractions and fantasies involve individuals of the same sex. For some, this awareness is experienced as undesirable or frightening. Others may be prepared to embrace their sexuality, but face the prospect of harassment or rejection from family members and peers.

The term *sexual minority* is sometimes used to encompass anyone whose sexual identity is nonheterosexual or whose gender identity does not match their biological sex. It is important to differentiate among some terms that pertain to sexual-minority individuals and that are sometimes confused with one another. *Sexual orientation* refers to the pattern of one's sexual attractions, fantasies, and behavior. Simply categorizing sexual orientation as "homosexual" or "heterosexual" is a gross oversimplification. People's attractions, fantasies, and behaviors range from exclusively homosexual to exclusively heterosexual, with all flavors in between. The term *sexual preference* is considered inappropriate, because "preference" implies a choice, a notion that is not consistent with the subjective experience of individuals whose sexual orientation is other than exclusively heterosexual. *Sexual identity* overlaps with but is distinct from sexual orientation. Sexual identity implies that one has adopted for oneself a label selected from those commonly available (i.e., gay, lesbian, bisexual, or heterosexual). In fact, many individuals who experience same-sex attractions or who engage in sexual contact with the same sex do not label themselves as gay, lesbian, or bisexual (GLB). In one study, 45% of youth who reported same-sex experience did not self-identify as GLB (Garofalo, Wolf, Wissow, Woods, & Goodman, 1999), a figure comparable to the 50% of adult males who reported same-sex experience but did not identify as gay or bisexual (Laumann, Gagnon, Michael, & Michaels, 1994). *Gender identity* refers to one's subjective experience of oneself as male or female. Some individuals (including adolescents) experience themselves as *transgendered,* which means that their subjective experience of gender does not match with their biological sex. Although transgendered youths are becoming more visible, we know even less about their development than we know about the development of GLB youth (Grossman & D'Augelli, 2006). Transgendered youth face unique challenges that include dealing with the societal disapproval for gender-atypical behavior, negotiating school policies regarding attire and restroom usage, and weighing the risks and benefits of gender reassignment (Lev, 2004).

Until the early 1970s, homosexuality was considered to be a mental illness. It was removed from the DSM in 1973, and replaced by the diagnosis "ego-dystonic homosexuality," which was assigned when a person experienced his or her same-sex desires as unwanted. This diagnosis was eventually eliminated in the early 1980s. Now, most mental health professional organizations, including the American Psychological Association (1998) and the American Psychiatric Association (1999), view homosexuality as a normal variant of human sexuality.

Contrary to unsubstantiated claims that sexual orientation is "a choice," a person's sexual orientation is discovered rather than chosen. In recent years, evidence has been accumulating to support a genetic and/or biological basis for sexual orientation (Hershberger, 2001). There is no evidence that early childrearing practices affect sexual orientation. Myths about a "dominant mother and absent father," once claimed to be the cause of male homosexuality, have been discredited (Ellis, 1996). Many individuals who later adopt a GLB identity eschewed gender-typical interests and activities as young children, but this pattern does not universally apply. There are many examples of gay men who were "jocks" and lesbians who enjoyed "girl games" as children. Nevertheless, the best early predictor of a later gay or lesbian identity is the experience of feeling different from peers, a feeling that often arises from a lack of interest in activities that are preferred by members of one's own gender (Savin-Williams, 2005).

THE DEVELOPMENT OF A GLB IDENTITY

Based on extensive interviews with late-adolescent males who identified themselves as gay or bisexual, psychologist Ritch Savin-Williams (1998a) documented the milestones that commonly occur in the process of embracing a GLB identity. While these milestones are by no means universal, they do give a general road map for the process that many GLB individuals follow.

As already noted, most GLB individuals recall *feeling different* during childhood, usually because they were not interested in the same activities that were preferred by peers of the same gender. For many youth, the feeling of being "different" hits home when they realize that they are not experiencing the same heterosexual attractions that their peers seem to be experiencing but instead are attracted to people of their own gender. *First awareness of same-sex attractions* among boys typically occurs around ages 10 or 11, although for some boys this experience occurs as early as age 8 or as late as age 13. While awareness of same-sex attractions tends to occur a bit later for girls, it is clear from these findings that GLB youth are beginning to notice sexual interest in the same sex by early adolescence. Some time might pass, however, before youths *label these feelings* as "homosexual" and even more time is likely to pass before they *label themselves* as GLB. In Savin-Williams's studies, boys typically adopted a gay or bisexual identity between the ages of 16 and 19, whereas girls did so between the ages of 17 and 21. Self-labeling as GLB can occur before the young person has experienced sexual activity with a member of the same sex. About 50% of boys and up to 80% of girls adopt a GLB identity before they have had sexual contact with a member of the same sex (Savin-Williams & Diamond, 2000). These statistics are important to remember when parents claim that their child can't "really" be GLB because they have not had same-sex sexual contact. Pushing youths to delay labeling themselves as GLB because they have not yet experienced same sex sexual contact can undermine the youth's subjective experience of their sexuality and prolong the process of achieving an integrated sense of identity.

At the same time, it is important to keep in mind that the process of identity consolidation remains fluid during adolescence, and this fluidity applies to sexual identity as well. Youths might adopt a sexual identity label and relinquish it later. This experience is more common for females, although it occurs for boys as well. In her studies of late-adolescent and young adult females, Lisa Diamond (1998, 2000) found that only 32% of self-identified adult lesbians reported exclusive sexual attractions for women, and 39% reported changes in sexual attractions over time. It is perhaps for these reasons that 60% of the women in Diamond's sample changed their sexual identity label (i.e., lesbian, straight, bisexual) at least once and nearly 50% relinquished a lesbian or bisexual identity at some point during their late adolescence or early adulthood.

While Diamond's findings do support the idea that sexual orientation can be fluid during adolescence, it is also important to note that the majority of women in Diamond's sample (over 60%) reported stable attractions for other women. Sexual orientation stabilizes by adulthood, but even in adulthood more fluidity is found for women than for men. While the majority of adult men who report same-sex attraction report attractions *only* for other men (Laumann et al., 1994), only 32% of self-identified lesbians reported that their sexual attractions were exclusively toward women (Diamond, 1998). Kinnish, Strassberg, and Turner (2005) reported that 79% of their sample of adult gay men always identified as gay or bisexual whereas only 45% of adult lesbians always identified as lesbian or bisexual. In contrast, 97% of adult heterosexual men and women had always identified themselves as heterosexual, and none reported ever having identified as gay or lesbian.

DISCLOSURE TO OTHERS

The process of adopting a GLB identity is influenced by many factors. Certainly, contextual factors play a big role. Fear of exposure or rejection by family or community can delay the process of coming to terms with one's sexual identity, while growing up in a more liberal family and more tolerant environment might make it easier for a youth who experiences same-sex attractions to embrace a GLB identity. The strength and persistence of one's attractions for same-sex individuals are also likely to play an important role. Adolescents who experience strong, persistent, and exclusive attractions for members of the same sex are likely to arrive more quickly at the conclusion that a gay or lesbian identity fits them than will those adolescents whose sexual attractions for the same sex are less strong or persistent.

A milestone in the process of adopting a GLB identity is disclosure of one's sexual identity to others. In Savin-Williams's (1998a) sample of college-age men, 40% had disclosed their gay identity to another person during high school. Typically, a peer will be the first to be told. Disclosure to parents usually follows disclosure to peers, and disclosure to mothers generally precedes disclosure to fathers. Although many families respond positively or at least reasonably, some young people experience rejection or abuse after disclosure to family members (D'Augelli, Hershberger, & Pilkington, 1998). In general, a positive relationship between the young person and parents prior to disclosure predicts a good outcome after disclosure (Savin-Williams & Dube, 1998).

Empirical research has thus far not determined whether disclosure of one's GLB identity to parents is beneficial (Savin-Williams, 1998b). While a supportive parental response is linked to better adjustment (Darby-Mullins & Murdock, 2007; Savin-Williams, 1998b), the direction of effect is not clear: Does parental support increase self-esteem, are young people with higher self-esteem more likely to disclose to parents, or does a third factor (e.g., positive family relationships) account for the association between parental support and the youth's adjustment? Although some have argued that "coming out" to parents is a necessary step in achieving self-acceptance (e.g., LaSala, 2000), Robert-Jay Green (2000) advocates a more conservative approach that takes into account the likely costs and benefits of disclosure to parents. Given the very real risk to some adolescents of parental rejection, caution in disclosing their GLB identity to parents seems prudent.

FAMILY ISSUES

In working with families with gay, lesbian, bisexual, or transgendered (GLBT) adolescents, it is important to be aware of some of the common reactions family members exhibit. Parents must face their own "coming out" process as they deal with the disclosure. LaSala (2000) documents some common parental reactions, including fear for the child's safety and future welfare, self-blame for "causing" the child's homosexuality, grief over the lost dreams of weddings and grandchildren, concerns about reactions of extended family members and friends, and the need to address their own inaccurate stereotypes and misinformation about GLBT individuals. Many parents benefit from participation in support groups such as Parents, Families, and Friends of Lesbians and Gays (PFLAG).

What appears to be a family crisis that is precipitated by a child's disclosure of his or her GLBT identity might not be related solely to the child's sexual identity. The disclosure can uncover weak links in the family structure that had until then remained untested. For example, a mother who becomes depressed after her daughter's disclosure of her lesbian identity might be reacting not only to the daughter's disclosure, but also to a weak marital bond and lack of emotional support from a husband whose peripheral role in the family "worked" as long as there were no major crises. Focusing attention only on helping the mother accept her daughter's disclosure will fail to address the underlying structural problem in the family. Attention must be directed to strengthening the marital relationship, helping mother get the emotional support she needs from father, and helping father provide it.

Therapists must also be alert to the presence of these issues even in apparently accepting and supportive families. Conflict-avoidant families might simply refuse to deal with the child's disclosure, or might be eager to provide reassurance so that the crisis of the disclosure can be minimized and the family can return to a comfortable predisclosure homeostasis. For example, in working with a family of an adolescent girl who had recently disclosed her lesbian identity to her parents, I noticed that the parents frequently cut off the daughter with frenzied expressions of support and reassurance that they "loved her." I wondered if the girl felt free to express to her parents her own doubts and insecurities about her future. Was she reading their eagerness to reassure her as a message that any distress on her part was not really acceptable to her parents, who might interpret her distress as disconfirmation of their perception of themselves as unconditionally supportive and accepting? Paradoxically, by anxiously and repeatedly reassuring her that they unconditionally accepted her, the parents were giving the girl the impression that she could not be angry or disappointed in them, that she could not talk about her own fears about how the world might react to her, or express her frustration at not being able to get as close as she wanted to the heterosexual girls to whom she was attracted. Therapy needed to go beyond simply helping the family adjust to the girl's disclosure and helping the girl deal with the new challenges she was facing. The conflict-avoidant culture in the family needed to be addressed by increasing the parents' tolerance for uncertainty and insecurity, and creating space for the girl to express all of her feelings without worrying about provoking anxiety in the parents.

SUGGESTIONS FOR WORKING WITH GLBT YOUTH

Here are some additional suggestions for working with adolescents who identify as GLBT or those who are questioning their sexual identity:

• *Avoid making the assumption that all youth are heterosexual.* Therapists who ask boys about their "girl friends" and girls about "boy friends" are communicating that the normative expectation is that the boy or girl is heterosexual. Youths who identify as GLBT or who are questioning their sexual identity could interpret questions such as these as evidence that the therapist is not open to discussion of same-sex attractions.

• *Deal with heterosexist attitudes.* Heterosexism is the belief that being heterosexual is intrinsically better than being homosexual or bisexual (Herek, 2000). Many therapists who claim to be accepting of GLBT individuals might still hold unexamined heterosexist biases. For example, a therapist might assume that the adolescent's same-sex attractions need to be explained, while not assuming the same for what the therapist considers to be normative heterosexuality. A therapist might discourage a youth from acting on his or her same-sex desires while not exercising the same policy for heterosexual youths. Therapists must also confront their own reactions to gender-atypical behavior, grooming, and attire.

• *Accept the adolescent's own label for himself or herself.* Adolescents who won't adopt a label of "gay" or "lesbian" are not necessarily "in denial." As Savin-Williams (2005) points out, the current cohort of sexual minority teens use a variety of labels, or no labels, to describe their sexual attractions.

• *Don't pressure the young person to disclose to parents.* As discussed above, some parents might react negatively to the youth's disclosure. Even if the therapist believes that the parents will react in a supportive way, it is important to explore carefully and patiently the teen's reasons for his or her reluctance to disclose to parents.

- *Don't get confused by reports of heterosexual attractions or behavior.* Many GLBT youth have had both same-sex and other-sex experiences (Savin-Williams, 2005). The fact that an adolescent reports heterosexual attractions or engages in heterosexual behavior does not mean that he or she will not eventually adopt a GLBT identity. There is also not a direct correlation between one's sexual behaviors and one's sexual identity. Many individuals, both young and older, report same-sex attractions and behaviors but don't consider themselves anything but heterosexual (Garofalo et al., 1999; Laumann et al., 1994). Moreover, as discussed above, sexual identity is fluid for many adolescents, particularly sexual-minority girls, who might report waxing and waning attractions for both sexes.

- *Don't assume that an adolescent can't "really" be gay or lesbian if he or she hasn't had same-sex experiences.* As discussed above, many adolescents and young adults who adopt a GLBT identity have not engaged in sexual activity with a member of the same sex. For these adolescents, the strength and persistence of their attractions, fantasies, and desires for members of the same sex form the basis for their sexual identity. The fact that they have not yet had an opportunity to actualize these desires and fantasies is not a crucial factor in determining who they are.

- *Don't assume that homosexuality is just about sex.* It's about sexual desire, but it's also about love, attachment, and romantic feelings. What clinches the decision to adopt a GLB identity for many young people is the experience of falling in love with a member of the same sex, whether or not the feelings are reciprocated and whether or not sexual activity has taken place.

- *Monitor risk.* Clinicians who work with GLBT youth should be prepared to assess continually for mood disorders, suicidal ideation, substance use, or other maladaptive reactions to the very real stressors in their lives. There is an elevated risk of suicide among GLBT adolescents, although the incidence of suicidality might not be as high as suggested by some early reports (Savin-Williams, 2001). Youths who experience high levels of generic stress as well as stress associated with being GLBT (e.g., victimization) appear to be at higher risk for suicide (Savin-Williams & Ream, 2003). Adolescents who are gender-atypical in their behavior, and so can't easily "pass" as heterosexual, are at higher risk, because they couldn't hide their sexual orientation even if they wanted to, and because they are frequently subject to teasing and hostility. On the other hand, it is also important to keep in mind that "storm and stress" is not a universal experience for GLBT teens. Only a minority of GLBT youth actually experience suicidal ideation—between 10% and 30% (Savin-Williams, 2005)—and most GLBT kids are well-adjusted. Buying into the stereotype that GLBT teens are unhappy and suicidal can lead GLBT teens who do not feel this way to question whether they really are GLBT since they aren't experiencing the *angst* they have been led to believe is universal.

• *Seek education and information.* Therapists who work with GLBT teens and their families must keep abreast of the current literature and the resources in their communities, including the availability of gay–straight alliances (GSAs) in local high schools. Therapists must be prepared to address misinformation and direct the family members to reliable resources. In particular, therapists must be prepared to address requests to "convert" the adolescent to heterosexuality. Many professional organizations oppose so-called conversion therapy as not only ineffective, but also unethical (Haldeman, 1994).

Making Moral Decisions

With increased independence and exposure to new experiences, adolescents face the challenge of deciding between "right" and "wrong." Expanding upon Piaget's theory, Lawrence Kohlberg (1963) presented a model for understanding how individuals at different ages and developmental stages make moral decisions. Kohlberg proposed that moral decision making progresses sequentially through six stages. Each stage is characterized by a principal rationale for making a particular moral decision. These stages are as follows:

Stage 1: To avoid punishment
Stage 2: To earn rewards for oneself
Stage 3: To receive approval from significant others
Stage 4: To obey rules and laws
Stage 5: To preserve the common good
Stage 6: To comply with universal and abstract ethical principles

Although Kohlberg's theory has been criticized as more applicable to boys than girls (Gilligan, 1982), his framework can be useful for assessing the sophistication with which an adolescent makes moral choices. For example, a boy who is primarily at Stage 2 will base decisions of "right and wrong" on whatever will earn him the better outcome. He'll return a lost wallet if there is a chance he'll get a reward; otherwise, he'd be inclined to keep it.

Because moral development progresses sequentially through these six stages, it would be futile to try to persuade this boy with arguments based on the common good ("We all need to help one another if we're going to live together in society") or universal moral principles ("Relieving the owner's anxiety over the lost wallet is more important than the inconvenience you would incur from trying to locate him or her"). A more realistic goal might be to help this boy move to Stage 3. One way to do so might be to help him see that the approval he'd receive from the wallet's owner is reason enough to return the wallet, even if no monetary reward were offered.

Many arguments between teenagers and parents regarding moral issues reach an impasse because a parent is using sophisticated Stage 5 or 6 arguments to persuade an adolescent who is at Stage 2 or 3. By using Kohlberg's framework to assess how an adolescent thinks about issues of right and wrong, a clinician can more effectively help families through these impasses.

Studies using Kohlberg's framework with adolescents have shown that very few adolescents are at Stage 4, and virtually none are at Stage 5. Colby, Kohlberg, Gibbs, and Lieberman (1983) found that only about 8% of 14-year-olds and 21% of 18-year-olds were at Stage 4. Their sample of 14-year-olds was almost evenly split between Stages 2 and 3, with a very small percentage at Stages 1 and 4. About 60% of 16-year-olds were at Stage 3, although a sizable minority (30%) was still at Stage 2 and a smaller minority (15%) was at Stage 4. By age 18, over 50% are still at Stage 3, and the rest are about evenly divided between Stages 2 and 4.

What these data imply is that it is not particularly unusual for young adolescents to cite tangible or social rewards as the prime determinant of what is the "right" thing to do. Young adolescents will voice opinions that they believe will earn them the most approval, and since young adolescents are more oriented toward their peers than toward their parents, the approval of the peer group will weigh most heavily. Even when adolescents move into Stage 4, the rules or laws they choose to follow might not be sanctioned by adults. For example, a 15-year-old boy who won't "rat" on a friend who has broken into a neighbor's home out of loyalty to his friend exemplifies Stage 4 reasoning in his invocation of the value "loyalty," even though adults might disagree that this value takes priority over the value of respecting personal property or honoring the common good.

It is also important to note that morality is not necessarily the same as social convention (Smetana & Turiel, 2003). Some decisions that adults frame as moral issues (i.e., right and wrong) might not be seen in that way by adolescents, who might view these issues as matters of social convention or personal taste rather than morality. For example, adults might view substance use, sexual behavior, and religious observance as moral issues while adolescents might view these issues as governed not by morality but rather by social standards. Conflicts can arise around who has the right to dictate these social standards. Adults who insist on framing these issues as "moral" will miss the mark, as the issue is actually one of autonomy rather than morality. Keeping in mind this distinction between moral and social standards can dispel the myth that adolescents are disinclined to respect moral standards. As Smetana and Turiel (2003) note, "[I]n straightforwardly moral situations, adolescents may generally think and act morally. That is, the overwhelming majority of adolescents routinely refrain from hitting, hurting, killing, stealing, maiming, acting dishonestly, or harassing others, though countless opportunities exist on a daily basis to do so" (p. 256).

Balancing Autonomy and Accountability

"So I skipped school again today. So what? Why do you care? I don't want you to care."—*A 15-year-old boy defending his truancy to his mother*

Adults and teenagers often disagree on the definition of "autonomy." Parents emphasize that autonomy requires responsibility, while kids define autonomy as freedom from adult authority. Many adults believe that teenagers are merely puppets of the peer group, but the available evidence does not support this belief. Peer conformity peaks in early adolescence (ages 12–14), but then declines (Berndt, 1979).

While adolescents are strongly influenced by peers in matters of dress, music, and choice of leisure activities, most young people defer to adults in those areas in which adults are perceived as having expertise, such as career choices and financial decisions (Wilks, 1986; Young & Ferguson, 1979). However, adolescents no longer see their parents as the all-powerful and all-knowing authority figures of childhood and are thus inclined to question parental opinions rather than accept them on faith (Steinberg & Silverberg, 1986).

Some parents are not prepared for these challenges to their authority. They might perceive the adolescent's challenges as disrespectful and become more authoritarian as a result. Their efforts to assert their authority over the teenager are met with more resistance, in a pattern that can lead to escalating power struggles that weaken the relationship between the adolescent and parents. As a result the adolescent is even less likely to consider the impact of his or her choices on the parents' feelings and more likely to gravitate toward sympathetic peers. A study by Fuligni and Eccles (1993) supports this idea: Adolescents who were most dependent on peer-group approval were those from authoritarian homes. Adolescents from homes in which parents encouraged independent decision making were less oriented toward peers and more inclined to accept their parents' guidance.

At the same time, autonomy must be balanced with accountability. As adolescents exercise more freedom in making their own decisions, they also must experience the impact of these decisions on themselves and others. Parents should avoid taking responsibility for the adolescents' decisions and allow natural consequences to occur whenever possible. Parents must go beyond expressing anger at the adolescent's apparent defiance and instead should communicate how sad, worried, or disappointed the adolescent's choices are making them feel. When denying requests, they should acknowledge and empathize with the adolescent's disappointment and frustration, thus demonstrating that they care about the child's feelings even if they are unable to gratify them. In so doing, the parents are balancing their role as authority figures with their role as attachment figures for their child. According to a model developed by Baumrind (1978) and Maccoby and Martin (1983), parents who follow this philosophy are known as *authoritative* parents. A large body of literature has supported the correlation between authoritative parenting and positive outcomes for adolescents (Steinberg, 2001).

Authoritative Parenting

According to Baumrind (1978) and Maccoby and Martin (1983), parenting styles can be categorized along two dimensions: *responsiveness* (warmth, support, nurturance) and *demandingness* (expectations for mature, responsible behavior). Crossing these two dimensions results in four parenting styles: *Authoritarian* parents are high in demandingness but low in responsiveness; *indulgent* parents are high in responsiveness but low in demandingness; *indifferent* parents are low on both dimensions; and *authoritative* parents are high on both dimensions.

Authoritative parents are not permissive. They have standards and expectations, and communicate these clearly to the adolescent. They set limits, but are open to negotiation. They avoid unnecessary power struggles and refrain from taking the adolescent's apparently irrational behavior as a personal affront. Authoritative parents freely offer guidance when asked but try to avoid protecting adolescents from the consequences of their own choices. Only when these natural consequences are likely to be severe or irreversible do the parents intervene with more immediate and ultimately less devastating consequences of their own.

Ann and Vince Rossi were examples of authoritative parents. When 15-year-old Frank announced that he was taking a part-time job after school, Ann and Vince discussed with him their concerns about the impact of the job on his schoolwork. When Frank's grades dropped after a few months on the job, Anne and Vince did not gloat or pontificate. Instead, they engaged Frank in a calm conversation about their concerns and offered a compromise: Frank could choose whether to cut back his hours at work, or he could spend one evening each weekend studying rather than going out with his friends. Not without some blustering, Frank chose the latter. By the next report card, Frank's grades had increased slightly but had not returned to where they were prior to his taking the job. What had become clear to Ann and Vince in the interim was that Frank was really comfortable with his academic performance and seemed to realize its potential impact on his future. They acknowledged that Frank was still performing well enough to achieve his goal to attend a state college. They admitted that foregoing a job in order to get higher grades was a value to which they were strongly committed, but that Frank was not. Frank ended the academic year with lower grades, but he had earned several hundred dollars that he applied to purchasing car insurance. He also appeared more mature and confident, which he attributed to his experiences on the job. Most importantly, he and his parents had maintained their warm and mutually respectful relationship, and in some ways had even grown closer.

Some caveats are in order. First, the whole notion that parenting can be categorized into a style is a bit of an oversimplification. Most parents use a variety of methods in disciplining their children, and to characterize a style may be too limiting. The Rossis did their share of yelling, but not too often. In the final analysis, what characterizes authoritative parents is an attitude about their relationship with their child rather than a particular set of skills (see Darling & Steinberg, 1993).

Second, the reciprocal influence of families and children must be taken into account. Families in which authoritative parenting practices prevail foster a climate of mutual respect and mutual trust (cf. Cook, 2001). Children who are raised by authoritative parents more willingly disclose information to their parents, and their willingness to do so makes it easier for their parents to monitor them (Kerr & Stattin, 2000). In contrast, parents who follow an authoritarian style are more likely to have children who are strongly oriented toward their peers and more influenced by their peer group (Fuligni & Eccles, 1993). Thus, it is likely that authoritative parenting and positive parent–child relationships evolve together over time.

Third, the family's ethnic and cultural background is relevant. While the benefits of authoritative parenting appear to cut across ethnic and cultural groups (Amato & Fowler, 2002; Steinberg, Lamborn, Darling, Mounts, & Dornbusch, 1994), authoritative parenting practices are less common in certain cultures (Chao, 1994; Yasui & Dishion, 2007).

Moreover, the apparent adverse effects of authoritarian parenting found among European American, middle-class families do not appear to apply to families from other ethnic backgrounds. For example, the distinction between authoritative and authoritarian parenting might not apply to Asian cultures, where strict limit setting coexists with strong family ties, physical closeness, and intense investment in the child's success (Chao, 1994). Rohner and Pettengill (1985) reported that Korean youths perceived parents as showing more warmth toward them when the parents were more (rather than less) controlling. While these families might be viewed as excessively strict and authoritarian from a Eurocentric perspective, the very high levels of warmth and investment in these families promote positive child outcomes. Thus, youngsters raised in certain cultural contexts might take a different view of parental control than those raised in the dominant culture.

Developing New Relationships with Peers

During the early years of adolescence, a boy or girl socializes primarily with small cliques of same-sex peers, and interaction between the sexes is usually limited to large-group activities. By middle adolescence, the composition of the peer group has shifted. At this age, mixed-gender peer groups become common, and some boys and girls are pairing off into couples (Dunphy, 1963).

Along with this change in the way social time is spent, adolescents are also beginning to experience themselves as more differentiated from the peer group. During early adolescence, the peer group functions almost as an extension of the self. Eleven-to-13-year-olds can't accurately distinguish what they think or feel from what (they believe) their friends think or feel. By age 14 or 15, teenagers begin to distinguish their own beliefs and feelings from those of their friends, and begin to feel more comfortable acting on their own beliefs and feelings. Since the youngster's peers are also going through the same process, the middle years of adolescence herald greater tolerance among the members of the peer group, and less anxiety over being seen as "different" by one's associates.

Kegan's "Evolving Self"

Robert Kegan (1982) has proposed a model that helps to explain the shift in the teenager's relationship to the peer group during mid-adolescence. According to Kegan, an individual develops through successive stages characterized by increasing complexity and sophistication in the way the person differentiates self from the world. The "self" is continually evolving as one gradually recognizes that experiences that were once considered part of oneself can be differentiated from the self and instead viewed more objectively.

According to Kegan, infants in the first 2 years of life (the *incorporative* stage) have difficulty differentiating self from the environment— what is "self," and what is "other" is not distinct in the mind of the very young child. Gradually, as children learn to differentiate self from the environment more accurately, they enter the *impulsive* stage, when they are bound to their own perceptions and see themselves as equivalent to their impulses rather than "having" these impulses. The 3-year-old wants what he wants when he wants it, and there are no other options.

As children gradually differentiate themselves from their impulses, so that they can observe these impulses as objects rather than as equivalent to the self, they enter the *imperial* stage. This stage, which corresponds to Piaget's stage of concrete operations, is characterized by an embeddedness in one's own needs and perceptions and an inability to appreciate that others might experience situations differently from oneself. The 8-year-old can wait patiently for her father to take her to the playground but can't appreciate that her dad does not find the experience as enjoyable as she does.

According to Kegan, the early years of adolescence are characterized by a transition from the imperial stage to the *interpersonal* stage. During this transition, teenagers gradually become aware that their peers have needs and desires of their own. However, adolescents at this stage have difficulty distinguishing their own needs, wishes, or interests from those of the peer group. In the early teen years, Kegan claims, kids have trouble telling the difference between how they think and feel and how they believe their peers think and feel. It is not that teenagers are putting their own needs and wishes aside in order to be accepted by the peer group. Rather, young teens have not yet developed the cognitive capability to differentiate their own thoughts and feelings from those of the group. A young adolescent's sense of self is so tied up with the perceived expectations of the group that he's unsure where the group ends and he begins. The 13-year-old can't differentiate between liking hard rock music because it appeals to him personally, or because his friends think it's "cool."

The emergence of a separate self that can evaluate the perceived norms and expectations of the group more objectively begins in the middle years of adolescence and is not complete until well into young adulthood. At this point, the young person enters the *institutional* stage, when a clearer sense of personal identity is crystallizing. The 16-year-old acknowledges with some pride that her passion for 1950s jazz music sets her apart from her friends, who are more interested in contemporary popular music.

Kegan's model implies that adolescents view themselves and other people in a way that is qualitatively different from the way adults do. Beyond a simple problem in "communication," adolescents and adults interpret the world in radically different terms. Parents might believe that their child is following the herd in order to be popular or to keep friends, when in fact the child simply has not yet developed a clear conception of self that is distinct from the peer group.

Kegan posits that the transition from one stage to the next is often associated with a repudiation of the meaning-making style of the stage that is being left behind. This observation can also account for conflicts between some parents and their teenage children. Parents who themselves are in transition between the interpersonal and institutional stages might react vigorously against an adolescent's embeddedness in the interpersonal stage, because they themselves are in the process of rejecting the "old self" that was interpersonally embedded. The teen's interpersonal embeddedness represents for the parent the way of making sense of the world that they themselves are repudiating in favor of the new institutional balance. Based on Kegan's model, we might expect that parents who are comfortably situated in the institutional stage or beyond would experience less difficulty empathizing with adolescents and moderating their reaction to them. It would seem, then, that the resolution of cyclical, escalating conflicts in some families might require a developmental shift in the parents in addition to a developmental shift on the part of the adolescent. Although Kegan does not explicitly recommend it, family therapy seems the ideal context for facilitating the simultaneous and coordinated development of both teenager and parents.

Table 2.2 summarizes the developmental issues, and typical and atypical behaviors of middle adolescence.

LATE ADOLESCENCE

Consolidating an Identity

If asked to identify the major developmental task of adolescence, most clinicians would probably say that adolescents are struggling to establish an identity. This point of view is derived from the writings of Erik Erikson (1950, 1959, 1968), who believed that the chief psychosocial task of adolescence was establishing a coherent sense of identity. According to Erikson, the task of consolidating an identity had to be successfully completed in order for subsequent development to proceed normally. Erikson also believed that the successful resolution of the identity crisis depended on the degree to which the adolescent had successfully resolved four earlier developmental crises: the establishment of *trust* (vs. mistrust) during

TABLE 2.2 Middle Adolescence (Ages 14–16)

Major developmental issues

- Handling sexuality
- Making moral decisions
- Balancing autonomy and accountability
- Developing new relationships with peers

Typical behaviors

- Greater awareness of the needs of others and a greater willingness to compromise
- In making decisions about right and wrong, less emphasis on obtaining tangible rewards and more interest in gaining the approval of significant others
- Increased interest in sex and curiosity about sex
- Shifting in peer associations and formation of couples
- Increased differentiation from the peer group; greater tolerance of differences and diversity among people
- Increased emphasis on being independent and free from parental rule
- The beginning of the moratorium—increased attention to defining one's identity, which includes exploration and experimentation in a variety of areas

Signs of problems

- By age 15 or 16, still seems to show many of the characteristics typical of a younger teenager (ages 11–13)
- Sexual promiscuity–although many adolescents at this age are sexually active, indiscriminate choice of sexual partners is not common
- Unusually anxious about sex (e.g., becomes nervous whenever sexual issues are discussed, claims to have no interest in sex)
- Doesn't seem to feel guilty when he or she does something that is clearly wrong or that hurts another person
- Has a very narrow range of activities (e.g., seems interested in little else but "hanging out" with same-sex peers; spending several hours a day playing video games or using the Internet)
- Appears to be a "loner," has no friends, and doesn't seem interested in associating with peers
- Associates exclusively with peers, avoids the company of adults, even those (e.g., teachers, coaches, employers) who have taken a personal interest in him or her

infancy; *autonomy* (vs. shame and doubt) during the toddler years; *initiative* (vs. guilt) during the preschool years; and *industry* (vs. inferiority) during elementary school.

Marcia's Identity Statuses

James Marcia (1966, 1976) developed a method of identifying an adolescent's position or "status" in the process of defining an identity. Marcia identified four possible "identity statuses" that are defined by the intersection of two dimensions. The first dimension describes how much explo-

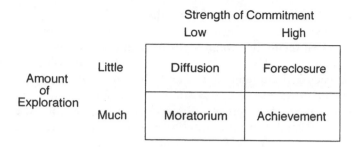

FIGURE 2.1. Marcia's four identity statuses.

ration the adolescent has engaged in prior to reaching a decision. The second dimension describes the strength of the adolescent's commitment to the decision. The resulting four statuses are depicted in Figure 2.1.

An example of an adolescent in *diffusion* might be one who shows little concern about the future and is focused almost entirely on immediate gratification. A boy who shows no interest in academics, sports, or the arts, who hasn't even a hazy dream about a future career, and who spends all his free time "hanging out" with peers who seem similarly adrift exemplifies the diffusion status. An example of an adolescent in *foreclosure* is one who is certain about his or her career choice and has never seriously considered other alternatives. Adolescents in *moratorium* are actively engaged in the process of exploration. They are considering a variety of alternatives and might frequently change their mind about their future goals. The moratorium status is a way station toward identity achievement. These adolescents eventually emerge with a clearly defined identity, at which time they would be classified in the *achievement* category. In contrast, adolescents in the foreclosure category have committed themselves to a decision without having first gone through a period of exploration or experimentation. They are likely to be relatively constricted and conservative. These youngsters face the risk that they might discover later in life that decisions they made during their youth no longer reflect who they are or who they want to be.

Over the years, considerable evidence has accrued in support of Marcia's model (Kroger, 2003). As expected, those classified into the achievement status are the most mature and successful young people. On the other hand, while the percentage of individuals classified into the achievement category increases with age, less than 10% of adolescents have reached the achievement status by high school graduation (Meilman, 1979) and about half can be classified into foreclosure or diffusion (Kroger, 2003).

There is general agreement that the diffusion status is associated with the least favorable adjustment. These are the youngsters who have not committed themselves to an identity definition, and who seem uninterested in doing so. These young people are most susceptible to negative peer influence and are unlikely to exhibit much motivation in school or other achievement-related areas. The diffusion status is associated with the greatest incidence of problem behaviors (Adams, Gullotta, & Montemayor, 1992) and difficulties establishing close and secure attachments to others (Zimmerman & Becker-Stoll, 2002). According to Erikson's framework, these adolescents have often failed to resolve one or more of the earlier developmental crises. For example, prior to adolescence, children must successfully establish a sense of industry, the confidence that they are good at something. Children who fail to do so, perhaps because of a learning disability or severe parental neglect, are poorly equipped to deal with the issue of identity, and so often fall into the diffusion status.

Family dynamics play a role in identity development. The achievement status is associated with secure attachments to the family (Kroger, 2003) and clear intergenerational boundaries (Perosa, Perosa, & Tam, 2002). Adolescents raised in homes where parents do not agree on parenting decisions are more likely to fall into the moratorium or diffusion status (Faber, Edwards, Bauer, & Wetchler, 2003). The households of foreclosed adolescents are often characterized by an authoritarian parenting style. While foreclosed adolescents describe themselves as close to their parents and supportive of parental values, they also tend to doubt their own ability to function independently of their families (Kroger, 2003; Perosa et al., 2002).

While Erikson's and Marcia's models have provided useful frameworks for understanding the process of identity development, there have nevertheless been some criticisms. Some have argued that the models do not apply to girls, whose sense of identity is typically intertwined with competency in relationships (Gallatin, 1975; Josselson, 1987). For girls, the process of identity development and the establishment of intimacy might coincide or overlap. The period of moratorium might therefore be longer for girls, since the successful establishment of an intimate relationship, for heterosexual girls at least, is contingent upon the boys catching up to them in their capacity for intimacy, which for boys is thought to emerge after an identity has been established. The confusing and conflicting societal messages regarding what is possible or "proper" for women to achieve can also complicate and prolong the process of identity development for girls.

It is also important to keep in mind that there are multiple aspects to identity, such as occupational identity, religious/value identity, gender identity, ethnic identity, and political identity. The process of establishing a position in each of these areas can follow different time frames and trajectories (Archer, 1989). For example, a young person who is gay or lesbian might not "come out" until well into his or her 20s, even though his or her identity might be secure in other areas. Similarly, it is conceivable that an adolescent might be in moratorium on some issues, foreclosure on others, and diffusion on still others, such as the high school junior who is actively exploring career options (moratorium), but has unquestioningly adopted his or her family's religious beliefs (foreclosure) and seems uninterested and unconcerned about politics (diffusion). Thus, the model shouldn't be used to categorize adolescents in a global sense, but rather to assess how young persons are dealing with important life decisions.

Helping Adolescents and Families Negotiate the Identity Crisis

Some parents mistakenly believe that adolescents should have a clear idea of their future career goals by the time they leave for college, even though the research indicates that only a small minority of high school graduates has reached the achievement stage. Under pressure to make a decision, some adolescents might cut short their moratorium and prematurely foreclose on a decision. In other cases, the adolescent has reached achievement, but the parents don't like the choice he or she has made. To encourage these young people to reconsider their decision and return to moratorium constitutes a developmental regression. Rather, it is better to help the adolescent explain to the parents the process by which the decision was made and help the parents listen and ask questions rather than try to convince the young person to reconsider.

What about adolescents in diffusion? It is important to consider the possibility that an adolescent might not be in diffusion in all areas. Sometimes, adolescents who appear to be in diffusion in one area (e.g., career goals) are in moratorium in other areas (e.g., personal values). In these cases, it might be possible to stimulate progress from diffusion to moratorium by asking questions about the area in which the adolescent appears to be in diffusion. For example, if the youngster is in diffusion in the area of career goals, therapists might ask questions such as the following: Where do you want to be in 5 years? How much money do you want to make? How do you see yourself spending your time? Which adults in your life seem to be happy about the career choice they have made? Which adults seem to be unhappy with their careers?

If the adolescent appears to be in diffusion in all areas, it might be beneficial to explore whether the adolescent could be engaged in a process of moratorium on at least one issue. If this approach is not successful, then it is possible that the adolescent might not have resolved the "industry versus inferiority" dilemma. These young people might not have a clear sense of their own strengths and weaknesses or might believe that they have no strengths at all. For example, an adolescent who has struggled in elementary and middle school might have abandoned any hope of academic success. Not perceiving any alternatives and reacting to parental demands for more commitment to academics, the adolescent simply avoids thinking about the future. In this case, it is important to help the adolescent identify and develop talents in areas other than academics, such as mechanics or art. Of course, following Erikson's framework, if the youngster has not resolved the "industry" crisis, it is possible that there have been problems at earlier developmental stages as well. Thus, therapists should start with the "industry versus inferiority" stage, and, if unable to make headway, proceed backwards through the earlier stages to explore where the youngster might be stuck.

Racial and Ethnic Identity

A particular challenge facing adolescents who are members of ethnic and racial minority groups is the development of a strong *ethnic identity* (Quintana, 2007). Jean Phinney (1989) proposed a model of ethnic identity development that is based on Marcia's model. According to Phinney, ethnic identity follows a developmental progression from *unexamined* (cf. Marcia's diffusion or foreclosure), through *ethnic identity search* (moratorium) to *achieved ethnic identity* (achievement). The stage of unexamined ethnic identity is characterized either by little interest in ethnicity and little thought directed to one's own ethnicity (diffusion), or attitudes regarding ethnicity that have been absorbed from parents or other adults (foreclosure). Movement to the second stage (ethnic identity search) is often provoked by an experience of oppression or discrimination that stimulates awareness of one's ethnicity (Cross, 1991; French, Seidman, Allen, & Aber, 2006; Phinney, 1990). At this stage adolescents are engaged in the process of learning about their own culture and participating actively in cultural events. Following this period of exploration, some young people progress to a clearer understanding and appreciation of their ethnicity (achieved ethnic identity). Development of a strong ethnic identity has been linked to more favorable psychological adjustment among members of racial and ethnic minority groups (Yasui & Dishion, 2007).

Another issue facing members of racial and ethnic minority groups is their relationship to the dominant or majority culture. Phinney and Devich-Navarro (1997) described several patterns of cultural identification, that is, ways in which adolescents conceptualize their relationship to the two cultures to which they are exposed. In *assimilation,* individuals give up their own cultural identification and identify entirely with the dominant culture. In *fusion,* the two cultures are combined to produce a "new" culture with which the individual identifies. In the *blended bicul-*

tural pattern, the two cultures are perceived as overlapping but not identical. Individuals who exhibit this pattern see themselves as occupying a middle ground between the two cultures and do not identify exclusively or more strongly with either one. This pattern is contrasted with the *alternating bicultural* pattern, in which individuals move back and forth between the two cultures, even though they might describe themselves as being more strongly identified with their own ethnic culture. Individuals who are unable to integrate their membership in two cultures exhibit one of two patterns. In the *separated* pattern, the individual identifies solely with one culture and rejects the other. In the *marginal* pattern, the individual identifies with neither culture and finds a position outside both of them. In research with African American and Mexican American students, Phinney and Devich-Navarro (1997) found evidence for the blended, alternating, and separated patterns, but no evidence for the assimilated, fused, or marginal patterns. African American students were more likely to exhibit the blended pattern while Mexican American students were more likely to exhibit the alternating bicultural pattern.

Family environment influences the development of ethnic identity. The attitudes of parents toward their own culture will have an impact on their children. Marshall (1995) found that parents who explicitly address racial topics in their parenting practices promote ethnic identity development in their children. However, provision of either too few or too many racial socialization messages to children could be detrimental. In a study of African American mothers and their early adolescent sons and daughters, children of mothers who supplied a moderate number of racial socialization messages were better adjusted than children whose mothers supplied a low or high number of such messages (Frabutt, Walker, & MacKinnon-Lewis, 2002).

Because studies of racial and ethnic identity are still in their infancy, it is difficult to reach firm conclusions about this topic. There seems to be a growing consensus that a strong racial and ethnic identity is beneficial, and that at least a moderate degree of socialization relevant to race is helpful in promoting a stronger sense of ethnic identity among children. There is some support for a model such as Phinney's to describe the development of racial identity, but it is also likely that variation exists both within and among different racial and ethnic groups.

Experiencing New Levels of Intimacy

Attachment to Parents

Early scholarship emphasized the need for adolescents to sever their emotional ties with parents, a process that has been termed "detachment"

(Freud, 1958). Adolescents were expected to repudiate their "infantile dependence" by rebelling against parental authority and rejecting their attachment to their parents. Teenagers who remained close to their parents were considered immature and fearful of growing up. Parents were advised to discourage an overly warm relationship with the teen, lest they impede the process of separation. Later, this notion was replaced by the idea that adolescents are faced with a more complex challenge: retaining their relationship with the significant adults in their lives while at the same time transforming these relationships to include a greater sense of personal autonomy. This process has been termed "individuation" (Blos, 1967).

In fact, adolescents neither detach from nor disengage from their parents. As adolescents grow older, their capacity for intimacy increases, and their relationships with both parents and peers become more intimate over time (Rice & Mulkeen, 1995). Strong relationships with parents continue to be important through adolescence into adulthood. In recent years, concepts derived from *attachment theory* have been applied to understand the evolution of the relationships between adolescents and their parents.

First proposed by John Bowlby (1988) in his studies of infants, the concept of attachment to parents has been extended into adolescence and beyond (Ainsworth, 1989). Bowlby maintained that the security of attachment bonds to primary caretakers during infancy fostered the development of *internal working models* that acted as templates for future relationships in life.

Four patterns that characterize an individual's attachment strategies have been described. A *secure* attachment is one characterized by confidence that the person to whom one is attached will be available when need arises. In contrast, a *preoccupied* attachment pattern is characterized by insecurity about the responsiveness of others, presumably related to inconsistent and/or unreliable behavior on the part of the parents. Those exhibiting a *dismissive* attachment pattern act as if relationships do not matter to them, because they had been unable to depend on their parents for security during their younger years. A fourth pattern (*fearful*), is sometimes observed, and applies to those who avoid getting close to others because of fear of rejection (Bartholomew & Horowitz, 1991). A considerable body of evidence has demonstrated that attachment security is related to favorable developmental outcomes (Allen & Land, 1999), while insecure attachment has been linked to both internalizing and externalizing problems during adolescence (Adam, Sheldon-Keller, & West, 1996; Allen & Land, 1999; Allen, Moore, Kuperminc, & Bell, 1998; Rosenstein & Horowitz, 1996).

Bowlby (1988) believed that internal working models were set in infancy and remained relatively fixed throughout life, but others have argued that these internal relationship templates could be revised in light of new information derived from interpersonal interactions later in life (Byng-Hall, 1995; Cook, 2000). This view has led to increasing interest in the manner in which particular family dynamics can promote strong attachment relationships (e.g., Hill, Fonagy, Safier, & Sargent, 2003). Cook (2000) found that working models could be affected by observable dynamics in the parent–adolescent relationship. Allen, McElhaney, Kuperminc, and Jodl (2004) found that adolescents who perceived their mothers as more supportive during disagreements made relative gains in their attachment security over a 2-year period, while those whose relationships were characterized by enmeshment and personalization showed declines in security. There is also evidence for reciprocal effects between symptomatic expression by adolescents and changes in their attachment security. While adolescents who exhibit symptomatic behavior tend to exhibit insecure attachment patterns, symptomatic adolescents also become less secure in their attachment to parents over time (Buist, Dekovic, Meeus, & van Aken, 2004). This finding suggests that relationships in families with symptomatic adolescents progressively deteriorate, as represented in the concept of the symptomatic cycle to be discussed in the next chapter.

Although peer relationships take on greater importance as children grow older, parents continue to be important in the lives of adolescents. While adolescents become less dependent on their parents, peers do not supplant parents as objects of attachment and intimacy (Allen & Land, 1999). In fact, adolescents who are strongly attached to both parents and peers are the best adjusted, while those who are weakly attached to both parents and peers are the least well-adjusted (Laible, Carlo, & Raffaelli, 2000). Moreover, the degree to which adolescents turn to peers for support is moderated by their attachment to their parents. Securely attached adolescents place relatively more importance on their relationship with their parents, while insecurely attached adolescents place relatively more importance on their relationships with peers (Freeman & Brown, 2001; Nickerson & Nagle, 2005). Moreover, among boys who associate with so-called "deviant" peers, the likelihood that the boy will engage in problematic behavior is lower if the attachment between the boy and his parents is secure (Vitaro et al., 2000).

What occurs during adolescence is the transformation of the nature of the relationship between children and parents. The relationship changes from one that is asymmetrical to one that is more symmetrical in terms of interpersonal power and authority (Allen & Land, 1999). Older adolescents want a close relationship with their parents, but expect parents to treat them more like equals and less like children who need protection and guidance. From the parents' perspective, showing respect for the older adolescent or young adult means knowing when to step back and refrain from offering unsolicited opinions. It also means being honest with the adolescent about how he or she is coming across to the parent, and expecting the adolescent to put energy into the relationship as well.

Intimacy with Peers

The nature of peer relationships continues to evolve during the later adolescent years. In early adolescence, the peer group functions almost as an extension of the adolescent's self, serving as a substitute family and a temporary referent for his or her emerging identity (Kegan, 1982). In the middle years of adolescence, the peer crowd expands to include both boys and girls and many adolescents pair off into couples or smaller cliques. As adolescence wanes into young adulthood, the importance of establishing an intimate bond with a peer increases.

Erik Erikson (1959) proposed that the next developmental step that follows the establishment of a coherent identity is the establishment of an intimate relationship with a peer, which usually occurs in the context of a romantic relationship. Erikson had placed the "identity crisis" before the "intimacy crisis," claiming that persons must know who they are before they can be truly intimate with another person. Feminist scholars such as Ruthellen Josselson (1987) have challenged this idea, arguing that women often consolidate their identity in the context of an intimate relationship with another person, typically a romantic partner. For girls, the tasks of consolidating an identity and developing the capacity for intimacy go hand in hand, strengthening one another in a process that extends well beyond adolescence into adulthood.

Both boys and girls have needs for intimate relationships, even though the genders may experience and express intimacy differently. While girls express intimacy through mutual self-disclosure, boys express intimacy with other boys through shared activity and time spent together (Buhrmester & Furman, 1987). Girls originally learn how to be emotionally intimate with same-sex friends, whereas opposite-sex relationships are more important for the development of emotional intimacy in boys.

The majority of heterosexual adolescents have experienced a "steady" relationship with romantic overtones by the end of high school (Bouchey & Furman, 2003). These relationships are neither short-lived nor trivial: Approximately 60% of adolescents over the age of 16 report a romantic relationship that has persisted 11 months or more (Collins, 2003). While dating has many benefits, including the opportunity to learn and practice interpersonal skills related to intimacy, there are also risks. The breakup of a romantic relationship is the single most common precipitant of a first episode of major depression (Monroe, Rohde, Seeley, & Lewinsohn, 1999). Since high school romances commonly end when one partner enters college (Savin-Williams & Berndt, 1990), college freshmen might be at particularly high risk for developing a depressive episode following a breakup because they are no longer living in proximity to other important attachment figures, namely, family members and high school friends. Since boys tend to depend more on opposite-sex relationships for experiencing intimacy and emotional closeness, it is not surprising that boys are four times more likely than girls to report feeling lonely during the first year of college (Savin-Williams & Berndt, 1990). These findings have been based on studies of heterosexual adolescents. We know very little about the manner in which gay, lesbian, and bisexual adolescents actualize their needs for emotional intimacy in a context where available partners might be in short supply (Diamond & Savin-Williams, 2003). What is clear, however, is that late adolescence is a period during which the capacity for intimacy evolves and the establishment and maintenance of intimate relationships with both parents and peers become important developmental challenges.

Leaving Home

In our culture, high school graduation is about as close to a "rite of passage" as we come. Graduating from high school marks the point at which the adolescent is expected to loosen ties to the family of origin and step into more independence, whether it be going to college, working full time, or enlisting in the military. This transition is sometimes fraught with turmoil for both the adolescent and the family. In Chapter 11, I discuss in more detail the problems associated with leaving home, but here I highlight only a few points.

The crisis of "leaving home" is not restricted to the period following high school graduation. It begins during the senior year of high school, when the end is in sight and the pressure to make post-high school plans mounts. Often, problems that emerge during the senior year of high school are linked to rough spots in the process of leaving home. Adolescents might not express their anxieties about leaving home, perhaps because of actual or imagined expectations on the part of parents and teachers. Thus, they show their reluctance to leave in other ways, such as "forgetting" college application deadlines, neglecting their schoolwork, or developing symptoms.

Whatever the specific nature of the problem presented to the therapist, it is important to inquire about the process of leaving home and invite the adolescent and other family members to express their feelings about the transition. When it becomes clear that the young person is

simply not ready to leave, then the therapist must take the lead in helping the family find concrete ways to ease the transition, such as part-time
employment, reduced college course load, or a precollege transitional
year of schooling.

How do we know whether an adolescent is really not ready to leave
home or whether he or she simply needs encouragement? The only way
to make this distinction is to listen carefully to the adolescent and to the
other family members. The boy or girl who has been making steady progress toward college, but who begins to fall behind in senior year, might
simply need encouragement. On the other hand, the young person who
seems to falter at any obstacle, or who repeatedly creates obstacles that
could easily be avoided, is probably not ready to leave. In these cases the
process of preparing to leave home might need to be prolonged. Much
of the work will involve coaching the parents to be supportive of these
efforts without being overly protective or too impatient. In Chapter 11
other suggestions for handling problems at this stage are discussed.

Table 2.3 summarizes the developmental issues, and typical and
atypical behaviors of late adolescence.

SUMMARY

We have covered a lot of ground in this chapter, so I want to close by
emphasizing what I believe are the most important points for a therapist
to keep in mind:

• Adolescence is not a time of inevitable turmoil. Serious or prolonged moodiness, withdrawal, aggression, appetite disturbance, or
oppositional behavior should be taken very seriously. Even if at first
glance it appears that a family is grappling with normal developmental
issues, it is far less risky to take a few sessions to get to know the family
before offering reassurance.

• Although adolescence is not tumultuous as a rule, there are nevertheless a series of normal developmental challenges that are encountered
during the second decade of life.

• During early adolescence (ages 11–13), the boy or girl faces the
challenge of coming to terms with the physical changes associated with
puberty and dealing with the reactions of others to his or her physical
appearance. They are beginning to develop the capacity to think and
reason more abstractly, but lacking experience with these new tools, they
are apt to apply them inconsistently. For many adolescents, this period
is one of intense self-consciousness. Self-esteem tends to drop, especially

TABLE 2.3. Late Adolescence (Ages 17–19)

Major developmental issues

- Consolidating an identity
- Experiencing new levels of intimacy
- Leaving home

Typical behaviors

- Greater interest in planning for the future and exploring options
- Increased capacity for intimacy; girls may seem more mature than boys in this area (see text)
- High school romances may be breaking up
- Fewer arguments with parents; daily struggles over rules and freedom have subsided, but adolescents at this age expect parents to show respect for their choices and their individuality
- Getting ready to leave home (e.g., college, job, military)

Signs of problems

- No plans for the future, and little interest in making them
- Still (or again) seems as moody and unpredictable as during the early years of adolescence
- Has shown no interest in dating (this could also be a sign that the adolescent is struggling with his or her sexual orientation)
- Avoids making postgraduation plans and bristles whenever parents bring up this topic
- Expresses the desire to go to college but is not taking the necessary steps (e.g., filing applications, taking SATs)

for girls who experience for the first time the need to suppress parts of themselves in order to be accepted by others. Finding a place among the peer group is of utmost importance at this age. For early adolescents, peers provide a reference point for their budding sense of identity and allow a smooth transition away from the emotional security of the family home. However, peer conformity is high at this age, because young teenagers are not yet able to distinguish their own thoughts and feelings from those of their peers. Intensification of pressure to behave in culturally prescribed "masculine" or "feminine" ways provokes the process of gender-identity development and creates difficulties for kids who don't conform to cultural gender stereotypes. Both boys and girls experience pressures associated with culturally prescribed standards for masculinity and femininity.

  • During the middle years of adolescence (ages 14–16), the boy or girl must make important decisions about how to express sexuality and how to decide between right and wrong. At this age, they are beginning to differentiate themselves from the peer group and are more willing to deviate from actual or perceived peer conformity. The same-sex peer clique expands to include both genders and some members are pairing off into opposite-sex couples. As adolescents become more independent, they must learn to balance autonomy with responsibility and accountability to others. This balance is fostered by parents who follow an authoritative style of parenting: warm, supportive, but firm in setting limits that are negotiated with the child.

• During late adolescence (ages 17–19), the consolidation of an identity becomes the primary challenge, along with the refinement of the capacity to experience and express intimacy. As high school graduation approaches, so does the transition to "leaving home," which for many young people and their families can be a stressful time.

In a nutshell, these are the major developmental milestones of adolescence. Keeping them in mind can help us hold realistic expectations of adolescents and provide reassurance to worried families. Some families, however, are not simply muddling through normal developmental issues. It is these families that we therapists are usually called upon to aid, and it is to these families that we turn in the later chapters of this book.

one another can enhance the effectiveness of biological treatments and in some cases may even obviate the need for these treatments.

FAMILY SYSTEMS AND FAMILY THERAPY

Family systems theory is built on the idea that a system composed of multiple members (e.g., a family) has certain properties. One of these properties is that the members mutually influence one another. This influence takes place in such a way that it is really not possible to identify cause and effect. Since the behaviors of the members of the system evolve over time, we cannot really say with certainty how any specific behavioral pattern (e.g., a symptom) began. While it is tempting to try to find the "cause" of a particular symptom, systems theory tells us that this is never possible. Rather the behaviors of individuals in a system shape one another, such that the behavior of any one member influences the behaviors of the other members of the system and is also influenced by them.

When talking about two people (a dyad) who are in an ongoing relationship with each other, the term *complementarity* refers to the way in which the behaviors of the members of the dyad "fit" with one another. For example, a parent criticizes an adolescent, who responds defensively, thereby eliciting more criticism from the parent. The more the parent criticizes, the more the adolescent feels compelled to defend herself, and the more she defends herself, the more the parent feels compelled to repeat and intensify the criticisms in an effort to "get through" to her. While we might be tempted to blame the adolescent's defensiveness on "low self-esteem" that resulted from parental criticism, systems theory takes a different view. The criticism of the parent and the defensiveness of the adolescent elicit one another, in such a way that it is merely arbitrary to identify one behavioral pattern as the cause or antecedent of the other.

This principle applies even when biological factors influence the behavior of a member of a system. Genetic and biological factors play a role in many psychological and behavioral symptoms, such as schizophrenia, major depression, bipolar disorder, and some anxiety disorders. However, even when biological factors are influential, they are not the sole cause of a particular behavioral pattern. Human behavior is profoundly influenced by environmental conditions, and one of the strongest influences on behavior is the behavior of another person with whom one has an ongoing relationship. Even the particular symptomatic presentation and severity of schizophrenia, for which genetic and biological factors are virtually certain, are influenced by the behavior of other members of the family. A behavioral pattern in families that has been called *high expressed emotion* (Hooley, 2007), characterized by a high level of overt conflict and criticism of the member with schizophrenia, has been linked to greater symptom intensity, higher relapse rates, and less compliance with medication. Tempting as it might be to assert that families who exhibit high expressed emotion *cause* the member with schizophrenia to behave more bizarrely, it is equally likely that the bizarre behavior of the schizophrenic member *elicits* the kind of responses characteristic of high expressed emotion. Rather than seeing either as cause or effect, systems theory asserts that they mutually shape one another and create a repeating pattern over time.

In order to understand the behavior of any one member of a system, one needs to take into account the behaviors of the other members of the system. Focusing on the behavior of a single individual in isolation offers a limited perspective and restricted options for helping to change this behavior. Taking into account the interpersonal context in which symptomatic behavior occurs opens up new possibilities for promoting change.

Let's take the example of a depressed adolescent. After gathering a family history, a therapist could reasonably conclude that there is a genetic or biological component to the depression, since many other family members have also experienced depression. These family members all experienced symptom relief from taking medications, so it would be reasonable to speculate that medications might be helpful to the depressed adolescent as well. It would also be reasonable to conclude that treatment methods based on cognitive therapy or interpersonal therapy could also help the depressed adolescent. None of these inferences would be unjustified. However, systems theory offers other possible avenues to promote change.

For example, upon meeting with the family, the therapist might notice that the parents are very protective of the depressed adolescent, answer questions for her, don't ask her own opinion, and ignore her when she does offer an opinion. The therapist might also notice that the adolescent, once ignored, withdraws and appears more depressed. This behavior elicits more caretaking behavior from the parents, and provides more evidence to them that the girl is not able to talk for herself.

From a systems perspective, then, additional interventions are available. The family therapist might work to alter the interactional patterns described above by paying attention to the girl, giving credence to her point of view, and encouraging her to disagree openly with her parents. Meanwhile, the therapist could discourage the parents from rescuing the girl when she seems to be floundering, and instead allow her space to figure out how to handle difficult situations on her own.

Thus, a family systems perspective opens up additional possibilities for helping the girl and the family get out of the position in which they appear to be stuck. A growing body of empirical evidence supports the effectiveness of family therapy for treating a variety of presenting problems (e.g., Bogels & Siqueland, 2006; Diamond & Josephson, 2005; Diamond, Serrano, Dickey, & Sonis, 1996; Eisler et al., 2000; Henggeler, Clingempeel, Brondino, & Pickrel, 2002; Kendall et al., 2008; le Grange, Crosby, Rathouz, & Leventhal, 2007; Liddle et al., 2001; McFarlane, Dixon, Lukens, & Lucksted, 2003; Miklowitz, Biuckians, & Richards, 2006; Robbins et al., 2008; Sexton & Alexander, 2002).

THE SYMPTOMATIC CYCLE

Fundamental to my approach to understanding and helping families with troubled adolescents is the concept of the *symptomatic cycle*. This concept describes how symptoms arise, evolve, persist, and eventually come to dominate the interactional patterns in the family.

Symptoms begin as relatively minor alterations in behavior that can be a response to many different factors, such as genetic vulnerability, developmental stress, or traumatic experiences. These minor behavioral changes occur from time to time in all adolescents and are usually transient. Some of the time, however, they evolve into lasting problems that defy solution. The crucial element in problem development is the way in which the family members respond to these behavioral changes that are characteristic of all developing adolescents (see Chapter 2).

Most families adapt to the developmental challenges associated with adolescence and flexibly adjust their responses to provide the adolescent with whatever he or she appears to need from them at that particular time. However, some families don't make these adjustments or misread signs that the adolescent is in distress. These families are prone to react in unproductive ways that can contribute to the development of serious symptoms.

The more the family members focus on the adolescent's troubling behavior, the more they are liable to see the youngster as "the problem." They will be less likely to acknowledge the adolescent's positive qualities or contributions to the family. This view leads the adolescent to feel misunderstood, resentful, and increasingly isolated from the rest of the family. In this context, symptomatic behavior is likely to persist and increase. As efforts to eliminate the symptom repeatedly fail, the family members feel more and more helpless and frustrated. Their preoccupation with the symptoms leads them to neglect other important aspects of their relationships with each other and thus promotes further deterioration in the family relationships. As the family relationships deteriorate, all family members, particularly the symptomatic adolescent, experience an increasing sense of isolation and alienation. In this context of isolation and alienation, symptoms persist and intensify (see Figure 3.1). This symptomatic cycle, whereby interpersonal disconnection fuels symptoms and symptoms fuel further disconnection, constitutes the basic process driving symptomatic behavior (Brendler, Silver, Haber, & Sargent, 1991; Hoffman, 1981).

For example, consider a family with an adolescent boy who exhibits temper outbursts. The parents might become so preoccupied with their son's outbursts that they neglect other relationships, such as their relationship with each other or with their other children. The more the parents focus on managing the boy's temper, the less they pay attention to his other qualities, such as his wit, intelligence, or vulnerability. In response, these positive qualities of the boy begin to fade from view, reinforcing the tendency to see him as "the problem." The family is now caught in a bind. Labeled as the problem, the boy feels misunderstood by his family, which increases his isolation from them and fuels his frustration and anger. As the outbursts continue and intensify, the other family mem-

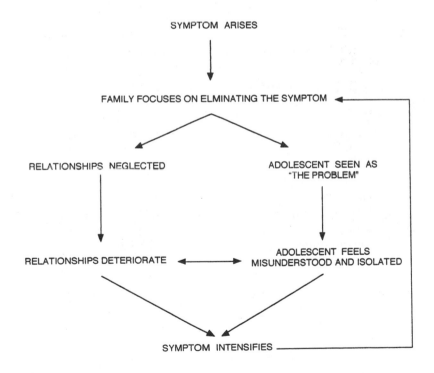

FIGURE 3.1. The symptomatic cycle.

bers find it increasingly difficult to see beyond them to the boy's other qualities, and are thus less equipped to help him find alternative ways of handling frustration and hurt. Deprived of his family's guidance, the boy continues to be susceptible to temper outbursts, thus reinforcing the family's focus on his explosive behavior.

CONSEQUENCES OF THE SYMPTOMATIC CYCLE

Constriction and Rigidity

In a systemic paradigm, an individual's "self" is seen as a fluid concept, changing as the context changes. Salvador Minuchin and Charles Fishman (1981) describe the self as "multifaceted" and maintain that different aspects of the self emerge in different contexts. The context pulls particular facets of the self to the foreground as other facets recede into the background.

Families who are locked in rigid patterns of interaction around symptoms are repeatedly engaging the same facets of each other. These facets exist in complementary and symmetrical relationships and are typically so pronounced that it is difficult to see beyond them to other, more positive facets.

For example, a father who insists on setting more limits on a symptomatic child might be perceived by the mother and other family members as overbearing and harsh. Other aspects of the father—such as his sensitivity, understanding, and nurturance—are neither activated nor reinforced in such a context. Similarly, to the extent that the father's harshness elicits the mother's overprotectiveness, her other facets, such as her capacity to discipline with gentleness, are not activated. These complementary facets of the parents are mutually activated in such a way that rigid patterns emerge.

The therapeutic task is to engage the untapped resources (facets) of each family member and use these newly engaged facets to help stimulate new interactional patterns. The therapist achieves this goal by utilizing his or her relationships with the family members to draw out new facets of each family member. As the therapist elicits new behaviors from each family member in the presence of the others, the family members have the opportunity to see each other differently, and thus interact differently. A new pattern begins to emerge (see Figure 3.2).

Arrested Development

As people develop, they discover more facets to themselves and learn to integrate these facets. The availability of a variety of facets permits

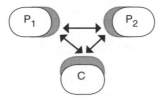

(1) The initial conditions in the family prior to therapy. The symptomatic cycle repeatedly activates the same facets of the parents (P_1 and P_2) and the symptomatic child (C).

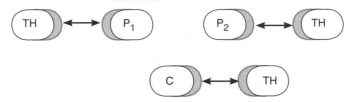

(2) The therapist (TH) engages in interactions with the family members that activate facets of the self that had not been activated by the symptomatic cycle.

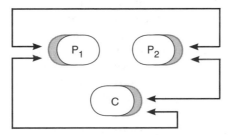

(3) The therapist then induces the family members into new patterns of interaction that activate the facets of the self that had not been activated by the symptomatic cycle.

FIGURE 3.2. Disrupting the symptomatic cycle.

optimal adaptation to a constantly changing environment. Families who are caught in symptomatic cycles repeatedly draw upon certain facets of themselves to the exclusion of others, a process that impedes the development of all family members who are participating in the cycle. Individuals lose touch with aspects of themselves that are not activated by the cycle. They become increasingly constricted and predictable, and less complex or flexible in their responses to one another. Since development is a process that aims toward increasing complexity, the constriction imposed by the symptomatic cycle impedes the process of development, not just for the symptomatic adolescent, but for all who participate in the symptomatic cycle.

While it is the symptomatic adolescent whose development is most obviously impaired, it is important to recognize that the developmental arrest affects all members of the family who participate in the symptomatic cycle. Since individual development and family development are inextricably linked and influence each other (Carter & McGoldrick, 2005), as one member of the system develops, others must follow suit or exert pressure on the changing member to revert to more predictable forms of behavior.

Even after the symptom remits, the therapist must be prepared to help the family adjust to the changes associated with the resumption of normal developmental processes. A depressed, withdrawn adolescent who becomes more argumentative and assertive after the depression lifts challenges the parents' ability to set reasonable limits that support the adolescent's autonomy. An adolescent who begins to express feelings more openly challenges the family's familiar ways of regulating conflict and anger. A formerly defiant adolescent who begins to handle independence more responsibly and requires less monitoring by his or her parents might no longer serve as a focus of common interest for parents who have drifted apart from one another over the years.

Families can vacillate between stasis and change. When the cycle is disrupted, development resumes, which creates anxiety and triggers the reemergence of the cycle. The return of the cycle can halt the developmental process once again. The therapist returns to disrupting the symptomatic cycle, only for the pattern to repeat. However, with each successful disruption of the symptomatic cycle, development moves slightly forward. The family members do not regress to their original positions, but to the state just prior to the reemergence of the cycle. Families can oscillate back and forth between reemergence of the symptomatic cycle and developmental progression, as they struggle to adapt to change. It is important to be patient and persistent in helping the family make these transitions. At this stage of treatment, it might be appropriate to consider couples therapy or individual therapy for one or more family members to help promote the developmental process and to complement the changes occurring in family therapy.

Mutually Reinforcing Narratives

Language is a powerful tool for shaping human experience. Over time, we begin to draw links and make inferences about ourselves, others, and the world and organize these inferences in the form of "narratives." The narratives then become templates for understanding future experiences and in so doing emphasize certain facts and deemphasize others.

In symptomatic families, narratives are rigidly organized and closed to new information. These closed narratives function as organizing schemas that promote selective attention to information that confirms the schemas. Family members seek out information that proves that their preferred view is the "right" one, thus reinforcing the original narrative and decreasing the likelihood that disconfirming information will be noticed. These views form a system of *complementary biased perceptions,* as family members are inclined to interpret each other's behavior in accordance with their original assumptions. As they act on these assumptions, they reinforce the complementary perceptions of the other family members, thus keeping the cycle active.

For example, the harsher parent selectively notices evidence that the other parent is "too lenient" and interprets this evidence as justification for his or her own harshness. Similarly, the more lenient parent selectively notices evidence that the other parent is "too harsh" thus justifying his or her own leniency. Direct challenges to their preferred beliefs can actually reinforce individuals' commitment to their beliefs by encouraging them to attend selectively to information that supports their position (White, 1983). Rather than listening to one another and giving credence to alternative points of view, family members might focus their energies on defending and justifying their own points of view.

It is important to help the family members take a different perspective on the problem that brought them to treatment. This is best accomplished experientially rather than through direct challenges or confrontation. One way to do so is to use the technique of *enactment*, described in the next chapter. It is also possible to use *reframing* to help family members view each other's behavior in a more complex light. For example, the therapist might suggest that the harsh parent is one whose love for his or her children and worry about their welfare drives him or her to set strict limits in an effort to prevent the children from making mistakes that could hurt them later in life. The lenient parent might be described as one who feels so much compassion for his or her children that he or she forgets that growing up means learning to live with not always getting what you want and learning to deal with situations that might seem unfair or unjust. It is also helpful to direct the family members' attention to those times when other family members are not behaving in accordance with their biased perceptions (White & Epston, 1990). In this way, it is possible to dislodge the system of complementary biased perceptions by suggesting alternative ways of interpreting each other's behavior or by eliciting new behaviors in the session and then helping the other family members to notice them.

COMMON PATTERNS IN SYMPTOMATIC FAMILIES

A number of patterns are commonly observed in families with troubled adolescents. Although the following list is not intended to be exhaustive, these patterns are among those most frequently encountered in work with symptomatic families. To illustrate these patterns, I will refer to the case of Mickey (father), Judy (mother), and their only child, 16-year-old Louis. In his initial phone call, Mickey explained that Louis's grades had recently dropped from A's and B's to C's and D's. The boy had become more defiant and was associating with a group of friends who were drinking and using drugs. Mickey claimed that he and Judy had a good relationship, but that they sometimes got into arguments about Louis. Mickey's job as a salesman required him to be away from home from Monday through Thursday each week. While he was traveling, Judy would call him almost every night to complain about Louis. Mickey would try to help by mediating the conflict or sometimes punishing Louis, though it was Judy who had to enforce the punishment.

Conflict Avoidance

Many families avoid airing conflicts openly for fear that they will have destructive consequences. Whenever conflicts threaten to emerge, they engage in behaviors that keep the conflict from surfacing. Perhaps a child's symptom helps to distract parents from conflicts with one another. Perhaps one parent withdraws from an interaction because he or she is fearful of engaging in direct conflict with the other parent or with the child. Perhaps a child "acts out" because he doesn't trust his parents enough to tell them directly how much they have hurt him. Perhaps bickering over minor issues distracts a married couple from addressing the major conflicts in their marriage.

One might hypothesize that Louis's defiant behavior keeps the parents' attention focused on him and thereby distracts them from addressing marital conflicts. While Mickey and Judy did not always agree on how to "handle" Louis, they both agreed that he was the problem. By focusing on him, they could ignore or minimize their conflicts with each other, such as the strain placed on the marriage by Mickey's job that required him to travel every week. It is important to note that Louis is not deliberately acting out to "protect" his parents (though this might be an unconscious motive) but that the family members are all participating in a pattern that keeps them stuck and prevents certain conflicts from being aired and potentially resolved.

Overprotection

In a sense, virtually any symptom exhibited by an adolescent could be framed as an example of immaturity or as a way to avoid accepting the responsibilities of growing up. Conversely, the parents' efforts to help the adolescent can reinforce the adolescent's dependency and immaturity by depriving the young person of opportunities to learn how to solve problems on his or her own.

For example, Judy insisted on checking Louis's homework to make sure that he had completed it, but this apparently helpful behavior prevented Louis from experiencing the consequences of his own choices and gave him the message that he was incapable of handling his school obligations on his own. In the case of Tina, discussed in Chapter 5, Rose's willingness to talk for Tina and interpret what the reticent girl "really felt," apparently intended as a way to show support for her daughter, actually reinforced the girl's helplessness and withdrawal and gave her the message that Mom didn't trust her to speak up for herself.

Disengagement and Abandonment

Families sometimes minimize problems, or at least fail to recognize the potential severity of them. Parents might be distracted by other obligations or interests, or in some cases might not be strongly attached to the child. This pattern might emerge in the session when the parents minimize or discount important statements made by the adolescent, when they drop out of conversations, or when they turn the conversation around to focus on their own needs. For example, a parent might be so focused on how much time and money the adolescent's "problem" is costing the parent that this issue comes up whenever the adolescent begins to verbalize a need or address a conflict. The adolescent then reverts to acting out, which not only obtains the attention he or she can't get through dialogue, but also passive–aggressively hurts the parent by costing more time and money.

A more subtle way in which abandonment might occur is in what I call the *"Tell me/Don't tell me" bind*. Overwhelmed and anxious about being blamed for the child's problem, the parent gives the youngster a double message: "Open up to me—but be sure not to say anything I don't want to hear." Trying to avoid upsetting the parent, the child withholds information, which only increases the parent's anxiety. For many kids, complete silence is their only defense against this bind. The parents might continue to pursue the kid, but in overt or subtle ways they give the young person the message that they are not able to handle the truth.

We'll see an example of the "Tell me/Don't tell me" bind in Chapter 5. While Rose claimed to want her daughter Tina to express her feelings, she kept interrupting Tina whenever she began talking, and appeared so anxious about what she might be about to hear that she covertly gave Tina the message that sharing her feelings was not a good idea. This bind was also active in Louis's family. Although his parents complained that Louis seemed distant and unwilling to talk with them, whenever he would express an opinion that they disagreed with they would cut him off and argue with him.

Escalation

Just because there is a lot of emotion in the room doesn't mean that people are truly connecting. In some families, conflicts quickly escalate because the family members provoke one another. While the parents might view the adolescent as provoking them, they are also provoking the adolescent. Deliberately or not, the parents might be saying or doing things that are increasing the adolescent's anxiety or frustration, rather than reducing the level of tension by staying calm and listening carefully to what the adolescent is saying. For example, one Friday night Louis came home an hour late. Despite being exhausted from having waited up for him, the parents decided to "have it out" immediately rather than wait until the next day when everyone was more rested. As soon as Louis entered the house, Mickey began screaming at him, Judy cowered in the background, and Louis screamed back. The conflict escalated to the point where Mickey threatened to hit Louis, Judy threw herself between them, and Louis stormed out of the house, not returning until the next day.

Constriction

One of the consequences of the symptomatic cycle is that families become trapped in repetitive patterns of interaction that impede their growth and development. In many families, they become so preoccupied with the symptom that they withdraw their attention from other aspects of their lives, including other children in the family. For example, Mickey and Judy stopped going out on Saturday nights so that they could stay home to supervise Louis. When they did talk with each other, the topic quickly turned to Louis. These were active, vibrant people with many interests, who had become so constricted in their lives that they were both on the verge of depression. The pattern was manifest in the room when the therapist noted that Mickey and Judy seemed estranged from one another, and could not maintain a conversation with each other for more than a few seconds without mentioning Louis. The more Mickey and Judy focused on Louis, the more exhausted they became, the less connected they felt to each other, and the more frustrated and helpless they felt about not being able to change Louis's behavior. As they continued to engage in more and more lecturing and other unsuccessful methods of trying to change Louis, the more discouraged and exhausted they felt because these methods weren't accomplishing anything.

THE PATTERN IS THE PROBLEM

In considering all of these patterns of interaction in families, it must be emphasized that these patterns do not *cause* the problem. Rather, it is more accurate to say that *the pattern is the problem*. A basic assumption of a family systems perspective is not that family dynamics *cause* symptoms, but rather that the symptomatic behavior of a family member is inextricably linked to the behavior of other members in the family, in such a way that assignment of cause and effect is arbitrary. A systemic view avoids getting caught up in discussions about antecedent causes and instead focuses on observations of interactional patterns that are taking place in the therapy room. Rather than relying on abstract terms to define problems (e.g., depression, poor impulse control, anxiety), which localize the problem *inside* a person or contained within the individual psyche, the family systems approach dissolves the dualism between *inside* and *outside*. Family interactional patterns influence the symptom, which in turn influences the family interactional patterns. Thus, the problem is *both* "inside" an individual person and also "outside," in that it is inextricably linked to the behavior of other people and how they are interacting with one another. The value of taking this perspective is that it opens up possibilities for intervention, as we will see in the next chapter.

SUMMARY AND WHAT'S NEXT

In this chapter, I provided an overview of my framework for understanding and helping families with symptomatic adolescents. Basic to this framework is the concept of the *symptomatic cycle*. Symptoms persist and intensify because the family members become so focused on eliminating or controlling the symptoms that they fail to attend to their relationships with one another. As these relationships deteriorate, family members grow farther and farther apart, and in this context of interpersonal disconnection and isolation symptoms persist and intensify. Consequences of the symptomatic cycle include increased constriction and rigidity, arrested development of all family members, and reinforcement of a system of complementary biased perceptions that helps to keep the cycle active. I also discussed several common patterns in symptomatic families: conflict avoidance, overprotection, disengagement/abandonment, escalation, and constriction.

In the next chapter, I discuss strategies and techniques that therapists can use to intervene in symptomatic cycles involving adolescents and their families.

4

How to Assess
and Treat Problems

In this chapter, I expand upon the concepts discussed in the previous chapter and propose a basic framework for working with troubled families. After presenting some general guidelines, I offer specific suggestions for building an alliance with the family, identifying symptomatic patterns, linking the problem to the pattern, and helping the family change the patterns of interaction that are linked to the symptom or presenting problem.

The basic principle guiding all intervention strategies is: *The therapist works to replace automatic, reactive responses between people with more thoughtful, planned responses.* Families who are caught up in symptomatic cycles engage in repetitive, unproductive interactions with one another that are motivated by a desire to find a solution but actually reinforce the problem that they are trying to solve. They react automatically to each other, rather than in planned, thoughtful ways. If they reflect on their behavior at all, they believe that their responses are logical and justified under the circumstances. In many cases, they haven't even considered the possibility that there could be other ways of acting.

For example, if an adolescent is depressed, the parents try to cheer her up. If a youngster seems immobilized by anxiety, the parents try to reduce stress by relaxing their expectations. If an adolescent repeatedly breaks the rules, the parents react by tightening the reins and "cracking down." In some cases, responses such as these might be helpful, and they might even succeed in solving the problem and bringing the family back to a comfortable stability. However, in families who come to therapy because they are unable to find their own solutions, what they experience as the "natural" and expected reactions to one another are actually making the problem worse. In the previous chapter, I referred to this pattern as the _symptomatic cycle_. Basically, the pattern and the problem have become inextricably linked, so that solving the problem requires a change in the interactional patterns in which the problem is embedded.

The goal of therapy is to alter these patterns. As explained in the previous chapter, therapists can accomplish this goal by using their relationship with each family member to encourage him or her to reflect on his or her behavior and experiment with new ways of behaving. As stated in the previous chapter, the therapist engages a hidden "facet" of a family member and encourages him or her to use this neglected aspect of himself or herself to try to change dysfunctional patterns and replace them with new patterns that create the potential for change.

GENERAL PRINCIPLES GUIDING
EFFECTIVE INTERVENTION

Have a Plan and Stay Focused

It is important for the therapist to adopt a focus for treatment and stick with it until there is convincing evidence that it will not net the desired result. In many cases, therapists simply need to be persistent in pushing for a particular change. The family's apparent "resistance" to the change is not, in and of itself, sufficient reason to abandon it. Although families and the people who make them up are complicated, therapists who refrain from taking a position because they are daunted by the family's apparent complexity run the risk of succumbing to paralysis.

Let's take an example. A therapist is consulted by two parents about their adolescent son who is staying out past curfew, refusing to help out around the house, neglecting his schoolwork, and arguing with his parents. The therapist observes the family for a while and notices that the mother dominates the session, the boy interrupts to defend himself, and the father barely participates at all. The therapist hypothesizes that the mother and father are not working together as a parenting team. To confirm this hypothesis and to observe how the mother and father interact, the therapist asks the parents to talk with each other and decide how they will respond the next time the boy comes home late.

The parents try to comply with this request, but within a few minutes, the mother is shouting at the father for "never having been there" in the past, declaring that the marriage is a sham, and threatening to leave if he doesn't shape up. In response, the father feebly defends himself and then just shuts down. Eventually, the mother turns to the therapist, announces that she is "tired of trying to make this marriage work" and launches into a history of the relationship that includes the fact that the father drank heavily until 5 years ago and the family has been on the verge of financial ruin several times.

The therapist now concludes that the "real problem" in the family has surfaced: The boy is acting out in order to distract his parents from the marital problems that threaten to tear the family apart. The therapist presents this hypothesis to the family and suggests a contract that involves working on the marriage. The therapist offers to meet individually with the adolescent from time to time to provide support and help him to learn how to exert more self-restraint. Six sessions later, nothing has changed. The marriage seems no better and no worse than before, the boy is continuing to break the rules, and the mother is muttering about not coming to therapy any more because "it's not helping." What went wrong?

Well, one thing that might have gone wrong is that the therapist too quickly abandoned the first hypothesis (that the parents were not working as a team) in favor of another, apparently more complex hypothesis (that the boy was acting out in order to regulate the degree of tension between the parents). What the therapist failed to notice, however, is what happened in the first session when he asked the parents to collaborate. While they initially complied, they did not complete the task. Instead, somewhere along the line, the conversation shifted from "what to do about the boy" to "what is wrong with this marriage." Although the latter might at first blush appear to be a "deeper" issue for this family, the next 6 weeks lead us to doubt it. In fact, the parents could go on for weeks ostensibly talking about marital issues, but they could hardly spend 5 minutes talking about parenting.

Perhaps the therapist might have noticed this early on and redirected the parents to the task at hand, with a comment like, "I'm sure there are many hurt feelings between you, and we can get into that later if you wish, but right now what I want you to do is to talk with each other about what to do the next time your son comes home late." The therapist might still entertain the hypothesis that the boy's acting out is a way of maintaining the family "homeostasis," but does not abandon the initial position in favor of this new hypothesis, at least not until it is absolutely clear that no progress will be made on parenting until the marital issues are addressed. Even so, before venturing into the new area of marital work, the therapist should have a clear hypothesis about the specific ways in which marital issues are interfering with parental collaboration and not lose sight that the original goal of treatment was to help reduce the boy's noncompliance.

In addition to having an overall focus for therapy, it is important to have a focus for every meeting with the family. This is not to say that therapists refuse to listen to what the family members bring up at the beginning of the session, but rather that therapists should be working at a different level, namely, one that addresses basic relational patterns (*process*) rather than specific issues or conflicts (*content*).

It is possible to work at the level of process through any piece of content the family presents, but the goal should always be to help the family develop *more effective ways of resolving conflicts* rather than arrive at a resolution of a specific issue. Thus, in the example above, if the parents are struggling with the decision whether to extend the boy's curfew by a half hour, the most important issue is not negotiating the specific hour of the curfew but rather helping the family find better ways of disentangling themselves when they reach such impasses.

Therapists need to plan out their responses to the family so that they avoid responding in a reactive and emotional manner. The term *induction* refers to the risk that therapists can get caught up in a family's symptomatic patterns, and as a result compromise their ability to help the family. To avoid induction, therapists must keep track of cycles and patterns without becoming part of them. The goal is to help the family members become better observers of their own behaviors and reactions to one another, and in so doing remove themselves from the emotional pull of the patterns in which they are caught. Therapists can help families in this way only if they remain free from the emotional pull of the patterns and avoid responding reactively to the family. Having a plan and a clear focus will help a therapist retain this position.

Focus on Changing Relationships and Patterns

Changing patterns means requesting people to change what they "do," not who they "are." Consider the family of Mickey (father), Judy (mother), and Louis (son) described in the previous chapter. Although I was tempted to view Mickey as pompous and overbearing, I realized that confronting him on these supposed personality traits was not likely to enlist his cooperation. Rather, I decided to suggest a specific behavioral change and ask Mickey to try it out. I asked Mickey to have a conversation with Louis during which he limited himself to questions that did not have "yes" or "no" answers. I offered this suggestion in a playful tone, hoping to reduce the family's anxiety and imply that the goal was to try out new ways of interacting with one another in an atmosphere of experimentation and exploration without necessarily expecting a particular outcome.

Toward this end, rather than describing family members with terms that imply stable *traits* (e.g., stubborn, weak, critical, demanding, rebellious), it is better to focus instead on specific *behaviors*, keeping in mind that a different behavior could be elicited if the context were to change.

Thus, while an argument with his son tends to elicit critical statements and an overbearing tone, a different kind of discussion could elicit different behaviors from Mickey, such as warmth, curiosity, and humor. It is the task of the therapist to create contexts that are likely to elicit these underdeveloped behaviors of the family members. These new behaviors then can serve as the seeds around which new patterns can crystallize.

For example, while Mickey appears critical and controlling at times, he also appears to care about his son and shows concern for his welfare. It is important to avoid the error of trying to decide what is "the truth" about Mickey. Is he critical and controlling *or* is he concerned and sympathetic? Putting questions such as these in either/or terms demeans Mickey's complexity and slips into the kind of dualistic thinking that the family systems perspective seeks to avoid. Mickey exhibits all of these qualities, and which one emerges at any particular time depends upon the interpersonal context and the questions the therapist chooses to ask.

Invite Collaboration

Whenever the family is successful (or even unsuccessful) in changing a particular pattern, it is good practice to invite the family members to reflect on the experience. Often, the family members will begin to identify ways in which their interactional patterns contributed to frustration or helplessness. Giving the family members an opportunity to offer their own observations conveys the message that the therapist values their perceptions and also stimulates the family members to become better observers of their own interactional patterns.

The therapist might explore with the family members what made it difficult for them to change, or what life experiences might be getting in the way of adopting new behaviors (e.g., Minuchin et al., 2007). Rather than offering specific ways in which the family members could change their behavior, the therapist could engage them in a conversation that explores their ideas for approaching the situation differently. This communicates respect for the family's struggles and facilitates a more collaborative relationship between the therapist and family members.

For example, during one of the arguments between Louis and Mickey, I interrupted and asked them, "Did you notice what just happened?" In asking this question, I hoped to jolt them out of their reactive pattern and encourage a more observant role. In response, Judy said, "This is the way it always happens. They can't talk to one another." Mickey and Louis nodded their heads in agreement. I then asked them, "How do you think it could go differently the next time you try to have a conversation?" Mickey suggested, albeit halfheartedly, "I guess I could try to listen better." At least this was a start: Mickey acknowledged that a change on his part could help, and the idea was more powerful because it came from him rather than suggested by me.

Refer Back to the Pattern

When the symptom appears to get worse, the temptation is to focus on the symptom. However, as discussed in the previous chapter, the more the family members focus on the symptom in an effort to change, control, or eliminate it, the more entrenched the symptomatic cycle becomes. Whether the symptom improves or gets worse, the therapist should always link this change back to the pattern of interaction among the family members.

It is important not to lose sight of the systemic formulation and not conclude that therapy is failing if there is a recurrence or worsening of the symptom. Linear, steady improvement is the exception, not the rule. Change occurs in fits and starts, and regressions or relapses are to be expected. Long-standing patterns are difficult to change, and even when they appear to have changed, it is possible that family members could test the permanence of the change by resuming an old behavior. Presenting this perspective to the family could help them stay the course when it appears that their efforts at change haven't produced the desired results quickly enough.

For example, following the interchange recounted in the previous section, I asked Mickey and Louis to resume their conversation. I requested, "Do it differently this time. Mickey, see if you could try to listen better, as you had suggested." Louis and Mickey resumed their conversation, but after a few minutes they were fighting again. I stopped them and pointed out to them that they were stuck in the same pattern: "Did you see it? It happened again. You got pulled back into the same pattern of arguing and struggling with one another rather than trying to understand one another."

Offer Encouragement and Accentuate the Positive

Family members who are caught in symptomatic cycles frequently feel discouraged and hopeless. What appears to be depression might be a manifestation of this hopelessness, exhaustion, and resignation. It is important for the therapist to remain upbeat and hopeful that the family members can change. Focus on what the family is doing right. Therapists must be alert to signs of strengths and resources within the family and seek to capitalize on these as a way of stimulating change. One way to communicate this idea to the family is to say: "There's a lot to work *on* in this family, but there's also a lot to work *with*."

Therapists should also be vigilant for any sign that the family is changing in the desired direction so that they can help the family members notice these changes and work to amplify them. When making a request for a change, it is helpful to use the "stroke and kick" method advocated by Salvador Minuchin (Minuchin et al., 2007, p. 7). First point out something that the person is doing right, or a benevolent motive that the person appears to have, then follow it with a request for change. For example, I said to Judy, "I really admire your restraint in sitting back and not jumping into the conversation too quickly, but I think you have a lot to offer and I'd like you to participate more actively." Needless to say, these compliments must be offered genuinely and refer to behaviors or qualities that the therapist truly appreciates or admires.

In the previous chapter, I described the system of *complementary biased perceptions* that keeps the family locked into their habitual patterns of reacting to one another. Because of their complementary biased perceptions, the family members are often blind to events that do not fit with their expectations of one another. Even when these events are called to their attention, they often discount their significance. For example, neither Mickey nor Judy could identify instances when Louis demonstrated care or concern for them. In another family, neither the father nor the mother could recall incidents when their daughter showed that she was competent and capable of acting age-appropriately, even though the girl was engaged in expertly sketching a profile of the therapist during this conversation.

Michael White (1986) has used the term *unique outcomes* to refer to those times when the problem is less severe or not present at all. The family members' selective attention to information that confirms their biased perceptions makes it difficult for them to notice these unique outcomes on their own. Yet, to the extent that unique outcomes go unnoticed, they are less likely to recur, thus setting up the conditions for a "self-fulfilling prophecy." It is useful to help the family members notice these unique outcomes and then invite them to construct new narratives around them. This process can dissolve the system of complementary biased perceptions by introducing new complexity to the shared family narratives.

Promote Moments of Engagement

While members of symptomatic families usually feel disconnected and estranged from one another, they still long for connection. Creating opportunities in therapy for the family members to experience an emotional connection with one another can stimulate hope that their relationships with each other can improve. These moments might be fleeting, but the therapist should call attention to them and amplify their significance as harbingers of greater changes to come.

For example, I noted that the father of an adolescent girl rarely spoke to her directly but instead addressed her indirectly through me or through her mother. To encourage direct contact between the girl and her father, I drew upon their mutual interest in art to suggest that they spend a day together at an art museum and then talk with each other about their reactions to the paintings they saw. After a number of experiences such as this in which the father and daughter come to know each other better, the relationship between them has grown to be far more complex than it once was: Now it is *sometimes* distant and *sometimes* close, and there is an opportunity for the father and daughter to build upon the latter "unique outcomes" to create a new narrative about their relationship.

The foregoing describes some general principles that can orient therapists toward the appropriate stance to take with families. In the following sections, I describe the process of conducting therapy in more detail.

HOW TO BUILD AN ALLIANCE WITH THE FAMILY

The first step is to build a working alliance with the family. This is accomplished by developing a relationship with each family member, getting to know them as individuals, and respecting their unique points of view. The process by which the therapist forges an alliance with the family has been called *joining* (Minuchin, 1974). Joining goes beyond simply building a context in which family members feel supported and safe to express their concerns. The family must also come to trust that the therapist has the skills and expertise to help them. The following suggestions for facilitating the process of joining with a family are based on those recommended by Minuchin (1974) and Haley (1987):

1. *Starting the session.* The process of joining with the family begins as soon as the therapist greets the family. I suggest starting the session with a brief "social" period, as recommended by Jay Haley (1987). The therapist chats casually with each family member and finds out a little bit about him or her, before jumping into talking about the problems that brought him or her to therapy. After making an initial contact with each family member in this way, the therapist then shifts to gathering information about the concerns that brought the family to treatment. A transitional comment might be, "Now I'd like to hear about the concerns

that have brought you here today, and I'd also like to hear from each of you what you'd like to accomplish here. I just want to go around and hear a little bit from everyone and then I might come back and ask some questions, OK? Let's start with you—what concerns have brought you here today?"

2. *Respecting the family's structure.* Based on initial information gathered about the family from the first phone contact or referral, the therapist can formulate a preliminary hypothesis about the family's current structure. In most instances, the therapist should begin by addressing one of the parents rather than the adolescent "identified patient," but there are exceptions. If the identified patient is an older adolescent, the therapist might address him or her first, particularly if the adolescent has already expressed a concern and is participating willingly in treatment. If one parent seems dominant and the other submissive or peripheral, it is best not to challenge this structure, but rather to address the dominant parent first as a way of acknowledging his or her role in the family. When there are no clear-cut reasons to suspect that one parent occupies this role, the therapist should consider first addressing the parent who did not make the initial phone contact, as a way of emphasizing that the views of both parents are important. The therapist might say, first addressing the parent who made the initial call and then turning to the other parent, "Since you and I talked a bit on the phone the other day, I'd like to start with you [turning toward the other parent]. What are your concerns?"

3. *Listening and tracking.* The therapist listens carefully to what each person says, paraphrases as appropriate, and accepts the person's point of view without challenge or comment. If one family member interrupts another, the therapist could use this opportunity to request that no one speak until the speaker has finished. If a family member (usually it's the adolescent) refuses to talk, the therapist should simply accept this fact and state, "OK, I accept that you don't feel like talking right now. I appreciate that you are here anyway, and I think you can get a lot out of listening as well as talking. Hearing what you have to say is important to me, so I might just keep checking in with you as we go along to see whether you have anything to contribute to the discussion." If one family member dominates the proceedings and launches into a monologue, the therapist might say "I appreciate that you have so much to say, and I definitely want to hear it, but right now I'd just like to get a brief description of your concerns, and then hear from the other people who are here. Now, what I've heard you say is ... [therapist briefly paraphrases what the family member has said]."

4. *Getting more information.* After obtaining a brief description of each family member's concerns, then the therapist might follow up with

more questions to help expand on certain topics. As discussed below, the therapist is interested in the particular way in which each family member describes the problem, and also in the ways that the family members have tried (unsuccessfully) to solve the problem in the past.

5. *Acknowledging strengths.* One of the problems in symptomatic families is that they become caught up in their problems and lose sight of what they are doing right. Therapists should take every opportunity to acknowledge strengths or to compliment the family on something they have observed that they (genuinely) like. It is important that therapists not view this as a technique and so feel forced to compliment the family on something trivial. Rather, it is our job to search for something about the family that we can genuinely compliment, and then do so. By acknowledging strengths, we imply that the family is capable of rising above their current problems and we communicate our confidence that we can help them achieve these changes.

One question that frequently arises is whom to include in the family sessions. In the initial session family members might directly or indirectly suggest that absent parties play a key role in the symptomatic cycle. These individuals could be members of the nuclear family, members of the extended family, or individuals outside the family who have engaged in significant interactions with the family members around the problem. It might be necessary to prolong the assessment phase of treatment until it is possible to arrange for these absent parties to attend a session. On the other hand, the therapist should not automatically assume that everyone in the family is a participant in the symptomatic cycle. Often, symptomatic cycles might involve only a subsystem of the family and not include everyone in the household, such as siblings or grandparents. While it is often useful to include these individuals in at least one assessment session to ascertain their role in the cycle, it is rarely useful to insist that they participate on a regular basis.

HOW TO IDENTIFY SYMPTOMATIC CYCLES

In addition to building an alliance with the family, during the first few sessions the therapist should also attempt to identify interactional patterns that are linked to the symptom or presenting problem.

Three sources of information are useful for identifying the symptomatic cycle: (1) the language used by each family member to describe the problem, (2) the history of the problem, and (3) direct observation of interpersonal interactions that take place in the therapy room.

Language: How Does Each Family Member View the Problem?

By carefully tracking how each family member talks about the problem and about each other, it is possible to gain insight into the symptomatic cycle and the system of interlocking narratives that supports it. By asking the question, "How do you see the problem?" the therapist can elicit from each family member his or her narrative about the problem, the person with the problem, and his or her relationship to the person with the problem. Thus, the therapist can uncover the unspoken and unquestioned assumptions each family member brings to therapy.

For example, a father of an adolescent girl with anorexia said, "My daughter is the problem. She has anorexia. She won't eat and keeps losing weight. There's nothing we can do to get her to eat."

This response implies several hypotheses about the father and his relationship to the problem. He sees the problem as residing within his daughter. He sees the problem as having a name, which he also describes more specifically in behavioral terms ("She won't eat and keeps losing weight"). He expresses impotence and frustration at his failure to help, but the phrase "*get* her" implies that he might be in a power struggle with his daughter.

In contrast, the girl's mother said, "I just hope that she finds the strength within herself to get well. She didn't ask for this disease. She doesn't want it. She just wants to get well."

Like the father, the girl's mother sees the problem as a "disease." She believes that the solution lies within the girl. Mother also makes several statements that imply that she has access to the girl's private thoughts and feelings. Meanwhile, the girl remained silent, thus implying assent, if not agreement, with the mother's assumptions about her.

When asked her view of the problem, the girl replied, "I don't know, it just happened." When the therapist pushed for more, the girl muttered a few inaudible words, then burst into tears. This behavior reinforced her mother's view of her as a helpless victim, who lacks the "strength within herself to get well."

In this example, it is clear how these narratives in the family reinforce and complement one another. Father says the girl "won't eat," while her mother implies that she "can't eat." While both the mother and father seem to agree that the solution to the problem resides within the daughter the father implies that one solution is to "get her" to eat while the mother implies that the solution must come from "within herself." As the father intensifies his efforts to "get her" to eat, the mother will undermine these efforts in order to support her view that the girl "can't eat" and that the solution, if it exists, lies "within herself." The girl herself remains noncommittal, though clearly presents herself as helpless. Her apparent powerlessness is deceptive, however: In her adamant refusal to eat or even to speak she renders both of her parents helpless.

History of the Problem: Which Solutions Have Already Been Tried?

Previous unsuccessful attempts at problem resolution tell the therapist what has not worked and how these solutions might have unwittingly exacerbated the problem. Often, problems crystallize because the family members are attempting to solve new problems by repeatedly using methods that might have worked for them at an earlier phase of development (Fisch, Weakland, & Segal, 1982). These attempted solutions do not solve the current problem because they neglect to take into account the need for a qualitative change in family organization. By carefully tracking the sequence of events leading up to the consultation, the therapist can gain insight into the patterns that have congealed around the problem.

For example, the family described in the previous section related that the current consultation was precipitated after the mother, in searching the girl's room, discovered empty bottles of ipecac (an emetic available in most pharmacies). Asked why she was in her daughter's room, the mother could respond only that she "suspected something was not right" and felt compelled to investigate. Noteworthy was the fact that the mother took unilateral action rather than consulting with the father. Asked what happened after the mother found the ipecac bottles, she responded that she confronted the girl, who became very upset. Mother didn't know what else to do, so in desperation she called the father and demanded that he take over, thus triangulating him into the conflict between her and her daughter. Father then proceeded to attack the mother, who defended herself against the father's attacks, while the girl wept silently in the background. Finally, the mother hung up on the father and called the girl's therapist (another triangulation). Sensing the mother's extreme anxiety and the danger involved in the girl's abuse of ipecac (which the girl had concealed from her therapist), the therapist suggested that the mother contact me (the "expert") for a consultation.

These events suggest the following pattern: Mother feels disconnected from the girl, and attempts to connect with her by violating a boundary. Then she confronts her daughter with the information she discovered and the girl collapses. Unable to deal directly with the girl the mother contacts the girl's father, who unhelpfully begins to criticize the mother. The parents get lost in their conflict, while their daughter's needs are neglected. Finally, the mother rejects the father and seeks out the girl's therapist, who recognizes that the situation has spiraled out of control and recommends a consultation with an "expert."

This pattern suggests that the mother and daughter are not able to regulate closeness in their relationship without involving a third party. It also suggests that the parents are unsuccessful in working collaboratively to help their daughter. Father appears peripheral, which is reinforced by the mother's efforts to distance him, a natural response to his hostility toward her. Father expresses his anxiety by attacking the mother, which only fuels further conflict and keeps the cycle going.

Direct Observations: How Do the Family Members Interact?

What distinguishes family therapy from other therapeutic approaches is the emphasis on patterns of interpersonal interaction. These repeating patterns, which usually occur outside the awareness of the family members, help to keep the symptom alive. Although what the family members *say* about the problem is important, the therapist must also attend to the *manner in which the family members interact* with one another. A technique that can be helpful in eliciting the patterns in the family is called *enactment* and was first described by Salvador Minuchin (1974).

The following steps can be followed to carry out an enactment:

• *Step 1.* The therapist must be alert for an opportunity for an enactment. Usually, this will occur when a family member is describing to the therapist a problem he or she is having with another family member who is also present in the room.

• *Step 2.* The therapist asks the family members if they would be willing to discuss this problem right now, while the therapist observes. To elicit the family's cooperation, the therapist might say that this method has been helpful to other families in the past.

• *Step 3.* Without further instruction, the therapist sits back and observes the interaction that takes place. The therapist should allow the interaction to proceed for several minutes and not intervene too quickly. The goal at this step is not to change the interaction, just to observe it. After a suitable period of time, or when the conversation breaks down because the family reaches an impasse, the therapist could say, "Let me stop you there."

• *Step 4.* The therapist invites the family members to reflect on the interaction that has just occurred. The therapist might ask, "How did you feel about what just happened here? Did you get what you wanted to get out of this conversation? Do you feel as if you resolved anything? If not, why not?"

• *Step 5.* The therapist then offers the family his or her own observations.

• *Step 6.* The therapist suggests a change in the pattern and asks the family to re-enact the conversation with the recommended change.

• *Step 7.* The family re-enacts the conversation while the therapist silently observes.

• *Step 8.* If the family is successful in changing the interactional pattern, the therapist points this out and praises the family on their flexibility and willingness to change. The therapist then explores with the family members other ways in which they could build upon the change they have already made. If the family is not successful in changing the pattern, the therapist points this out to them and explores with them what made it difficult for them to change. At this point, the therapist has an opening to offer the family a reformulation of the problem that links the symptom to the pattern, and then can suggest that treatment be focused on altering the pattern. This is a crucial stage. By agreeing to work on changing their patterns of interaction rather than trying to change or control the "problem" adolescent, the family members have demonstrated that they are capable of seeing beyond the symptom and instead attend to their relationships with one another.

As an example, let's return to the case of Mickey, Judy, and Louis. In the first session, Mickey began complaining to me about Louis's recent drop in grades and his association with a new set of friends that the parents didn't like. I noted that this presented an opportunity for an enactment (Step 1). Rather than addressing me, I asked Mickey to address his concerns directly to Louis (Step 2). Louis did so, but after a few minutes, the conversation broke down. Mickey was verbally berating Louis, who sat silently with a scowl on his face, and Judy acted as if she wasn't even in the room (Step 3).

I asked the family to share with me their experience of what had just happened, starting with Judy (Step 4). She said, "It's just like this at home," and Mickey and Louis concurred. I then offered my perspective (Step 5):

> "I'd like to tell you what I observed. What I observed is that the conversation started out well. You, Mickey, addressed your son directly, telling him what your concerns were regarding his failing grades and his new friends. You, Louis, tried to explain to your father your views on why your behavior has changed in this way. But then I think the conversation broke down, because you, Mickey, interrupted Louis and started lecturing him about what he was doing wrong. In response, you, Louis, just shut down and it looked to me that you stopped listening to your father. Meanwhile, you, Judy, just sat on the sidelines and didn't participate in the conversation."

I added (Step 6), "I'd like you to try it again, but this time I'd like you to do two things differently. First, I'd like all three of you to participate in the conversation. Second, Mickey and Judy, I'd like you to keep your comments short, and instead try to involve Louis in the conversation by asking questions and listening to his answers."

In their reenactment, Mickey and Judy started out by asking Louis some questions, but after a few interchanges Judy again withdrew, Mickey started lecturing, and Louis shut down (Step 7). I interrupted them at this point and pointed out what I had observed (Step 8). I then said to them:

"I think it is very difficult for you to change this pattern, but I believe it is this pattern that is keeping you from reaching a resolution to the problem that brought you here. This is what I see happening: Judy and Mickey, you two are really not working together as a parenting team, so you are only half as effective as parents as you could be. I think you, Mickey, get frustrated with Louis and you don't know what else to do but try to talk him out of the behaviors that you believe are harmful. Louis has heard these arguments many times before, so he just shuts down and doesn't listen. This frustrates you even more, Mickey, and Louis just keeps up what he has been doing. You see, the more you try to get Louis to change, the more he resists your efforts to change him. Louis begins to resent you and you begin to resent Louis. However, people are more likely to change when they care about other people's feelings and want to change in order to please them. Right now, Louis is angry, and he's not about to change to please you because he's angry at you. I'd like to recommend a different approach. I'd like to work with you on changing these patterns. I'd like to help you to strengthen your relationships with each other so that you can engage in more productive problem solving. That means we have to change the pattern that I just observed. It would be helpful if we all could agree that this is going to be our goal. The problem is this pattern, not Louis and not Louis's behavior. I believe that if you successfully change this pattern, then Louis will change his behavior on his own."

SETTING THE COURSE FOR TREATMENT

As illustrated in the example above, an outcome of an enactment is to show the family how their presenting problem is connected to the ways in which they are interacting with one another. This constitutes a reframing of the problem. When the family comes to treatment, they view the adolescent or the adolescent's behavior as the problem. Via an enactment, the therapist helps the family to see that the problem is actually much broader than one person's behavior. To paraphrase what I stated to Louis's family: *The problem is the pattern, not the adolescent* or *the adolescent's behavior.* The family will be more receptive to a reframing of this type if they have experienced it themselves through an enactment. The therapist then suggests that treatment be focused on changing this pattern, and expresses the conviction that changing the pattern will lead to a change in the adolescent's behavior.

Here's another example derived from a family struggling with eating disorder, a case that will be discussed in more detail in the next chapter. After observing that the divorced parents were so caught up in their battle with one another that they were ineffective in helping their daughter (Tina), I offered the following reframe:

> "Tina is losing weight and can't eat because she feels isolated and alone, unable to express her true feelings to anyone. She is wasting away not only from lack of food but also because of the absence of nurturing and sustaining relationships in her life. This deprives her of the valuable help you both can offer her to grow and become the young adult she is capable of becoming."

This reframing includes the following elements:

- A statement of the problem ("Tina is losing weight and can't eat").
- A hypothesis about why the problem is present ("because she feels isolated and alone, unable to express her true feelings to anyone").
- A link between the problem and the relationships in the family ("She is wasting away not only from lack of food but also because of the absence of nurturing and sustaining relationships in her life").

This formulation frames the problem in a way that deviates from all of the problem definitions circulating in the family. For example, the father had described the problem as "not eating and losing weight," while the mother had emphasized Tina's helplessness in the face of an unwanted disease. The metaphors of growth and sustenance were used to extract a similar theme from both the mother's and father's accounts by linking Tina's weight loss to an inability to derive sustenance from the relationships in her life.

After presenting the formulation, the therapist then proposes a plan for solving the problem. It is not necessary to spell out this plan in great detail, but it should state clearly that the goal of treatment is to change the relationships in the family. For example, I proposed the following plan to Tina and her parents: "If you are interested, I will work with all of you, as a family, to give you the chance to begin building more sustaining relationships, so that Tina may begin to grow again."

This plan is brief but to the point: It states that the goal of therapy will be to change the way the members of the family relate to one another ("to begin building more sustaining relationships, so that Tina may begin to grow again"). Weight gain is linked to improved relationships in the family, consistent with the formulation that Tina was "wasting away ... because of the absence of nurturing and sustaining relationships in her life."

TECHNIQUES FOR CHANGING PATTERNS

What Leads to a Change in a Pattern?

A pattern changes when at least one participant in the pattern makes a conscious and deliberate effort to change the way he or she responds to the other participants in the pattern. Moreover, the participant who commits to this change also commits to maintaining the change despite pressure from the other participants to return to more familiar ways of behaving. If we accept that the pattern has taken hold of the family, and has done so by bending their perceptions of one another like a massive object bends light or a lens affects the perception of the size of objects, then it follows that the other participants experience disorientation when one participant in the pattern changes. To resolve their own confusion, they could exert overt or covert pressure on the person who has changed to revert to his or her former ways of behaving. From the perspective of the family members, the pattern is not the problem. The problem, in their view, is the behavior of the symptomatic person, and their own actions are simply natural and expected responses to this behavior. When one person chooses to disengage from this pattern, the other family members, who are comfortable maintaining their usual ways of behaving, might feel unsupported or disregarded.

For example, let's say that Mickey and Judy decide to take a break from their mutual focus on Louis and instead decide to spend time with one another by going out for the evening. Although we hope that Louis uses this opportunity to prove to his parents that he is able to follow the rules without their direct supervision, this outcome is by no means certain. If Louis gets into trouble while his parents are out of the house, it seems like a natural reaction for Mickey and Judy to conclude that they had erred by leaving Louis alone, and consequently redouble their efforts to supervise him. Some therapists might even hypothesize that Louis "acted out" in order to prevent his parents from being alone with one another because this might give them an opportunity to fight or discover that they don't have much in common. A simpler interpretation is that Louis lacks experience being on his own, and as a result he makes an error in judgment when his parents take a step back. In any event, if Mickey and Judy were to return to their habitual ways of behaving, the pattern would be reinforced. They need to take a risk and try something new. Rather than deciding that they can't leave Louis alone, they might decide instead that Louis would receive a consequence for his mistake, and next time they go out for the evening they would arrange for another responsible adult to supervise Louis. In this way, they maintain the new pattern of direct engagement in the marital subsystem while still discharging their responsibilities as parents.

The unproductive arguments and bickering that occur between adolescents and their parents provide another example. The pattern might go something like this: (1) The adolescent makes a request; (2) the parent denies the request; (3) the adolescent challenges the parent's decision and tries to get him or her to change it; and (4) the parent enters into a debate with the adolescent, which escalates into shouting and mutual recriminations. In effect, the adolescent and the parent are reacting to one another, and neither one seems to be able to step out of this pattern. This pattern can be broken if the parent could remain calm, avoid participating in an emotional argument with the adolescent, and instead empathically acknowledge the adolescent's disappointment with the decision without agreeing to change the decision.

The adolescent, however, is not likely to find this response reassuring, since the bottom line is that she does not get what she wants. In the past, she might have found that she is more likely to get what she wants when she engages the parents in an argument, so she redoubles her efforts to bait the parents and thus incite them to react. To change this pattern, the parents must make a conscious and deliberate effort to refuse to react and instead stay calm regardless of what the adolescent says or does in response.

So, to reiterate: A pattern changes when one participant makes a conscious and deliberate effort to change, and stays committed to maintaining this change in spite of the pull to revert to his or her typical ways of acting. The trick, of course, is how to bring this about. Simply requesting a change is not enough. So how do we convince the family members to change in spite of their reservations? In the following sections, I discuss some techniques that might be helpful toward achieving this goal.

Direct Instruction

Teaching about Systems

Explaining to families the role of the symptomatic cycle and how it contributes to their problems can help motivate them to pay attention to their interactional patterns rather than follow them automatically. Therapists who are accustomed to thinking systemically might assume that these principles are obvious to families, but this is rarely the case. Explaining the tenets of systems thinking, including the notions of circular causality and complementarity, could help family members understand why a commitment to unilateral change is necessary in order to disrupt the patterns that contribute to the problem. Diagramming or writing out the steps in the symptomatic cycle can help to keep the focus on the pattern. Explaining the reasons why the therapist might not focus directly on eliminating the symptom but rather on changing the interactional patterns might help the family members stay the course when they are discouraged if the symptom does not abate quickly enough.

Teaching Skills

In some cases, family members might be receptive to direct instruction in effective communication and conflict resolution skills. For example, teaching principles of effective discipline could help to break a cycle whereby parents who feel powerless lash out harshly and then relent, thus giving the child the message that they need not be taken seriously. Coaching family members in ways to listen better helps to encourage the expression of true feelings that lead to validation from the other family members rather than defensiveness or hostility. An adolescent who has a quick temper might be motivated to learn skills to help her tame her temper and respond in a more modulated way.

Many families can benefit from a review of *active listening* skills (Nichols, 2004). Parents who react impulsively whenever an adolescent challenges them can be reminded that listening does not mean agreement and an immediate response is not required of them even if the adolescent pushes for one. Rather than responding to the *content* of what the adolescent is saying (e.g., "Why *can't* I stay out until midnight?") the parent can instead respond to the *emotion* behind the adolescent's statement (e.g., "I can tell you're really disappointed that we won't let you stay out late"). To slow down the rapid-fire exchange that often occurs during family conflicts, family members might be taught to *paraphrase* what they have heard and refrain from speaking until the other person has finished.

Family members might also be taught how to be better *observers* of their interactions with one another. They might be instructed to keep track of how often a particular pattern occurs, or to "step out" of the stream of bickering to watch it more objectively and dispassionately from the "banks of the stream." As encouraged by cognitive-behavioral methods of intervention, family members might benefit from articulating the hidden assumptions and "dysfunctional beliefs" that impel them to feel and act in ways that invite undesired reactions from others.

Using Complementarity

When trying to encourage another person to change, it is tempting to try to attack the problem behavior head on, for example, by confronting the person, trying to convince the person to mend his or her ways, arguing with the person, or punishing him or her. These methods might be effective in some circumstances, but they represent a limited repertoire of options for encouraging change in another person. Furthermore, one of the factors that helps to sustain the symptomatic cycle is the attempt to control other people and force them to change. As we have seen, these attempts at interpersonal control are ineffective, because the person who is the target of these change efforts is likely to resist the efforts to coerce him or her to change, and because family relationships are damaged by the intense preoccupation with the symptom and neglect of other aspects of the relationship. Once the relationship is damaged, persons from whom change is desired are even less likely to change, because they are less motivated to please the other person and instead divert their energies into asserting their own autonomy.

All family members who are participating in the symptomatic cycle need to change their behaviors if they are to develop more effective ways of relating to one another. It is often the case, however, that family members will minimize the changes they themselves need to make and instead focus on changes they desire from others. The principle of *complementarity* can provide a way out of this dilemma. According to this fundamental principle of systems, two or more individuals who are in frequent contact with one another tend to shape each other's behaviors over time.

For example, a parent who complains that she can't trust her adolescent daughter anxiously monitors the daughter for any signs that she is trying to deceive her. The more the mother monitors her, the more the daughter feels compelled to avoid the mother and keep secrets from her. To deal with her daughter's deceptiveness, the mother might bribe her, bargain with her, threaten her, or otherwise try to cajole the daughter to be honest with her. These methods fail because the daughter continues to evade the mother's control. The therapist might proceed by helping the mother to see that her methods have not been effective in reducing the lying, but instead have eroded their relationship. The mother's anxious monitoring of the daughter might be framed as an example of overprotection that helps to keep the daughter young by encouraging her to focus her attention on ways to avoid her mother rather than ways to monitor and control her own behavior. By pointing out the complementarity, the therapist can help the mother find other ways of calming her anxiety, such as meditation or using the support of her husband or other family members. More positive ways of building contact between the mother and daughter could be developed. These can be framed as more mature ways of providing the girl with the attention she craves rather than serving as a living prosthesis for the girl's unreliable self-control.

Many impasses in relationships can be traced to complementarity. The example above is a *pursuit–withdraw* cycle, whereby the more the mom pursues the daughter, the more the daughter withdraws and evades, thereby inviting more pursuit. Another example is the *attack–defend* cycle, whereby the more one criticizes another, the more the criticized person feels compelled to defend against the criticism rather than consider it seriously. The more the criticism is rebuffed, the more the critic feels compelled to push his or her point. In both of these examples, either party can break the cycle, and it is often the more active party (i.e., the pursuer or the critic) who holds the key to change. The motivation can come from an appreciation of the ineffectiveness of the pattern, and a commitment to change oneself in relation to the other rather than trying to force or convince the other person to change.

The principle of complementarity also applies to the therapist's efforts to elicit change from a family member. For example, a family with an unruly son had two parents who seemed to lack a sense of humor, which is an essential survival tool for living with difficult adolescents. The parents rarely smiled and spoke in a monotonic voice using sophisticated words the son did not appear to understand. The parents seemed genuinely mystified that their son ignored virtually everything they said. I was tempted to point out to the parents that their ponderous and pompous attitude alienated the boy, but decided instead to try a less direct approach. I began joking with the boy, gently teasing him and accepting his ribbing in return. I began to invite the parents into the playfulness, not by challenging them directly, but rather including them in the banter. Eventually, the parents joined in, lost their heaviness, and the overall tone of the session became lighter and more relaxed.

By adopting a complementary position to a facet of a family member that the therapist wishes to bring to the foreground, the therapist can help facilitate a change in family interactions. As explained in the previous chapter (see Figure 3.2), the therapist uses the relationship with each family member to coax or elicit new behaviors that are not typically part of the family interactions. When these new behaviors are expressed, there is an opportunity for family members to see a hidden facet of each other, and thereby open up the rigidly closed system of complementary biased perceptions.

For example, when I interrupted an angry argument between Louis and his father, the boy snapped at me. Rather than confronting the boy on his behavior, I instead asked, "Did I say or do something to insult you?" Louis immediately softened, responded that I had not done anything to offend him, and addressed me in a more reasonable tone. By not confronting Louis but instead inviting him to talk with me directly about his apparent displeasure, I hoped to elicit a more mature aspect of Louis that was not usually in the foreground, and then use this experience to help the parents see Louis in a different light.

Sometimes a family member will balk at the idea that he or she might need to change his or her own behaviors, and instead insist that the purpose of consulting a therapist was to enlist the therapist's expertise in changing the behavior of the identified patient. A family member might ask, "Why do I have to change, if I'm not the one with the problem?" Here's a suggested response:

> "I understand your point, but I believe that it might actually be easier for you to change than it is for your child to change. If you change, she will also change. The issue is not who is to blame or who is responsible for the problem. The issue is achieving the goal you said you wanted to achieve—eliminating the problem, and improving the overall quality of life in the family. Maybe your daughter is unable to change on her own. Maybe she doesn't see the value or the importance of changing. In any case, you are able to change, and you do see the value of change, so it makes sense for you to do whatever you can do to try to elicit change from her. The methods you have been using have obviously not been working, or they would have solved the problem and you wouldn't be here. You are here because you are looking for new solutions and I am asking you to try a new approach."

Encouraging Direct Communication

Families who are stuck in symptomatic cycles do not communicate effectively with one another. They don't listen to one another, and react to one another automatically rather than thoughtfully. They don't ask for what they want and they do not express their true feelings, either because they don't think it will be well received or because they are so focused on the behavior of the other that they don't pay enough attention to themselves to listen to their own feelings.

One way to encourage direct communication is by asking the family members to talk *with* one another rather than *about* one another. When a father tells a therapist about his son's frustrating behavior in the presence of the adolescent, the therapist can ask the parent to talk directly to the boy about his concerns. When a mother asks the therapist for advice on how to respond more effectively or how to be more helpful to her daughter, the therapist could suggest that the mother ask the daughter directly what would be helpful to her.

Working with Emotions

Another way to facilitate direct communication among family members is to elicit and call attention to emotions that are not directly expressed. A parent who is frustrated by an adolescent's angry defiance can be helped to see the anxiety and pain that lie behind the adolescent's anger. An adolescent who takes dangerous risks and acts out defiantly against the parent's rules can be helped to see the fear and hurt that lie behind the parent's anger. The therapist can use techniques from emotion-focused therapy (Johnson, 2004) to help to amplify the unexpressed painful emotions beneath the surface. Sometimes, these emotions will not emerge in the family session and individual sessions might be necessary to help the person identify and articulate the emotions.

This approach is particularly useful in families in which there is a high level of conflict and where anger is the dominant emotion that is expressed. In these families, it is helpful to try to access the "softer" emotions that lie behind the anger. People who have emotional bonds with one another become angry when they feel hurt, abandoned, or betrayed. When a family member appears to be overwhelmed by feelings of anger, the therapist might ask whether the person is feeling any other emotions as well. If the person denies feeling any softer emotions, then the therapist suggests what he or she might be feeling: "I mostly hear anger in your voice, but I also hear a little sadness, too. Do you think that, along with feeling angry, you might also be feeling sad?"

When the person acknowledges sadness, then the therapist can help to amplify this feeling, by calling attention to it and asking questions about it. Then, turning to the other family members, the therapist might ask, "What is coming up for you as you hear your son talk about how sad he has been feeling? What feelings are you having when you hear him talk about this?"

Changing the emotional tone of a family interaction is a powerful way of changing the patterns of interaction. Exposing a concealed emotion is a way of uncovering a hidden facet of a family member, and it calls attention to qualities that the other family members might have failed to notice. It alters the system of complementary biased perceptions because it enriches the way the family members see each other, and provides an opportunity to invite the family members to engage in new ways of interacting with one another. This technique is particularly useful when working with defiant adolescents and is discussed further in Chapter 8.

Uncovering and Challenging Assumptions

People are often not aware of the assumptions that they take for granted. Therapists can listen carefully for evidence of these assumptions, and when they occur they can point them out to the speaker and ask him or her to reflect on the validity of the assumption. For example, the therapist might point out to an anxious mother of a reckless teenager that she seems to assume that her daughter is incapable of handling the consequences of her own behavior. What contributed to this assumption? Does she believe that it is really true? If not, what is a more reasonable assumption? What behavior would be more in keeping with this revised assumption?

Therapists should be aware of and be prepared to challenge their own implicit assumptions. One common assumption is that a family member is "incapable" of change. Seeing the family member this way, the therapist might avoid challenging him or her, and instead try to elicit change only from the other family members. This marginalizes the family member who presumably can't change, contributes to his or her isolation from the rest of the family, and thus makes it more (rather than less) likely that the problematic behavior will continue. As mentioned above, therapists should avoid characterizing family members using terms that imply stable characteristics, and instead focus on behavioral descriptions in context. The therapist should also always be alert to signs of strength or resources that can make what might appear to be an impossible change a possibility.

Separating People from Their Problems:
Externalizing the Problem

Michael White and David Epston (1990) have pointed out that families come to therapy with "problem-saturated" narratives that selectively exclude attention to the "unique outcomes," that is, times when the problem is less severe or absent. They have developed a technique that enables the family to deconstruct their problem-saturated narrative and replace it with a new narrative that encourages more attention to the unique outcomes. Toward this end, White and Epston have advocated a technique known as *externalizing the problem.*

When using this technique, the therapist and family members give the problem a name, such as "anorexia" or "depression," that distinguishes the problem from the person seen by the family as "being" the problem. The problem is identified as an external force that is oppressing the entire family and the therapist asks the family to unite against it.

For example, in a family struggling with an adolescent girl's unhealthy eating habits and severe weight loss, the therapist frames the problem as "anorexia," but does so in a way that implies that the problem is controlling the behaviors of all members of the family, not just the girl who is not eating properly. The therapist can then invite the family members to explore how they might be enabling this problem to dominate their lives, and identify ways that they could undermine the problem's effects on the family.

White and Epston's technique challenges the family members' unquestioned assumptions about the problem. They become more aware of ways in which their interactions are shaped by the problem and how they can help each other stop "cooperating" with the problem. Essentially, if the family members accept the idea that the problem is an external influence on them rather than an attribute of a single family member, then the system of complementary biased perceptions that sustains the symptomatic cycle can be altered.

Unbalancing

In this technique, originally described by Salvador Minuchin (1974), the therapist attempts to break a rigidly entrenched cycle by taking the side of one participant in the conflict, and challenges the other participant in the conflict to change.

For example, the more a mother intercedes between the father and daughter, the more doggedly the father tries to wrestle back control by adopting a heavy hand. The more heavy-handed the father is, the more the mother feels compelled to protect the daughter from him. The daughter sees her mother as the more sympathetic parent and avoids her father, which further increases the father's sense of isolation.

Of course, the pattern is a complementary one, with each party supporting and encouraging the response from the other that he or she doesn't like. But the purpose of unbalancing is to break this cycle by upsetting the balance. Since both sides of the complementarity are equally true, the therapist simply punctuates the interaction in a particular way by adopting one of the two sides of the conflict. In using this technique, the therapist states that he or she agrees with one of the conflicting parties, and insists that change must start with the other party changing. For example, the therapist might say to the father:

> "I agree with you. You won't be able to take a softer hand with your daughter until you feel that your wife is stepping up to the plate and being a co-parent with you. As long as she continues to protect your daughter from you, she gives her the impression that you are a monster rather than the sensitive, caring man that I have come to know in these sessions. So, I think your wife needs to change. She needs to stop interfering in your relationship with your daughter and allow you to show your daughter that you truly care about her and want the best for her, even if sometimes you are too harsh."

For this technique to be effective, it is important to plan in advance how it will be utilized. It is also essential to believe that the chosen punctuation is just as accurate as the alternative, and is selected for a strategic reason, not because it is more "correct." A clear hypothesis about the family structure is also necessary in order to choose which punctuation to emphasize. Unbalancing is most likely to be effective when the therapist "sides" with a family member who is marginalized in the family interactions or whose viewpoint is overtly criticized by other family members. In the example above, unbalancing by taking the mother's side could further alienate the father and could reinforce the coalition between the mother and daughter. While the father's harshness might make it seem as if he is a very powerful member of the family, in actuality he has little power because the mother–daughter coalition prevents him from having much influence.

Assigning Tasks

Frequently it is helpful to assign a task to be carried out between sessions. In order for this intervention to be effective, the following principles should be kept in mind:

• *The task should be within the family's ability to complete successfully.* This means that the task should not take an excessive amount of time nor represent a significant alteration in the family's usual routine.

3

Basic Concepts

In this chapter, I present basic concepts for understanding the evolution and persistence of problems in families. In the next chapter, I discuss intervention strategies and techniques based on these concepts. In the chapters that follow, these ideas are applied to specific presenting problems, such as eating disorders, depression, and defiant behaviors.

A CORE ASSUMPTION

My framework for helping troubled adolescents and families is built on the core assumption that the interpersonal context of the adolescent, in particular the family, plays a crucial role in the development and maintenance of symptoms. The relationship between adolescent adjustment and family functioning has been well documented in the literature (e.g., Buist et al., 2004; Cook, 2001; Crockett et al., 2003; Farrell & White, 1998; Freeman & Brown, 2001; Fuligni & Eccles, 1993; Kroger, 2003; Laible et al., 2000; Sheeber, Hops, Alpert, Davis, & Andrews, 1997; Vitaro et al., 2000). While other contexts, notably the peer group and the school, become important during adolescence, the influences of these other contexts are mediated by the quality of the adolescent's relationship with the family.

While the approach discussed in this chapter concentrates on work with the family, it is understood that biological factors can contribute to the emergence of some severe symptoms such as psychosis and major depression. It is not my intention to deny the importance of these factors, but rather to focus on the role of family interactions in the development and maintenance of symptoms. Altering unproductive interactional patterns and introducing the family members to new ways of relating to

- *The task should be directly related to the treatment goals.* Since the goal of family-oriented treatment is to stimulate a shift in relationship patterns, effective tasks should involve more than one person in the family. For example, a mother and daughter who are working to improve their relationship might be assigned the task to go out to lunch together, or a father and son whose interactions are competitive rather than cooperative might be given the task to work on a household project together.

- *The task should build on a change that was observed during a session.* The task should evolve from an interactional shift that occurred during the session and used to reinforce the change that occurred. If the family members were unable to engage in the new behaviors during the session, it is unlikely that they will be able to do so on their own. For example, to encourage a parent to listen to a child's feelings without feeling compelled to argue with the child, do not assign this as a task unless the parent was able to perform the behavior successfully in the session. Doing so will almost certainly result in failure and frustration and might make it even less likely that the parent will risk attempting the new behavior in the session. Assigned tasks should flow naturally from the rhythm of the session and reinforce what has already occurred rather than break new ground.

- *Always follow up on an assigned task.* If a task had been assigned, it is important to ask about the task at the beginning of the next session. Failure to do so conveys the message that the assignment was not important, and family members are less likely to comply with task assignments in the future.

- *Explore reasons why the task was not completed.* If the family has not carried out the task, or carried it out incompletely, this issue should be discussed, but not in a way that blames the family or emphasizes their failure. The discussion should be an exploratory one and focus on the factors that prevented the family from carrying out the task. Failure to complete the task should not be attributed to "resistance" or lack of motivation on the part of the family members. Rather, failure to complete the task should be attributed to external factors or to internal emotional states such as fear or sadness rather than defiance or oppositionality. For example, if a mother and daughter did not go out to lunch as assigned, their failure to do so might be attributed to fear that conflict might erupt or fear of experiencing sadness about how distant their relationship had grown in recent years.

- *Assign paradoxical tasks sparingly, if at all.* Assigning paradoxical tasks was once a popular method of intervention in family therapy (Weeks & L'Abate, 1982). Properly designed paradoxical tasks can be effective, but they must be based on a sound theoretical formulation. It is also important that a convincing rationale be given when a paradoxical task is assigned, in order to increase the chance that the family members will comply with the task.

It was once common to prescribe that the family "not change" as a paradoxical maneuver to invite them to rebel against this directive. However, simply prescribing "no change" without giving a rationale for the prescription is likely to alienate families who expect therapists to help them to make changes they can't make on their own. This prescription could be presented with the rationale that the therapist has not yet completed the assessment of the family, and in order to be able to understand the problem better he or she would like them to try to keep things as constant as possible by not changing anything prior to the next session.

Prescribing the symptom, that is, asking the symptomatic adolescent to engage in the symptom deliberately, is sometimes assigned with the expectation that the youngster will "recoil" and rebel by not exhibiting symptomatic behavior. In some instances, this expectation might be fulfilled. On the other hand, paradoxically prescribing a dangerous symptom poses ethical and legal dilemmas, not to mention loss of trust on the part of family members who are fearful of the symptom. In the case of symptoms that are not dangerous, it might be useful to present the paradoxical symptom prescription as an "experiment." For example, an adolescent who claims to have no control over his obsessive worries might be asked to worry at specific times of the day, whether he feels like it or not, as an "experiment" to see if this approach increases or decreases the intensity of his worries.

Prescribing the symptom might also be used when trying to make a point about interactional patterns. Adolescents might be encouraged to display a symptom "deliberately" to test how committed their parents are to the new ways they have adopted to respond to the symptom. Sometimes the symptom might be prescribed to highlight how the symptom actually "helps" the family. For example, an adolescent might be instructed to "look more depressed" if he noticed that his mother was sad and lonely and his father was not attentive enough to his mother, but "act happier" if he noticed that his father was being sufficiently attentive to his mother's sadness. If a task such as this one is assigned, it is important that the therapist has already shared with the family the hypothesis that the son's depressed appearance might be related to the interactional pattern between the parents. Otherwise, a prescription such as this will appear to have materialized "out of the blue" and the family members might feel manipulated by the therapist.

it is essential to offer confidentiality to a minor, they should obtain an explicit agreement to that effect from the parents before meeting with the child alone.

At the beginning of therapy, I inform the family that there are circumstances in which confidentiality will not apply (e.g., immediate danger to self or others, child abuse) and explain that in these instances I might unilaterally decide to disclose confidential information in order to protect someone from serious harm. I then discuss the ground rules for individual sessions. I tell the family that keeping important secrets from one another could jeopardize our work together. Whenever I meet alone with a family member, I ask if he or she would permit me to share any information we discuss with the other members of the family if I believe it would be helpful to do so. If family members request confidentiality, I will usually agree, but I tell them in advance that I might encourage them to reveal the confidential disclosure to other members of the family if I believe that keeping the information secret would seriously compromise my ability to help them as a family. I suggest that they not tell me anything that they would absolutely not consider revealing to other family members. If a family member expresses the desire to have confidential sessions on a regular basis, I will first evaluate the basis for this request and if it appears appropriate I might refer that person to a colleague while I continue to work with the entire family.

Individual Sessions Early in Therapy

It can be helpful to request a private session with a family member to explore in more depth a topic that the therapist believes is not appropriate to discuss in the presence of the entire family. For example, a therapist might learn in the first sessions with the family that a father received a medical discharge from the service for combat-related stress, or that a mother was hospitalized for depression before she was married, and might want to gather more information about these experiences to determine if they are important to the family's current situation.

Individual sessions early in treatment can facilitate the process of joining with a particular family member. As I have emphasized throughout this chapter and the previous one, therapists must utilize their relationships with each member of the family to stimulate new interactional patterns among the family members. Thus, a strong relationship with each member of the family is crucial if the therapist is to engage this person in the process of change.

In some cases, the therapist might find it difficult to join with one or more members of the family in the context of the family session. For example, a peripheral father comes reluctantly to an initial session scheduled by the mother, who proceeds to dominate the session and interrupts whenever the therapist attempts to connect with the father. One possibility is to block the mother's interruptions and persist in trying to engage the father in the family session. This approach, if used in the first few sessions before the therapist has built a solid relationship with the mother, could offend her and could result in her dropping out of therapy. Yet, to ignore the father reinforces his peripheral position in the family. The therapist might decide to request an individual session with the father so that the therapist can concentrate on his or her relationship with the father without the distraction of worrying about his or her relationship with the other family members.

Often, an individual session or two early in therapy is necessary to engage an adolescent in treatment. Many youngsters come to therapy reluctantly and expect the therapist to take the parents' side. Meeting individually with the adolescent is a good way to communicate that the therapist is interested in him or her as a person and is committed to making therapy a valuable experience for the youngster. If the adolescent is particularly resistant to the idea of participating in therapy, it is important to explore the basis of this resistance and try to identify a concrete way that the adolescent could benefit from participating in the process (e.g., fewer school suspensions, fewer restrictions at home, earning back the trust of the parents).

Individual Sessions in the Middle Phase of Therapy

After the therapist has identified the symptomatic cycle and negotiated a goal with the family members, the subsequent sessions focus on disrupting the cycle and encouraging new interactional patterns among members of the family. The therapist utilizes his or her relationship with individual family members to encourage them to restrain themselves from their usual ways of responding and instead experiment with new ways of solving problems. While most of this work can and should take place in the family sessions, it is also helpful at times to meet individually with a member of the family.

For example, in working with a family in which a father relies on authoritarian methods of discipline and recoils from even gentle challenges in the family sessions, the therapist might meet alone with the father to help him understand that his reactions to the therapist's challenges are making it difficult for the therapist to be helpful to the family. Rather than confronting the father directly, the therapist might frame the father's aversion to the therapist's challenges as a sign that their relationship is not as strong as it could be. The individual session can be used to strengthen the relationship with the father and to secure the father's assurance that he will allow the therapist to challenge him in future family sessions.

Periodically, the therapist should meet individually with the adolescent to maintain the connection with the youngster. Even when the therapist has joined successfully with the adolescent early in treatment, it is prudent to keep checking back in with the young person, especially if the family sessions have focused on supporting the parents' authority.

For example, the therapist might meet alone with an adolescent to coach her in ways of communicating her opinions to her parents more effectively. Or, if the therapist believes that it is necessary to confront the adolescent about something, the therapist might first ask her to decide whether she wants the therapist to be honest with her or whether she prefers the therapist to hold back and not risk offending her feelings. Many adolescents will be more receptive to hearing confrontations when they don't have to risk losing face in front of the other family members and when they believe that the therapist cares enough about the relationship to be honest, even at the risk of offending them.

I want to stress that the most effective use of these individual sessions during the middle phase of therapy is not to work on issues that the family members identify as personal or private. This work is best delayed to later in treatment (see below). The purpose of these individual sessions is to use the relationships that had been forged during the early phase of therapy to challenge a family member to change in ways that will help disrupt the symptomatic cycle. The best challenge is one that is couched in terms of the relationship with the therapist, that is, the therapist requests a personal commitment from the family member to try something new for the sake of the relationship with the therapist and whether or not another family member changes also. For example, in a private session the therapist asks an authoritarian father for a personal commitment to try less punitive methods of discipline, a commitment that is not made to anyone but the therapist and that is not contingent upon anyone else in the family changing.

Individual Sessions Late in Treatment

Once the symptomatic cycle has been disrupted, the individual development of each family member is free to resume. Signs that individual development has resumed include the following: (1) the adolescent begins to engage in age-appropriate activities at higher frequency, (2) the adolescent begins to bring up developmentally appropriate issues at family sessions, and (3) the parents begin addressing the change in their marital relationship that is ensuing from the family life cycle progression.

Once the symptomatic cycle has been disrupted, the formerly symptomatic adolescent might face challenges that are developmentally normal but for which he or she is inadequately prepared because his or her own developmental process had been delayed by the cycle. Individual sessions with the adolescent could be beneficial at this point to help address the developmental changes directly.

The metaphor of "multiple selves" or "multiple voices," proposed by Richard Schwartz (1987, 1995), can be useful at this juncture. Each aspect of the person (i.e., facet of the self) could be labeled as a "self" or "voice" and the characteristics of this part of the self delineated and explored. Through this process, adolescents learn to reflect on their behavior, which makes them less likely to react impulsively. For example, in the case to be discussed in more detail in the next chapter, the symptomatic adolescent Tina was encouraged to get to know the parts of herself that we identified as "anorexia," "bulimia," "the little girl," and "the young adult." In so doing, she embraced a way of thinking about herself as a complex person who could tolerate ambivalence and avoid reacting impulsively to anxiety.

It is important to note that it is not just the symptomatic adolescent who faces developmental issues. The development of all family members is free to proceed once the symptomatic cycle is disrupted. It would be an error to focus attention strictly on the developmental issues of the postsymptomatic adolescent while neglecting to consider the disorientation that other family members might be experiencing once development resumes. Parents might need help with the complementary developmental challenge of redefining their role as parents of a developing teenager. For example, as I worked with Tina to promote her development as a young adult, I also worked with her mother to help her adapt to these developmental changes.

BENEFITS AND RISKS OF CONSULTATIONS

Sometimes a therapist who feels stuck with a family considers calling in a consultant to help resolve the impasse. For example, a psychiatrist might be engaged to prescribe medications, or a psychologist hired to conduct psychological testing. Calling in a consultant (e.g., for medication or psychological testing) at a time when the therapy is stuck runs the risk that the consultant will be triangulated into a conflict between the family and the therapist (Carl & Jurkovic, 1983).

Before calling in a consultant, it is important to examine the motives for doing so. Is the therapist attempting to find an ally to join in a coalition against the family? Does the therapist want to terminate therapy but is reluctant to address this issue directly with the family? Does the therapist feel frustrated or angry at the family for their noncompliance and invites a consultant to defuse the conflict rather than deal with the conflict directly?

One of the ways to avoid this pitfall is for the consultant to meet with the therapist in the presence of the family. The roles of the therapist and the consultant should be clearly negotiated, and the family apprised of these roles. If a consultant is engaged to dissolve an impasse between the therapist and family, it must be clear to all parties that the purpose of the consultation is to address this impasse. In these cases, it should be understood in advance that the consultation might result in changes in the way the problem is defined or changes in the goals of treatment.

An example of effective utilization of a consultation is described in the next chapter, when psychological testing was used to stimulate an adolescent's curiosity about the many facets of herself. Another example is described in Chapter 9, when effective collaboration with a prescribing psychiatrist led to better communication between the mother and the psychiatrist. In Chapter 10, I describe several ways that therapists can work effectively as consultants with schools.

SUMMARY

In this chapter, I proposed a number of techniques that can be used to assess and treat problems in families with adolescents. The basic principle guiding all intervention strategies is: The therapist works to replace automatic, reactive responses between people with more thoughtful, planned responses. I proposed six *general principles for effective intervention:*

1. Have a plan and stay focused.
2. Focus on changing relationships and patterns.
3. Invite collaboration.
4. Refer back to the pattern.
5. Offer encouragement and accentuate the positive.
6. Promote moments of engagement.

I offered suggestions for building an alliance with the family and identifying symptomatic patterns by attending to language, history, and direct observations. I then discussed a number of techniques to help family members change their habitual but unproductive patterns of interacting with each other. These techniques included (1) direct instruction, (2) using complementarity, (3) encouraging direct communication, (4) working with emotions, (5) uncovering and challenging hidden assumptions, (6) separating people from their problems, (7) unbalancing, and

(8) assigning tasks. I also discussed when and how to conduct individual sessions and the benefits and risks involved in requesting a consultation.

In the chapters that follow, I illustrate how these principles can be applied to a variety of presenting problems. We begin with eating disorders, because I believe the case discussed in that chapter provides a clear example of the ideas I have covered in the preceding chapters, and helps to flesh out these ideas a bit more.

5

Eating Disorders

Frail and bird-like, Tina reminded me of the little waif on the posters for the musical *Les Misérables*. Carrying only 83 pounds on her 5-foot 4-inch frame, Tina looked much younger than her 16 years. She clutched a sketch pad under her left arm and a pencil dangled from her right hand. Her hair, with the wispy, thinned quality often seen in young women with anorexia, hung forlornly over her face. Her eyes had the vacant look of a young woman trying to numb some unbearable pain.

Rose, Tina's mother, sat at her right. Her close-cropped red hair framed a face marked with worry for her daughter. Her eyes were glued on Tina, and she sat as if poised to spring up at any moment to defend her daughter from unseen dangers. Her left hand clutched the right arm of Tina's chair. Though I knew that Rose worked full time as an elementary school teacher and had raised two children with no assistance from their father or from other family members, I could see no sign of this competence in her hopeless face. She moved as if checking every motion, restraining herself from gesturing too broadly or calling attention to herself. Her voice, hesitant, tremulous, and always on the verge of a sob, told me she was suffering, though her words were never about herself, only Tina.

At Tina's left sat her father, Bill, who had only recently resumed seeing her after 10 years of infrequent and sporadic contact. In his face, I read frustration and mistrust. This was a man who "didn't believe in therapy." He didn't have to tell me (although he did, immediately upon meeting me); I could guess. He warily entered the room, well behind Tina and Rose, then perched on the edge of the seat on Tina's left, grasping the right arm of her chair in a gesture that appeared more desperate than supportive. Tina squeezed into

108

the center of her seat as if shrinking from contact with her parents, who almost literally seemed to be pulling her in opposite directions.

I already knew part of their story from the phone call with Rose that preceded our session. Tina had been losing weight for the past 18 months and was now on the brink of medical crisis. Tina and Rose had been living alone for the past 2 months, since Tina's older brother, Jeff, had moved to California to pursue a career in film-making. Three years previously, Rose's second marriage ended when her husband of 5 years left her. Ten years previously, Rose and Bill divorced after 8 years of a marriage that was miserably unhappy for both of them. Less than a year after the divorce, Bill remarried and now had a son by his second marriage.

Bill did not challenge Rose's bid for custody of the children. After 2 years of gradually decreasing contact, the children stopped visiting Bill, aside from the occasional weekend during summer and winter vacations. They had not communicated until 6 months ago, when Rose contacted Bill out of desperation when Tina's pediatrician told Rose that Tina had anorexia. Following the advice of the pediatrician, Rose immediately sought therapy for her. Tina saw her therapist individually twice a week, but continued to lose weight. Eventually, she stopped going. Bill phoned Rose several times a week, berating her for allowing the problem to get out of hand. One week before our meeting, Bill threatened to take Tina home with him and force her to eat until she gained weight. Then Rose panicked when she found empty bottles of ipecac serum in Tina's room. She phoned Bill, who lambasted her for "mishandling" the situation. After an argument that ended with Rose hanging up on Bill, she turned in desperation to Tina's former therapist, who suggested that Rose contact me.

A disturbingly high percentage of adolescents, both girls and boys, engage in unhealthy weight loss strategies. In one study of over 4,000 adolescents attending public schools, 58% of girls and 33% of boys reported unhealthy weight control behaviors (Neumark-Sztainer, Wall, Story, & Perry, 2003). Some of these youngsters develop a full-blown eating disorder, and most of those who do are girls. Boys and men make up only about 10% of clinically diagnosed cases of eating disorder, and these are predominantly cases of bulimia and binge eating (Ricciardelli & McCabe, 2004).

Because eating disorders are more common among girls, much of the literature on eating disorders has focused on females. However, the factors that promote disordered eating are similar for both boys and girls (Keel, Klump, Leon, & Fulkerson, 1998; Ricciardelli & McCabe, 2004). Boys who pursue patterns of disordered eating generally do so in pursuit of a more muscular appearance. In this respect, their motives are similar to those of girls who are desirous of transforming their bodies to conform to culturally idealized standards of attractiveness.

Eating disorders are complicated to treat, and this chapter is not intended as an exhaustive or comprehensive discussion of the treatment of eating disorders. Rather, my goal is to present some general guidelines for working with families of adolescents with an eating disorder. The case that is the centerpiece of this chapter was chosen not necessarily because it is representative of all cases of eating disorders, but rather because it presents a good illustration of the application of the model and techniques discussed in Chapters 3 and 4. I also acknowledge that some cases of eating disorder are too severe to treat on an outpatient basis and require the intensity of an inpatient setting, particularly if the eating disorder is chronic, the symptoms are life threatening, or there has been little improvement after a reasonable course of outpatient therapy.

Empirical research has demonstrated that family-based treatment methods are effective for adolescent eating disorders (Wilson, Grilo, & Vitousek, 2007). The principles discussed in this chapter share much in common with one of these approaches, the Maudsley model (Krautter & Lock, 2004; Lock, le Grange, Agras, & Dare, 2001), but it also incorporates ideas originally proposed by Minuchin, Rosman, and Baker (1978), as well as some other theoretical perspectives on eating disorders that are briefly reviewed below.

PERSPECTIVES ON EATING DISORDERS

Psychodynamic Perspectives

Early psychoanalytic accounts viewed anorexia as a defense against the threatening sexual impulses reawakened by puberty (Waller, Kaufman, & Deutsch, 1940). Later accounts emphasized two themes in the development of eating disorders: fears of maturity and struggles over autonomy.

Arthur Crisp (1983) believed that individuals with anorexia unconsciously equated physical maturity with rejection and abandonment. Hilde Bruch (1982, 1988) described the girl with anorexia as engaged in a struggle to assert herself in a stifling family context. According to Bruch, the future anorectic's mother does not empathically understand the needs of her infant. Thus, the mother responds to the child based on her own needs rather than those of the child. As a result, the child fails to discriminate among her own perceptions of bodily sensations and emotional states. Some empirical research has provided support for this idea. A tendency known as "poor interoceptive awareness" has been found to be associated with the development of eating problems in girls (Leon, Fulkerson, Perry, & Early-Zald, 1995).

According to Bruch, the mother discourages the child's autonomy because she is dependent on the child. Eventually, the child embodies what she believes others expect of her rather than how she herself feels. Bruch recommended a modification of the psychoanalytic process that placed less emphasis on insight into the symbolic significance of the symptom and more emphasis on helping patients discover their true selves: "They need to face their problems of living in the present, reconstruct what had gone on during the preillness period, and understand how their experiences interfered with their developing a sense of self and competence" (Bruch, 1982, p. 1536).

Feminist Psychodynamic Perspectives

Feminist psychodynamic theorists have challenged the emphasis on autonomy in traditional psychoanalytic theory and maintain that eating disorders arise when young girls are confronted with social pressure to reject a way of life based on relatedness in favor of one based on independence, which for many girls is equated with isolation (Steiner-Adair, 1990). Janet Surrey (1991) associated eating disorders with the "loss of voice" experienced by young girls when they reach adolescence and are faced with the demand to conceal their real needs in order to preserve relationships with others.

Some feminist theorists have also challenged traditional psychodynamic theory's emphasis on the mother as primarily responsible for the development of eating disorders in the child. These theorists point out that the mothers themselves were often recipients of poor parenting in their own families, which diminished their capacity to care for their children. In addition, feminist theorists point out that the relationship between the father and the mother influences the mother's relationship with the infant. Marital distress can distract the mother and make her less emotionally available to the infant. Eating disorders, then, should be viewed not so much as emerging from the mother–child relationship system as from the triadic relationship system involving both parents and the child. In support of this claim, empirical research has documented the role of poor father–daughter relationships in the development of eating disorders (Cole-Detke & Kobak, 1996; Evans & Street, 1995; Mueller, Field, Yando, & Harding, 1995). In addition, there is evidence that a positive father–daughter relationship can buffer the negative effects of other risk factors for eating disorder, such as early pubertal timing (Smolak, Levine, & Gralen, 1993; Swarr & Richards, 1996).

Sociocultural Perspectives

Since over 90% of those with eating disorders are female, it has been argued that women are more likely than men to be exposed to risk factors for eating disorders, particularly those that originate in cultural gender-role definitions (Halmi, 1995). Gilbert and Thompson (1996) reviewed four theories that have been proposed to account for the higher incidence of eating disorders among women:

1. *Culture of thinness.* By extolling thinness as essential to happiness and promoting images of emaciated women, patriarchal society seeks to control women by rendering them powerless.
2. *Weight as power and control.* Women submit to cultural pressures to focus on their appearance in order to achieve a greater sense of control over their lives.
3. *Anxieties about female achievement.* Eating disorders represent attempts by successful women to escape from the negative stigma associated with women's achievement by adopting compensatory measures that will make them look more "feminine." Other women focus on weight control as the only area in which they feel competent.
4. *Eating disorders as self-definition.* Traditional gender roles promote an underdeveloped sense of self in women and thus make them more vulnerable to social expectations regarding their appearance. A related perspective is the idea that a young woman's desire for nurturance evokes guilt that is expressed in the form of an eating disorder.

One problem with sociocultural explanations is that these factors alone cannot account for the prevalence of eating disorders. All women in our culture are exposed to these media images and messages, but only a minority develops eating disorders. While cultural and peer pressures toward thinness might play a role, they must interact with other factors.

Family Systems Perspectives

Minuchin's Model of the Psychosomatic Family

Advocates of a family systems approach to eating disorder have focused on the here-and-now transactional patterns in the family rather than on early mother–infant interactions. Minuchin et al. (1978) proposed that families with anorexia commonly manifest four characteristics:

1. *Enmeshment.* Relationships in these families are characterized by a lack of appropriate emotional distance and overinvolvement in each other's lives. Families exhibiting this pattern often engage in "mind reading" (e.g., when a parent says what the daughter is thinking without the daughter having spoken) or "mediating" (e.g., when a parent serves as a go-between for the daughter and the other parent).

2. *Overprotectiveness.* Members of families with anorexia are overly protective and solicitous of one another. They are scrupulous about hurting each other's feelings and may go to great lengths to avoid overt conflict. These families are so sensitive to signals of distress in each other that they intervene too quickly to alleviate tension, thus impeding the capacity of the family members to learn how to handle stress on their own. As a result, the autonomy of each family member is compromised, and the interdependence of the family members on each other is reinforced.

3. *Rigidity.* These families are committed to maintaining the status quo. They find change threatening and often deny the need for change. Adolescence poses a particular challenge for these families, since they are unable to modify the family structure to permit increasing autonomy for the adolescent.

4. *Involvement of the symptomatic adolescent in parental conflict.* One of the ways that parents in anorectic families avoid overt conflict with each other is by detouring the conflict through the symptomatic adolescent. They divert attention away from their own conflicts in order to devote more energy to taking care of their daughter, who encourages this pattern by appearing helpless and emaciated. The daughter can be triangulated between her parents in such a way that she is unable to express herself without being perceived as taking the side of one parent against the other.

Anorexia as Maintaining Family Homeostasis

Other family systems theories claim that anorexia arises in families as a way of preserving a rigid family homeostasis. Peggy Papp (1983) recommended that therapists first identify the ways in which the anorexia functions to stabilize the family and then utilize paradoxical interventions to provoke change. The Milan School (Selvini-Palazzoli, Boscolo, Cecchin, & Prata, 1978) took a similar approach in assigning a "positive connotation" to the symptom and paradoxically restraining the family against change. Later, Selvini-Palazzoli and Viaro (1988) identified the "family game" that presumably led to the development of the eating disorder. From this perspective, the symptom is seen as a strategic move on the part of the patient to achieve more power, but at the same time the patient becomes a pawn in the game and is used by other family members to their own strategic advantage. Selvini-Palazzoli and Viaro recommended working individually with the patient to help her extricate herself from the game.

A Family Developmental Model

Proposing an integration of psychodynamic and family systems theories, Stern, Whitaker, Hagemann, Anderson, and Bargman (1981) linked anorexia to problems of separation and individuation, but noted that all members of the anorectic family, not just the patient, are developmentally arrested. They recommended that the therapists or treatment team function as surrogate parents to the anorectic family in order to create the optimal "holding environment" that will facilitate the process of separation and individuation. Specifically, the therapists must take leadership in setting the conditions for therapy, thus communicating that they will not allow the patient to act self-destructively, and then within this context challenge the family to accept initiative in taking the risks involved in change.

Narrative Approaches

The narrative perspective attributes the development and maintenance of an eating disorder to the family's way of describing and explaining their experiences. An early version of this model was Michael White's (1983) exploration of the role of rigid family belief systems in anorexia. White claimed that girls develop anorexia in response to rigid beliefs and role prescriptions that exert tight constraints not just on the girl with anorexia but on all family members. He proposed that successful treatment requires challenging the constraining influences of these beliefs by rendering them and their consequences explicit to the family.

Later, White (1987) proposed a process of detailed questioning that was designed to free the family from the constraining effects of their beliefs and open up new possibilities for viewing self and others. Ultimately, White (1993) developed the technique of "externalizing the problem" that led to exploration of the ways in which "anorexia" had taken over the patient's and family's life ("mapping the influence of the problem"), searching for times when the patient or family were able to resist the problem ("unique outcomes"), and then building upon these unique outcomes to create new narratives about self and others ("reauthoring").

White's colleague, David Epston, helped to found the "Anti-Anorexia League," an archive of personal accounts from persons who had been treated for anorexia and who had discovered ways of subverting the effects of the "knowledge and practices upon which the anorexia nervosa depends" (White, 1993, p. 27).

Empirical Support for Family Therapy

Although there has been inconsistent empirical support for the notion that the characteristics described by Minuchin et al. (1978) are typical of all anorectic families (e.g., Blair, Freeman, & Cull, 1995), there is support for the efficacy of family therapy for treating eating disorders in adolescents (e.g., Eisler et al., 1997; Lock, Agras, Bryson, & Kraemer, 2005; Robin, Siegel, Koepke, Moye, & Tice, 1994; Russell, Szmulker, Dare, & Eisler, 1987). Minuchin et al. (1978) reported on a sample of 50 anorectic families treated with structural family therapy ranging in duration from 2 to 12 months. At follow-up (ranging from 1 to 7 years), 86% of the cases had recovered normal eating patterns, stabilized body weight within the normal limits for height and age, and had satisfactory adjustment in family, school, work, and peer relationships. Lock, Couturier, and Agras (2006) reported that 89% of adolescents diagnosed with anorexia who were treated with family therapy were above 90% of ideal body weight at long-term follow-up. In a study employing family therapy to treat bulimia, 49% no longer met diagnostic criteria for bulimia at 6 months follow-up (le Grange et al., 2007).

PRINCIPLES OF TREATMENT

My approach borrows from many of the above ideas, but I emphasize a particular theme: Treatment of families with anorexia must be informed by the awareness that profound isolation and disconnection lie beneath the apparent enmeshment in the family (Sargent, 1987a). Although the family members appear to love and care for one another, their acceptance of each other is highly conditional. Each individual is constrained within narrow limits of acceptable behavior, with rejection, guilt, or abandonment being the price for moving beyond these limits. Only certain facets of the self may be presented to other family members, since the emergence of new facets of the self threaten the bond of enmeshment. Facets of the self that do not fit into these prescribed patterns must be hidden or denounced. As a result, all family members become frozen in the process of development.

These patterns were apparent in Tina's family. Although her parents hovered over her during the session, Tina avoided direct contact with them. Rose spoke for Tina as if she could read her daughter's mind, while Tina passively encouraged her mother by remaining silent. Rose described their relationship as close, and I believed that she genuinely experienced it as such, but I wondered how Tina could become so emaciated, and how she could have engaged in secret purging if she and her mother were really as close as Rose described.

Any changes in the relationship, especially those that accompany adolescence, threaten the family and lead to efforts to counteract these changes. As a result, control substitutes for genuine connections. Fearful of losing the rigidly enmeshed attachment to which they have become accustomed, the family members rely on overt and covert methods of controlling one another. Ironically, the efforts at control only contribute to further isolation and disconnection, as the family members attempt to avoid each other's efforts to control them. Direct requests for change are not possible because these requests pose the threat of conflict.

As discussed earlier, some theorists have described anorexia as an extreme effort to assert self-control in a system in which normal autonomy is discouraged. While there is validity to this assertion, it is also true that the adolescent with anorexia exerts a powerful influence over the other family members through the symptom. It was tempting to view Tina as a victim of controlling parents. However, it was also true that Tina's apparent helplessness was exerting a powerful influence on her parents. One had just to look at the pained expression on Rose's face to see how much Tina's self-starvation had worn her down. Pain and fear also lay not far below Bill's hostile demeanor. He knew that Tina could die, and he was terrified because he had no idea how to prevent it.

The Symptomatic Cycle

The cycle begins when a girl starts to restrict her food intake as a way to manage the stresses connected with the developmental transition into adolescence. Perhaps she is uncomfortable with the way her body looks, perhaps she is fearful of sexuality, or perhaps she is struggling to earn the acceptance of peers. Whatever the specific nature of the stress, because of the injunction against change and conflict in the family, she submerges her true feelings and distracts herself by becoming preoccupied with food and weight. By restricting her food intake, she slows down and eventually reverses the physical changes associated with puberty. She loses her curves and her menses stop. She has managed to hold back the hands of time, and, at first, it appears that the family is calmer. No longer are the family members faced with the need to adjust their relationships to accommodate the new adolescent in the family. But they eventually begin to notice that something is wrong.

Their daughter is not eating and she is beginning to look very thin. At first, the parents and other family members try indirect methods to encourage the girl to eat, such as preparing special dinners or finding excuses to be with her during meals. But, by focusing exclusively on the girl's eating and weight, they fail to address the processes in the family that contributed to the problem in the first place. Eventually, the parents abandon the indirect approach and confront the girl on her eating habits. Then the battle shifts to a struggle over food and weight. The parents demand that she eat. She refuses, partly because she has now experienced one arena in which she can maintain control, partly because she has no other ways of managing stress.

Some parents try to get their daughter to open up to them, to share with them the terrible feelings they assume are behind such a terrifying symptom. But in the process the parents only reinforce the "Tell me/ Don't tell me" bind (see Chapter 3). They really don't want to hear anything that will upset them. They want to be reassured. The girl knows this and denies that she has any problems, or distracts her parents by raising trivial issues. In some cases, the girl herself might have lost access to her true feelings, having submerged them for so long.

The family is now stuck in a full-blown symptomatic cycle. The more control the parents exert over the girl's eating habits, the more she resists. The more earnest their pursuit, the more she shrinks from them, fearful that they might discover something about her that could devastate them. The parents might divert attention from other conflictual issues in order to focus on the girl's condition. Or, as in Tina's family, conflicts between the parents might now be detoured through the symptomatic child. As the girl loses more weight, the parents' arguments about how best to help her intensify. As each parent focuses on winning the conflict and thus exonerating him- or herself, the girl loses more weight, which only fuels more parental conflict.

The Symptomatic Cycle in Tina's Family

Figure 5.1 depicts the symptomatic cycle in Tina's family.

Already depressed as a result of her second failed marriage, Rose was not enthusiastic about Tina's growing up. She herself had a stormy adolescence marked by intense conflict with both of her parents. Tina had learned to read her mother very well over the years of their enmeshed relationship. She knew that Rose really couldn't handle hearing that she was angry at her for not taking better care of herself, for working too hard, and then rationalizing her constricted life as a gift of love for her

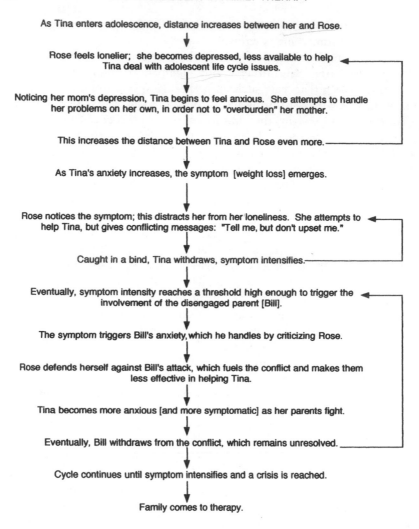

FIGURE 5.1. The process of symptom development in Tina's family.

children. Tina noticed how much more unhappy her mother appeared when Tina began to spend more time with her friends and less time at home. She began to focus on her weight and diet as a way to distract herself. When Rose asked her why she wasn't eating, Tina would mollify her with vague answers intended to divert attention away from her eating patterns and avoid upsetting her mother.

At first, Rose tried to handle Tina's eating problems on her own. She had read about anorexia and believed that it reflected underlying problems that could not be expressed any other way. Rose began to badger Tina to confide in her, anxiously reassuring Tina that she could handle whatever Tina might say. Rose did not realize that she was putting Tina in a "Tell me/Don't tell me" bind.

As Tina lost more and more weight, Rose, in desperation, called Bill, hoping that he might know what to do, even though Bill had had little contact with Tina or Rose over the past several years. When Rose explained that she was trying to help Tina by being supportive and caring, Bill interpreted her behavior as overly indulgent. He berated Rose for being too soft and blamed her for "allowing" Tina to get so thin.

Rose had forgotten how furious she felt when Bill criticized her. The anger, submerged for all these years, returned, and she counterattacked by blaming Bill for not being more involved in Tina's life and implying that this was the cause of Tina's eating disorder. As the battle of mutual blame raged on, Tina continued to lose weight. As is typical, this unproductive process continued until a crisis was reached. In this case, Rose learned that Tina had been vomiting, and then, on searching her room, discovered ipecac serum. Bill threatened to take Tina to his house and force her to eat. Conflict had reached explosive proportions.

Overview of the Treatment Process

Medical Backup Is Essential

Before initiating family therapy, it is essential to arrange for a thorough physical examination by a physician who has experience treating adolescents with eating disorders. The girl might have a medical condition such as Crohn's disease or colitis that has been misdiagnosed as anorexia or that could complicate the treatment of a coexisting eating disorder. Once medical reasons for the weight loss have been ruled out, the role of the physician is to monitor the girl's weight and if necessary to hospitalize her if her weight drops below a medically safe level. I recommend that the minimum weight specified by the monitoring physician be a condition for continuation of outpatient therapy. Should the girl drop below this weight, the physician hospitalizes her on a medical unit and keeps her there until she gains enough weight to be safely discharged.

Steps in Treatment

Family therapy then proceeds through the following steps:

1. *Negotiating a treatment contract.* While acknowledging the severity and potential lethality of the symptom, the definition of the problem

must be expanded beyond a narrow focus on weight gain and must call attention to the repetitive patterns of interaction in the family that have failed to successfully challenge the symptom or enabled it to continue. Successful resolution of the problem must be linked to changes in the patterns of interaction in the family.

2. *Encouraging parental collaboration.* With the problem now reframed, the next step is to encourage the parents to work together to help the girl to gain weight. The therapist gives the parents the task of deciding on a (reasonable) weight goal for the girl and a consequence if she fails to achieve it. While the therapist must be prepared to offer guidance on strategies for helping the girl to gain weight, the main purpose of this intervention is to provide the parents with a concrete issue around which their ineffective style of dealing with conflicts can emerge and be directly addressed. Success in helping their child gain weight requires the parents to join together to strengthen the executive subsystem and to create a clearer intergenerational boundary (Minuchin et al., 1978).

3. *Addressing unresolved conflicts.* The main focus of the therapy sessions is on uncovering and addressing unresolved conflicts in the family. The process of improving relationships among family members requires the therapist to establish a strong relationship with each family member individually, and then build on these relationships to encourage them to take risks and experiment with new ways of relating to one another.

4. *Handling relapses.* As a result of the process of negotiating the contract and encouraging parental collaboration, the girl will usually gain weight. However, after a while, it often happens that she stops gaining weight or loses some of the weight she had gained. This "relapse" is an important juncture in the treatment process. The therapist must respond to the relapse in a way that discourages the reemergence of the symptomatic cycle and instead keeps the focus on the relationships in the family.

5. *Supporting individual development.* After family therapy has successfully helped the family members address unresolved conflicts and change their patterns of relating to one another, a new phase of treatment begins. Now, freed from the symptomatic cycle, the development of the family members resumes. At this stage, individual sessions with the adolescent and/or other family members can be helpful to promote individuation and to encourage the transformations in family structure necessitated by the adolescent's growth in maturity.

6. *Supporting the transformation.* In the final phase, the therapist becomes less central and takes the role of supporting family members'

efforts to resolve their own difficulties. By now, family members have acquired more flexible ways of dealing with problems and interact with one another in qualitatively different ways.

STEP 1: NEGOTIATING A TREATMENT CONTRACT

How Do the Family Members View the Problem?

The therapist must attend to differences in the ways in which each family member describes the problem and its cause. Bill expressed the belief that Tina was using anorexia as a way to get his attention. Consequently, he expected that Tina would resume eating when he started spending more time with her. When this didn't happen, he revised his hypothesis: Tina was a victim of inadequate parenting by Rose. If Rose had taken charge, as a parent should, Tina would never have lost so much weight. His threat—to take her home with him and force her to eat—vividly expressed his view that the solution to the problem was taking control of Tina.

Rose, on the other hand, viewed Tina as a victim of a disease that she never wanted: "She didn't ask for this illness." Rose was convinced that Tina wanted nothing more than to be "happy and healthy." For Rose, the solution was for Tina to find "the strength to heal herself." Rose was not sure how Tina might find this strength, but she definitely did not believe that forcing Tina to eat was the answer. In fact, she believed that girls often fell prey to anorexia if they felt that their autonomy was being taken from them, as would be the case if Bill attempted to force her to eat.

There are certain common elements in each parent's account of the problem. First, both parents saw the problem as inside Tina, and neither parent saw him- or herself as part of the problem. Second, both parents saw Tina as a victim: Bill believed Tina was a victim of Rose's inadequate parenting, and Rose believed that Tina was a victim of an illness that had taken control against her will.

Each parent also had diametrically opposed ideas for solving the problem: Bill believed that Tina needed more structure, such as he could provide if he took over parenting and forced her to eat; Rose believed that Tina needed more space, that is, more opportunity to discover who she was and thereby "heal herself." The more Bill insisted on structure, the more Rose blocked his efforts, since she believed that Bill's approach would only make the problem worse. From Bill's perspective, Rose's attempts to undermine his efforts to take charge represented the root of the problem: Rose was too weak and too dependent upon Tina's approval to exercise the necessary authority as a parent. Because these positions were complementary, they reinforced one another in an endlessly repeating cycle (see Figure 5.2).

Tracking the Interactional Patterns

During the first session, Rose and Bill each tried to convince me of the validity of their own view of the problem, thus inviting me into a coalition against the other parent. When I asked them to reach consensus about how to help Tina, they promptly resorted to shouting at one another. When family members engage in heated arguments during sessions, therapists might feel pulled to intervene to prevent the conflict from escalating. However, doing so puts the therapist in a triangle between the arguing parties. Rather than interceding to stave off conflict, it is more effective to help the parties resolve conflicts on their own.

Instead of intervening as mediator, I interrupted Rose's and Bill's argument with a question about the process: "How long have you two been fighting like this?" The purpose of this question was to direct the parents' attention away from the content of their conflict (i.e., who is right and who is wrong) and instead focus on the patterns they were enacting. They answered almost in unison: "We don't fight. We just

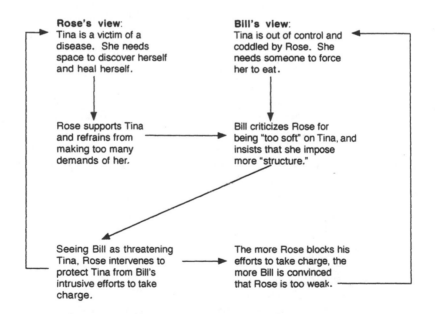

FIGURE 5.2. The system of complementary perceptions in Tina's family.

don't talk to one another." In other words, Rose and Bill regulated the intensity of the conflict between them through conflict avoidance. This strategy left the conflicts unaddressed and made it more likely that arguments would erupt again the next time they had contact with one another.

Redefining the Problem

It is important to define the problem in a way that expands the focus of concern beyond food and weight, without neglecting the important fact that the adolescent is starving herself. The severity and potential lethality of the symptom must be acknowledged, but it also must be linked to the interactions in the family. Each person in the family (including the symptomatic adolescent) must accept a role in the solution.

Insisting that family members take responsibility for solving the problem does not mean blaming the parents for the child's symptom. In fact, emphasizing this point is essential in order to promote a strong therapeutic alliance. The issue is not how the eating disorder came about, or who is to "blame" for it, but rather how the family members can work together to remove the problem from their midst. Externalizing the problem in this way, as is recommended by proponents of the narrative model and by the Maudsley team (le Grange & Lock, 2007; Lock et al., 2001), can help defuse the family members' defensiveness and mobilize their motivation to work on the problem.

It is also important to help the family members adopt an expanded view of the problem, one that goes beyond an exclusive focus on eating and weight. "Anorexia" is defined not simply as a problem involving eating and weight loss, but one that stimulates and is sustained by a particular pattern of family interactions. Thus, resolution of the problem of "anorexia" requires the family members to change the ways they typically interact with one another.

For example, toward the end of our first session together, I offered Tina's family the following formulation:

> "Tina is losing weight and can't eat because she feels isolated and alone, unable to express her true feelings to anyone. She is wasting away not only from lack of food but also because of the absence of nurturing and sustaining relationships in her life. This deprives her of the valuable help you both can offer her to grow and become the young adult she is capable of becoming. If you are interested, I will work with all of you, as a family, to give you the chance to begin building more sustaining relationships, so that Tina may begin to grow again."

I waited for a response. Would the family members accept this formulation? Would they acknowledge that their relationships had deteriorated? Would they agree that the state of their relationships had contributed to Tina's weight loss?

After a few seconds of silence, Bill spoke up: "Yeah, that's what I've been saying. Tina needs to tell her mother what's been bothering her all these years."

Before Rose could defend herself, I responded, "Yes, that will be part of what will need to happen. But, Bill, how do you think that your relationships with Tina and Rose could change?"

With irritation in his voice, Bill replied, "I'm willing to do anything to help Tina."

"Do you have any specific ideas about how you could be more helpful to her?" I asked.

He answered, almost predictably, "No, that's why I'm here. You're the expert. You tell me what she needs."

Not taking the bait, I asked, "Why do you think that Tina can't tell you what she needs from you?"

Bill squirmed, then shot back, "I don't think there's a problem between Tina and me. I think the problem is between Tina and her mother."

I had no right to expect that this would be easy. Bill was giving me the message that I shouldn't expect too much of him. If I pursued him too vigorously, he might leave and not come back, just as he had done years ago, when he cut himself off from Rose and the kids. I decided to take a less confrontational tack.

"Well, maybe you're right," I said. "Maybe there really isn't a major problem between you and Tina, though I wonder if she wishes that you and her mom wouldn't fight so much. Anyway, would you be willing to come to family sessions to see whether there is something that you and Tina could work on together, or whether there might be something that you could do to help Tina and Rose improve their relationship?"

I wasn't really surprised when Bill replied, "Well, I don't know how often I can come. I work full time, and I have a wife and kid, you know. My wife Ginny loves Tina, and she would do anything for her, but I've got to think of Billy; he's only 4, he needs me at home."

"I understand. So how often do you think you could come to sessions? Would you be able to come twice a week for a while?"

Sounding more annoyed now, Bill replied, "Look, I told you that I have other obligations. I'll tell you what. I'll come when I can."

Trying to get some kind of commitment from Bill, I suggested, "OK, let's look at our schedules and see what we can come up with."

In the end, Bill agreed to return for a family session in 1 week.

I turned to Rose next: "Rose, do you have any ideas about how you and Tina need to change your relationship?"

She looked at Tina, then back at me: "I only wish I knew. I only wish she could tell me."

I took this as an opening: "Then let's begin there next time. Tina [she raised her eyes halfway from the floor], would you think about that question so that we could talk about it next session? Would you think about ways in which you would like your relationship with your mom to change?" I took Tina's trembling nod as consent, then moved on to the next step.

Some readers might wonder why I am advocating Bill's involvement in decision making when the parents have been divorced for many years and Rose has been the primary parent. My rationale derives in part from general principles, and in part from the unique dynamics of this family. In general, children are more likely to thrive when their parents, divorced or not, can work together on parenting decisions. While there are divorced families where this goal is more an ideal than a reality, it is still important to do whatever is possible to reduce the conflict between the parents and try to promote better collaboration. I also had other reasons for wanting Bill to be involved in the sessions. First, he had only recently taken a more active role in Tina's life, and I wanted to support that role. Second, I believed that Tina would benefit from a closer relationship with her father. Third, Bill had warned me, through his threat to take Tina home with him and force her to eat, that he wanted to have a role in solving the problem. I wanted to give him a role that was collaborative with Rose, rather than one that was in opposition or in competition with her.

STEP 2: ENCOURAGING PARENTAL COLLABORATION

After finalizing a contract with the family that focuses on the goal of working on relationships, the next step is to ask the parents to agree on a target weight for the next family session. This intervention is supported by empirical research demonstrating the effectiveness of putting the parents in charge of helping their daughter gain weight (Wood, Flower, & Black, 1998).

After making a point of expanding the focus of the problem beyond food and weight, it might seem contradictory to bring weight back into the picture. Indeed, this would be the case if the therapist implied that achieving the target weight was the only goal of treatment. But this is not the primary purpose of the request. Instead, the chief focus of concern is the *process* by which the parents decide on the target weight and the consequences for not achieving it. Putting the parents in charge of the girl's weight gain challenges them to put their differences aside and work together for their daughter's welfare. It is a way to shore up the parental executive subsystem and create boundaries between the parents and the daughter. Now, if Tina doesn't gain weight, it is not Rose's fault, as Bill had implied, but rather a shared responsibility.

In setting expectations regarding weight gain, it is important that the therapist help the parents do so in a way that does not alienate the girl or minimize the intensity of her struggle. Parents cannot use this intervention as a way to punish or humiliate the girl. Rather, they must accept the challenge to oppose the symptom while supporting the girl. In doing so, they must communicate their care and concern for the girl and respect for the intense anxiety she will experience as she attempts to comply with parental expectations. The parents must set and maintain firm limits while acknowledging the girl's pain and communicating to her their unwavering commitment to her. For the girl to give up such a powerful symptom, the attachment to the parents must become stronger, so that her relationship with them and the sense of security she experiences in that relationship can take on more importance than the demands of complying with an eating disorder. This can happen only if she truly feels that her parents understand her and respect her.

I presented these ideas to Tina's family in this way:

> "I have found it helpful if parents could make it clear in a very concrete way that they expect their daughter to do her part if they are going to do their part. One way of doing this is to set a target weight. It's Tina's job to gain the weight, and it's your job to help her in whatever way you can. From my experience, I've found that a gain of 2 or 3 pounds a week is realistic. Rose and Bill, I'd like the two of you to decide how much weight you would like Tina to gain by our family session next week."

Most parents are relieved that the therapist hasn't forgotten why they came to therapy in the first place. They usually don't take long to arrive at a target weight. In this case, it was Bill who suggested that they set 2 pounds as the goal: "I'd be happy with that. At least it's a step in the right direction, and I think she could do it." Rose agreed.

I moved on: "Now, can you both tell Tina that you expect her to gain 2 pounds by next week, and that the two of you will help her do this any way you can?"

They complied; first Bill and then Rose. Tina remained silent, eyes downcast. I expected the next question, and it was Rose who asked it: "What if she doesn't gain 2 pounds?"

"That's a good question," I replied. "Why don't you talk with Bill about what will happen if Tina doesn't reach the target weight."

Rose turned toward Bill, and he responded before she could ask him his opinion: "I think there should be some kind of consequence, like maybe she would have to be grounded." Admittedly, this was not a very creative idea, but I remained silent. Without responding to Bill, Rose looked at me for my reaction.

"If you like that idea, Rose, could you talk with Bill about how long Tina would be grounded?" I suggested.

Bill jumped in again. "I think she should be grounded for the whole weekend, and she should have to stay in her room, in bed even, so that she doesn't work off calories."

Rose retorted, "And how am I going to make sure that she does that?"

More agreeable than I had expected, Bill answered, "We'll just have to see. If she doesn't do what we tell her, you and I will have to talk about what to do next."

With this glimmer of hope that Bill might be willing to collaborate with Rose, I punctuated their agreement and moved on, setting up a time to meet with Rose and Tina in 2 days.

STEP 3: ADDRESSING UNRESOLVED CONFLICTS

Once the parents have agreed on a weight goal, the basic structure of treatment has been set. The next step is *to help the family members address the unresolved conflicts that have contributed to the symptomatic cycle.* As John Sargent (1987a) has pointed out, isolation and disconnection lie beneath ostensibly close or even enmeshed relationships among family members who are struggling with anorexia.

The "rule" of conflict avoidance restricts the family members from saying what they truly think or feel. Each family member must operate within a narrowly prescribed range of acceptable behavior lest conflict erupt. The conflict avoidance, intended as a way to maintain closeness, has the opposite effect. Family members "walk on eggshells" and can't be honest with one another. As a result, the family members become more isolated and disconnected from one another, and more resentful about having to conceal parts of themselves in order to be accepted.

It is important to note that all family members are imposing these constraints on each other: No one is victim; no one is villain. While Rose and Bill might have imposed conditions on Tina for their approval or acceptance of her, Tina is also imposing conditions on her parents. By taking on the role of the helpless, emaciated child, she communicates her fragility and constrains her parents from pushing her too hard or confronting her. As an example, note that Bill did not attack Tina directly for not eating, but instead attacked Rose.

In the context of these constricted relationships, the family members repeatedly engage certain facets of themselves at the expense of others (see Figure 3.2, p. 65). But these untapped and underutilized parts of themselves can provide the way out of the cycle. To gain access to these hidden resources, the therapist must connect individually with each member of the family and then build upon these relationships to encourage the family members to take risks with each other that can open up new possibilities for growth and change. The next section illustrates how this process unfolded in the relationship between Tina and Rose.

Conflict Avoidance and the "Tell Me/Don't Tell Me" Bind

We began where we had ended our first session: Rose would talk with Tina about how their relationship needed to change. I reminded Tina that I had asked her to think about this question in our first session.

Rose began: "OK, honey, how would you like things to change between us?"

Tina, looking only a little less forlorn than in the first session, spoke in her characteristic whisper, "I don't know."

I silently gave Rose credit for persisting. "Come on, now, honey," Rose pleaded, "I really want to know. Please, tell me. Come on."

This time Tina didn't even bother to reply. She simply pulled her legs up to her chest and kept her eyes glued to the floor. Rose looked at me helplessly. I didn't say anything and Rose got the message that she should persist.

More frantically now, she demanded, "Tell me, tell me, tell me! What did I do? Or didn't do? Or should have done? Tell me, damn it!"

Tina simply whimpered in reply. Rose turned to me, "Give me a bag for my head."

I was puzzled: "What do you mean?"

"She can't look me in the eye to tell me how I failed her as a mother," Rose said, "so I'll wear a bag over my head, so that she doesn't have to look at me."

Though the idea sounded absurd, and I wasn't really sure that Rose was serious, it did speak to the lengths that Rose would go to help Tina.

I responded, perhaps a bit too firmly, "She has to look at your face while she tells you this."

Once again, Rose turned toward Tina. "Come on now, Tina," she begged. "We've been through this so many times."

Perhaps to rescue her mother from me, Tina found her voice: "I know, I know, I guess it was all those rules."

Given a crumb of content, Rose jumped on it. "What rules? Tell me, what rules? To make your bed? To do your homework? What rules? I want to know. What rules didn't you like?"

I interjected, "Rose, try to listen."

Stronger than I had seen her before, Rose contradicted me: "Yeah, but I don't want generalities, I want specifics. What rules, Tina?"

For the first time, Tina came alive, if only for a moment, "That's what I mean! You talk too much, and all you had to say was, like, one word!"

"OK, then, I'm listening," Rose assured Tina, with only a little less tension in her voice. "Come on then, I'm listening."

Tina retreated again, burying her face in her knees. Rose, unable to go on, burst into tears: "I can't do this anymore."

Here, we see a rigid pattern that was enacted between Tina and Rose over and over again. As Rose became more anxious about finding a way to connect with Tina, Tina became more withdrawn, which intensified Rose's anxiety. When she tried to be more assertive, Tina rebuffed her, withdrew, or expressed anger in an immature way. Rose reverted to the role of Tina's protector, but this only served to enable Tina to stay immature and helpless. In order to engage Tina in an age-appropriate relationship, Rose needed to gain access to the competent parts of herself.

It is essential to keep in mind that the more competent aspects of Rose (and Tina) are not missing; they are simply untapped. It is not that Rose and Tina lack these qualities, that they are deficient in some way, but rather that they have lost access to them. Salvador Minuchin would say to families, "You are richer than you know," communicating his belief that family members have within them untapped resources for growth and change (Minuchin & Nichols, 1993, p. 47). It is important to see beyond the immediate behavior of each family member to strengths that are not readily apparent and then help to create a context in which these strengths will emerge. Once this happens—once a family member experiences an aspect of him- or herself that had previously been inaccessible and invisible to both self and the other family members—an opening is created for new patterns to replace the old. These new patterns can elicit from other family members untapped facets of themselves, thus leading to the creation of new ways of interacting.

I decided that the next step would require me to establish individual connections with Rose and Tina, so that I could use my relationship with each of them to bring about a change in the way they related to one another. For the next session, I decided to meet first with Rose alone, and then with Tina alone, to try to reach those aspects of them that were hidden from each other. Then, I would use myself as a catalyst to stimulate a new relationship between them.

Connecting with Rose

To elicit Rose's competence, I decided to approach her as an authority on her daughter and request her assistance in helping me understand Tina. This request served a twofold purpose: First, it communicated respect for Rose as a parent; and second, it framed the purpose of our meeting not as "therapy" for Rose, but rather as an invitation to collaborate with me to help Tina. To respond to my request for a consultation, Rose would have to draw upon her competence as a parent. In doing so, she would experience an underdeveloped aspect of herself.

As I anticipated, Rose initially related to me in the same anxious, insecure manner that characterized her behavior in the family sessions. I had to remind myself that my goal was not to change Rose, nor to repudiate these parts of her, but rather to see beyond them to her hidden strengths.

Through the session, Rose spoke frantically with a pleading tone in her voice, a poignant demonstration that she was starving for a connection with someone who was willing to listen to her. At first, she depicted Tina as a helpless victim of anorexia and fear: "Tina has always been afraid of expressing her feelings. She can't help it."

I encouraged Rose to see beyond Tina's helplessness: "How do you think we can help her take the risk to open up?" The "we" was deliberate. It was intended to reassure Rose that she would not have to do it alone and that I would be there to help her.

Rose looked thoughtful, then tentatively said that she could understand why Tina was so fearful—because of the conflicts in the family.

I prodded, "And her silence contributes to the conflicts, too."

A glimmer of recognition flashed in Rose's eyes as she slowly began to realize that many of her fights with Bill revolved around disagreements over what would be "best" for Tina, who rarely spoke up to express her own feelings or opinions. Rose recognized that she had neglected to listen to Tina in the past. She had become so distracted by keeping Bill at bay, so intent on convincing Bill that her view of Tina was more accurate than his, that she had never really heard Tina's voice. Rose came to this realization slowly and without self-reproach. As she talked, her voice became calmer and she appeared to relax. Her tired, worn look was replaced by a hopeful smile. The competent, secure facet of Rose had come to the fore.

Finally, I asked, "So what does all of this have to do with the present?" The purpose of this question was to connect the experience Rose was having with me back to her relationship with Tina.

Rose took off her glasses, as if to ponder this question. Then, a flash of insight: "You mean, right now, today? I guess, I guess I need to *listen* to her, don't I? I really need to listen and not talk so much. I have to let her know that no matter what she has to say, I can hear it, I can take it."

Connecting with Tina

My next task was to coax Tina to emerge from her cocoon and express her feelings more directly. Once this had been achieved, I would bring Rose and Tina together and utilize my relationship with each of them to help them have a more productive conversation than the one they had in the previous session.

So constricted in her immature, withdrawn self, Tina was not easy to engage. I felt myself getting frustrated with her and thought to myself, "This is how Bill must feel."

Tina decided to use the opportunity to be alone with me to plead her case. She talked about her desire to be thin, since it made her feel more attractive. Her only complaint was that she felt "controlled" by her family, because they would not leave her alone to decide when or what to eat.

Mustering my patience, I listened for a while, and then commented that she seemed to be very unhappy.

Tina burst into tears: "I'm miserable."

I pursued: "And about what besides having to gain weight? Is there anything else that is making you so miserable?"

Over the next several minutes, through her tears, Tina expressed her frustration that her parents "fought all the time," her anger at her father for the way he treated her mother, and her worries about her mother, because she seemed so unhappy.

Finally, Tina cried, "I wish she would stop worrying about me and worry about herself for a change."

Although I was tempted to hear this statement as another ploy on Tina's part to be left alone to lose weight, I instead chose to hear it as Tina's suggestion for what needed to change in her relationship with Rose: "So I guess there are things that need to change in your relationship. Let's talk about that, so that you'll be prepared for the session tomorrow, when we get back to that conversation between you and your mom."

I sensed that we had just touched the tip of the iceberg, but at least it was a start. We talked for another 20 minutes, during which Tina began to formulate some ideas for her conversation with Rose.

Helping Rose and Tina to Connect

In the next session, we got right down to business. Reminding Rose of our conversation the day before, I suggested that she again ask Tina to talk with her about what was upsetting her, and what needed to change in their relationship. I reminded Tina to respond to her mother with the voice she had discovered in our session the day before.

During the ensuing conversation, whenever Rose's or Tina's newly discovered voices receded, I intervened to elicit them again. Initially, Tina needed coaching to tell her mother about her worries, and I needed to remind Rose to listen and accept Tina's fears without responding protectively or defensively, without feeling compelled to soothe Tina or solve her problems for her. Gradually, as Rose and Tina grew more confident in this new pattern of interaction, I found that I could take a less central role.

STEP 4: HANDLING RELAPSES

Relapses are inevitable in the treatment of anorexia. After the weight gain has been jump-started in response to the parents' joining forces, a period usually follows when the girl gains weight. Eventually, however, she tests the limit by stopping or reversing the weight gain. How will the family handle this relapse? Will they revert to old patterns, or will they respond differently than in the past?

Relapses test the resolve of both family members and the therapist. Will the therapist abandon the contract? Will the therapist desert the family? Will the therapist reduce his or her own anxiety by referring the girl for individual therapy or hospitalization? Will the therapist shift the focus back to the symptom and away from the family relationships?

Framing the Relapse

An essential principle in responding to relapses is *to resist the temptation to focus attention on coming up with new strategies to "get" the girl to eat*. To do so could reinforce efforts to "fix" the symptom while family relationships are neglected. Instead, the relapse should be linked to interactions in the family. When the therapeutic contract was originally negotiated, the symptom was connected to family interactions and resolution of the symptom to changes in family interactional patterns. In the case of Tina, her weight loss was framed as a response to the absence of nurturing relationships with her parents. The relapse, then, must be framed in a way that connects it to these same family relationship issues.

The manner in which the therapist frames the relapse depends on whether the girl loses weight, remains the same, or gains weight but fails to gain the amount the parents had specified.

Loss of weight is obviously the most serious occurrence. If the girl loses some of the weight she had gained over the previous weeks, it is important to ask what, if anything, was different in the current week that might have contributed to the weight loss. Evidence of regression in family relationships should be given the most significance, and the weight loss should be connected to these regressions. If the family relationships have changed, then the weight loss could be framed as an expression of the girl's fear that the change in the relationships could have unwanted consequences for her or for the other family members. These negative consequences can be explicitly discussed and the girl encouraged to express her feelings about them verbally rather than through the indirect medium of refusing to eat.

If *the adolescent neither gains nor loses weight,* the simplest way of framing this occurrence is to suggest that she is testing how her parents will respond. Will they recognize that it is not as serious as a weight loss, while still acknowledging that she did not meet the goal? Many parents fail to differentiate between a failure to gain weight and a loss of weight, though, in fact, the latter is more significant. The split between the parents, with one taking a more permissive stance and the other a more punitive stance, will often be brought into sharp relief at these times. It is important to challenge the parents to respond to the failure to gain weight in a way that does not lead to conflict between them and instead demonstrates respect for each other's positions. The parents must be discouraged from criticizing or attacking the girl, as this is simply another way of triangulating the girl in conflicts between them. While "ganging up" on the girl might make the parents feel closer to one another and relieve them of any guilt they might be feeling for failing to help her gain the required amount of weight, parental criticism has been found to impede successful treatment (le Grange, Eisler, Dare, & Hodes, 1992).

Another possibility is to frame the failure to gain weight as a sign that the girl is beginning to assert herself. The way in which this frame is presented depends upon the stage of treatment. Early in treatment, when little net weight has been gained, the girl's failure to gain weight should be interpreted as an inappropriate expression of autonomy, and the parents should be supported in treating it as such. Later in treatment, when the girl has demonstrated that she can gain weight and the parents have demonstrated that they can respond effectively, it is appropriate to lend more support to the girl and encourage her to speak up in favor of her own freedom of choice rather than use her refusal to gain weight as a way to convey this message to her parents.

A third possibility is that *the adolescent gains some weight, but less than the amount specified by the parents*. Assuming that the parents had set a realistic weight goal, the girl must be given credit for having gained some weight, while her failure to reach the goal must also be acknowledged. It is best to encourage the parents to discuss how to handle this situation, after they have listened to the girl's side of the story. It is necessary to monitor closely the process that unfolds between the parents and intervene to block intrusions by the girl or attempts by either parent to triangulate the girl into the conflict between them.

Failure to gain the full amount of weight can be framed as ambivalence on the girl's part. On the one hand, she feels safe enough to gain some weight, which means that the family has demonstrated some changes. On the other hand, she is afraid to trust her parents completely. Acknowledging this dilemma could lead to a fruitful discussion about power issues in the family and the girl's sense of her own boundaries.

On the other hand, the girl may say that she failed to gain the full amount of weight because she was "afraid of getting fat." This claim could be handled in the same way. Why did the girl choose this method of handling her fear, rather than turning to her parents for support? The focus should not be on the girl's anxiety, that is, what is "inside" of her, but rather on how the family members can help her deal more effectively with the anxiety she will inevitably feel when gaining weight. In other words, it is expected that change will evoke anxiety. But what will help the girl to deal with the anxiety in ways other than restricting her food intake will be a relationship with her parents that helps her feel more secure.

For example, Tina met the goal of 2 pounds of weight gain by the date her parents had specified. I framed this apparent success as evidence that the family relationships, particularly those between Tina and Rose, had begun to change, and that Tina was eager to do her part to convince her parents that they were on the right track. At the end of the session, I again asked the parents to decide how much weight Tina should gain over the next week, and they decided that 2 more pounds would be appropriate.

By the next session, however, Tina had gained only 1 pound. I asked Rose and Bill to talk with one another and decide how to handle this situation.

Rose began by explaining to Bill that Tina had been working hard, and that she thought they should acknowledge her efforts. Noticing that Bill was seething and probably viewing Rose's idea as another example of her overprotectiveness, I jumped in to forestall an angry explosion. I pointed out that Tina's failure to gain 2 pounds was a test of Rose's and Bill's willingness to listen to each other and find a different way of responding to Tina rather than protecting her or criticizing her. I reminded them that she began to lose weight in the first place because of the absence of sustaining relationships in her life. The fact that she gained 1 pound might mean that she was cautiously optimistic about the changes that her parents had made, but that she was giving them the message that the changes were not enough. We would need to discuss this issue in more depth, but first it was important for Rose and Bill to decide how they wanted to respond to Tina's failure to gain the required 2 pounds. I suggested that an appropriate response on their part should acknowledge three things: (1) Tina had gained some weight this week, (2) she had failed to meet the goal her parents had specified, and (3) her weight fluctuations were related to the amount of progress the family members were making in changing their ways of relating to one another.

Developing a Plan Based on the Frame

In response to my little speech, Bill suggested that rather than grounding Tina for the entire weekend (the original consequence for failing to gain weight), she should be grounded for 1 day, and that Tina could select the day. Rose looked doubtful—after all, Tina lived with her and she would be responsible for enforcing the consequence. On the other hand, I thought that Bill's compromise sounded reasonable. I debated whether to intervene to support Bill or whether to allow Rose and Bill to continue struggling together. I decided on the former, since I felt that my relationship with Bill needed to be stronger, and perhaps I could bolster our connection by supporting him.

I stated that I believed that Bill's suggestion was a good one, and that it addressed the first two points I had made. I wondered if we could also address the third point. I asked Bill if he would be willing to spend some time alone with Tina, perhaps on the day that Tina would otherwise be grounded. Anticipating an objection, I immediately reminded him that the grounding was not really a punishment, but rather a way of communicating to Tina that they as parents were serious about holding the line on their agreements.

Bill responded that he thought it was a good idea to spend a day alone with Tina, but he wanted her to be grounded as well—he apparently felt that some punishment was still necessary. After some discussion, we finally agreed that Tina would spend the afternoon of the "grounding" day with Bill and then return home and not be allowed to go out that evening.

Deciding not to push it, I encouraged the family to go with this plan and congratulated them on arriving at a reasonable compromise. Since Tina and Rose had made progress on their relationship, I believed that the failure to gain weight could be interpreted as a message that Tina and Bill needed to work on their relationship. By agreeing to spend time alone together, it would help to strengthen the connection between them and perhaps help Tina feel more secure about gaining weight the following week.

STEP 5: SUPPORTING INDIVIDUAL DEVELOPMENT

Development, which is a process of differentiation and expansion of self, is arrested by the symptomatic cycle. As I discussed in Chapter 3, when a family is caught in a symptomatic cycle, certain aspects of each family member are repeatedly activated, while other aspects are underdeveloped. Once the symptomatic cycle has been disrupted, development is free to resume. Emotionally, the adolescent might be profoundly immature for his or her chronological age, because the normal course of development had been arrested by the repeated activation of certain facets of him- or herself at the expense of others.

On Monday morning following Tina's weekend visit with her father, I met with her privately to talk about the visit. For the first time, Tina was relaxed and smiling. She stated that she felt that she was "over anorexia" because she had gained weight over the weekend and was not feeling "guilty." Speaking quickly and perhaps a bit too anxiously, she went on to describe her time with her father, emphasizing how much she enjoyed spending the day with him, particularly since they had not had any arguments. At the beginning of the visit, Bill had apologized to Tina for all the times he had blown up at her, and Tina had replied, "It's no big deal." The matter was then dropped, and they spent the rest of the day wandering separately through the art museum. At the end of the day, they met in the lobby. Bill drove Tina home, and dropped her off in front of Rose's house without walking her to the door.

Hearing this, I was faced with a dilemma. Obviously, Tina was experiencing success over the changes she had made and excitement about the potential she now saw in the relationship with her father. She appeared more relaxed, more animated, and more like a typical 16-year-old. She had gained weight and was talking about anorexia as if it were no longer the most significant aspect of herself. I wanted to share Tina's joy, congratulate her on her efforts, and celebrate with her.

However, I noticed that Tina had neglected to mention whether she and Bill had carried out the task to talk about their relationship, and I suspected that they had not done the task. Rather, it appeared that Tina and Bill had tacitly agreed to avoid conflicts in order to have a "nice" day together. Furthermore, Tina's statement that she was "over anorexia" because she had gained a few pounds seemed naive, to say the least.

Embracing the Anxiety

I decided to challenge Tina, both to explore further her experiences over the weekend but also to see how well she could handle being challenged. I asked her to explain exactly what changes had occurred in her relationship with her father. Tina evaded my question. She hastened to reassure me that she was certain that her father now "totally" supported her, but I persisted, repeating my question four times in the course of the conversation. Eventually, unable to answer and unsuccessful in distracting me from my question, Tina burst into sobs.

The anxiety that Tina was experiencing derived from my pushing her to define herself, to declare her feelings, and to justify her point of view. Although I sympathized with the depth of her pain, I interpreted what was happening as a positive sign. Perhaps for the first time, Tina was experiencing directly the anxiety associated with defining herself, an anxiety that is entirely age appropriate.

Freed from the symptomatic cycle, Tina's development was now unblocked, leaving her subject to the discomfort and uncertainty associated with the developmental changes all adolescents must experience. However, rather than submerging her pain and confusion or expressing it symptomatically, she was experiencing it and expressing it directly and verbally in a way that could lead to new possibilities for resolution.

A Helpful Metaphor

I decided to stimulate Tina's process of self-exploration by introducing the metaphor of "internal voices," similar to that proposed by Richard Schwartz (1987, 1995). Throughout development, significant people in one's life become internalized as different "voices" that can influence one's feelings and behaviors. Meanwhile, complementary aspects of the self emerge as separate voices that carry on a silent dialogue with the internalized voices of significant others.

The process of putting words to the internalized voices reinforces the differentiation of the voices from each other and stimulates the development of an aspect of the self that can view these voices objectively. Implicit in this notion is the idea that one can gain more control over these voices (i.e., impulses, urges, demands), but not by silencing them. Rather, one begins to experience a greater sense of personal agency only when one listens to the voices without feeling compelled to react to them. The challenge to integrate apparently contradictory aspects of the self that arise in different contexts is an age-appropriate developmental task of late adolescence and young adulthood (Harter, 1999).

The process I was encouraging in my work with Tina paralleled the one that had taken place within the family. Just as I had encouraged the family members to listen nonreactively, to hear and respect one another, I was now encouraging Tina to hear and respect the voices within her. One of my goals was to help the family members become more tolerant of conflict and disagreements. Similarly, in helping Tina to embrace the different aspects of her developing self, I was hoping to increase her own tolerance for conflict within herself.

As Tina and I explored her different voices, she came to label them "The Anorectic," "The Bulimic," "The Little Girl," and "The New Part"; the latter representing the voice of the young adult that she discovered she was becoming. As do many adolescents who are just beginning to experience freedom from their symptoms, Tina initially wanted to stifle the anorectic and bulimic voices, which had been so powerful in the past. However, were she to give in to this temptation by silencing these voices and suppressing these aspects of herself, she could risk subjecting herself to the culture of conditional acceptance that had helped to sustain the symptomatic cycle in the family.

My goal was to help Tina listen to these voices without feeling pulled to react to them. I wanted to encourage her to view these voices objectively, without allowing any single voice to drown out the others. I hoped that Tina might eventually discover that all of these voices had something important to say to her that could help her define herself in a more complete and, ultimately, more realistic way.

Constructing Tasks to Further Self-Understanding

It is helpful to arrange experiences outside of the sessions that carry on the process of self-discovery and self-acceptance. For example, I encouraged Tina to develop her artistic talent in a way that could lead her to connect with others, rather than as a way of putting distance between herself and other people, as she so often did. I suggested that she volunteer to give art lessons to young children at her local community center. I also encouraged her to use her artwork, rather than her symptoms, as a way to express her inner pain, and to use her artwork as a medium for exploring how to integrate the different aspects of herself.

Psychological testing can be another resource to help adolescents become acquainted with their many voices. Unlike the traditional model of psychological testing, in which the psychologist administers tests to uncover hidden pathology, I advocate the use of psychological testing to uncover hidden strengths and to advance the course of therapy. Properly timed, a referral for psychological testing can be a powerful intervention (Ziffer, 1985).

In Tina's case, after a few weeks during which she steadily gained weight, I arranged for a psychological consultation as a way to engage her more actively in the process of self-exploration. The psychologist administered a battery of standard psychological tests (Minnesota Multiphasic Personality Inventory, Rorschach, Thematic Apperception Test), but rather than interpreting the test results as an "expert" on Tina, she engaged Tina in a collaborative process of exploring what her test responses might tell her about herself. The psychologist was also invited to a family session to support Tina in explaining to her parents what she had learned about herself from the psychological testing.

Preparing the Family to Accept Change

As I pointed out in Chapter 3, it is best to postpone work on developmental issues until the symptomatic cycle has been disrupted and new family patterns have begun to emerge. In many cases, the symptomatic cycle arose in the first place because the family was not able to manage the stresses associated with the developmental transition into adolescence. Working prematurely on developmental issues can frustrate both the therapist and the adolescent, since each developmental step the adolescent takes can feed back into the cycle and reactivate it. The family members must be helped to adapt to the developmental changes that are taking place.

To address this concern, as I met with Tina to help her get acquainted with the many aspects of herself, I also met separately with Rose to explore the facets of her new role as the mother of a 16-year-old girl. In one of these meetings, Rose discovered an aspect of herself that she described as "the part of me that cherishes the little girl." At first, she was tempted to deny this part of herself out of fear that she might discourage Tina from growing up. However, just as I had discouraged Tina from silencing any of her voices, I discouraged Rose from silencing this voice. I encouraged Rose to accept this aspect of herself as the part of her that could remind her that Tina was no longer a "little girl" and could encourage her to find new ways of nurturing Tina that were appropriate for a 16-year-old.

STEP 6: SUPPORTING THE TRANSFORMATION

In a few short months, Tina and Rose had undergone a remarkable transformation. Tina's transformation was evident in her body: She had gained 15 pounds, had styled her hair, and dressed in designer clothes

WHEN TO CONDUCT INDIVIDUAL SESSIONS

Some family therapists insist that the entire family come for every session and refuse to meet with individual family members even when a family member requests a private meeting. I believe, however, that individual sessions can be a useful adjunct to family therapy by helping to complement the work being done in the family sessions. What is important is not who is physically present in the room but rather how the therapist is thinking about the problem and the patterns that maintain it.

At the beginning of therapy, individual sessions can help the therapist assess the contribution of an individual family member to the symptomatic cycle and to facilitate the process of joining with a particular family member. In the middle stages of therapy, while the therapist is focusing efforts on disrupting patterns, individual sessions can be used to challenge a family member to change. In the later stages of therapy, after the symptomatic cycle has been disrupted, individual sessions can help family members meet the challenges associated with the resumption of their developmental process.

The Issue of Confidentiality

Before meeting alone with any member of the family, the therapist must decide whether information disclosed in a private meeting will be held in confidence. There are arguments for and against the practice of offering confidentiality to individual family members. Family members (especially adolescents) might be more willing to disclose important information if the therapist agreed not to report this information to the other members of the family. On the other hand, a therapist who is told a family secret risks being inducted into a coalition with the family member who revealed the secret and could lose the trust of the other members of the family as a result. Family members could get in the habit of holding back in family sessions and instead use confidential individual sessions with the therapist to express feelings or thoughts that the therapist believes should be brought up in the family session.

However the therapist decides to resolve the issue of confidentiality, it is essential that all family members understand the conditions under which information disclosed in individual sessions might be reported to other members of the family. This issue must be discussed explicitly with the entire family before the therapist meets individually with any one family member. It is important also to keep in mind that in many jurisdictions parents have the right to insist that the therapist disclose information obtained in a private session with a minor child. If therapists believe

We continued to meet at increasing intervals for the next 6 months, and then Tina stated that she did not feel a need to continue coming for regular sessions. Rose and Bill agreed with her. By now, at 17, Tina was a healthy young woman on the threshold of adulthood. Though she did not have a steady boyfriend, she dated regularly and had an active social life. She had decided to apply to college and major in art. Rose had also grown. She had begun to think about dating again and had attended a few community dances.

PITFALLS AND COMPLICATIONS

Subtle Undermining of Parental Authority

Although it might appear that the parents are working as a team, the girl might not gain weight. In this case, it is possible that one of the parents might be subtly undermining the other. For example, one of the parents (typically the father) remains peripheral and by default delegates to the other parent (typically the mother) the responsibility for supervising the girl's eating. The girl resists when her mother tries to help her to eat. In desperation, the mother might modify the original expectation, and the girl might then eat, which reinforces the mother for having made the modification. However, since the girl is not taking in the required number of calories, she fails to gain weight. Sometimes the mother does not tell the father or the therapist that she had modified the plan, for fear of being criticized.

One way to test whether this process is occurring is to review with the parents in detail their plan for helping the girl to meet the weight goal. If one parent appears to be insufficiently involved, then that parent might be given primary responsibility for helping the girl to eat. A family "lunch session" (Minuchin et al., 1978) can be held to assess the subtle dynamics among the family members. By bringing food into the session, the parents can enact before the therapist the unsuccessful ways in which they have been trying to help the girl eat, and the therapist can intervene to change these patterns.

Occasionally, another family member who has not been an active participant in family sessions might be undermining the efforts of the parents to take charge. For example, a grandmother might be siding with the girl against the parents. A sibling might collude with the girl by helping her deceive the parents about her eating. Sometimes, someone outside the family is undermining the parents. For example, a boyfriend might enable the girl to continue losing weight or undermine efforts to reestablish connections with the parents by monopolizing the girl's time. It is even possible for another member of the professional team to undermine the parents either overtly (by giving the girl advice without consulting with the parents) or covertly (by communicating disdain of the parents or the primary therapist).

It is beneficial to invite these other individuals to family sessions to encourage a stronger alliance with them and to intervene directly in the patterns of undermining. When it is not possible to insist on participation from someone outside the family, an alternative is to coach the parents on ways to recognize the influence of external parties and to block their interference.

Weak Alliance with the Adolescent

In working to support parental collaboration and authority, it is important not to neglect the therapeutic alliance with the adolescent. Doing so risks marginalizing the adolescent by communicating that her thoughts and feelings are not important. In response, the adolescent might assert herself by resisting treatment. On the other hand, developing an alliance with the adolescent does not mean entering into a coalition with her against the parents. Rather, it means expressing interest in her as a person in her own right with aspects to her identity that are separate from the eating disorder. It is important to communicate empathy and respect for the adolescent's struggle to meet parental expectations without implying that these expectations are unreasonable. As discussed above, the technique of externalizing the anorexia and treating it as separate from the adolescent and family can help to strengthen the alliance with the adolescent.

Highly Critical Families

Although conflict avoidance is common among anorectic families, some families exhibit the opposite pattern and engage in intense criticism of the adolescent and each other. Continual bickering serves the same function as burying conflicts: The bickering parties snipe at one another but rarely engage in serious discussion of each other's points of view with the intention of reaching accord. While conflict avoidance helps to maintain the illusion of closeness, bickering helps to maintain the illusion of separateness.

Empirical evidence suggests that high levels of parental criticism interfere with the success of treatment (le Grange et al., 1992). Thus, reducing parental blaming, criticism, and attacks is essential. Some techniques for doing so include:

1. *Reframe the parents' criticism as an expression of their anxiety and helplessness.* Join with the parents around their care and concern for the girl, and the intense fear they experience at the prospect of losing her. Empathize with their plight, and then gradually help them to express the anxiety directly rather than through criticizing the girl.

2. *Externalize the problem.* Begin separating the girl from the eating disorder by talking about "the anorexia" as an external force that has invaded the family. Explore with each family member how "the anorexia" has affected him or her personally. The temptation to criticize the girl could be framed as a tactic that the anorexia uses to keep the family divided. Help the parents join with the girl and the therapist in a campaign to reclaim their lives from the grip of anorexia. By avoiding the temptation to criticize the girl they can display resistance to the anorexia's attempts to dominate their interactions.

3. *Conduct separate and parallel sessions with the parents and the girl.* With parents who exhibit high levels of criticism and who do not respond to the previous two interventions, it might be necessary to proceed by meeting separately with the parents as a couple and individually with the girl. There is empirical support for the effectiveness of this type of "separated" family therapy for families where there is a high level of criticism (Eisler et al., 2000). By meeting separately with the parents as a couple, it is possible to empathize with their feelings of anxiety, hurt, and frustration without the risk of being perceived by the girl as "siding" with them against her. The parent sessions can then be used to build an alliance with the parents and help them develop constructive ways to encourage the girl to gain weight. As the parents begin to feel supported by the therapist, conjoint sessions with the parents and the girl can be reintroduced.

Another Family Member Becomes Symptomatic

Sometimes symptoms that are exhibited by one family member help to stabilize the family by preventing even more disruptive forces from being unleashed. This might be the case if another family member becomes symptomatic when the child with an eating disorder improves. In more than one family I have treated, the mother became severely depressed after the girl achieved a normal weight. In these cases, the girl's individuation from the family left the mother bereft, as the father was emotionally unavailable to her and she lacked other social supports. Work had to be done to prevent the girl's regression in the service of stabilizing the family system while the mother's emerging symptoms and need for substitute sources of support were also addressed. Along with encouraging the girl's individuation, other supports for the mother had to be mobilized.

In one family, the mother became suicidally depressed and anorectic after the originally symptomatic daughter recovered and moved out of the house to attend college. The mother's depression was not only a reaction to the years of emotional distance between her and her husband, but also served to maintain distance from the father, who became increasingly frustrated at her rebuffs of his efforts to comfort and console her. It gradually became clear that the mother had fallen out of love with the father many years before, even though the father continued to have strong feelings for her. Fearful of hurting the father and disrupting the family, the mother concealed her feelings. As their daughter grew older and more independent, it became more and more difficult for the mother to keep her feelings hidden. The emergence of the eating disorder helped to keep this parental conflict from surfacing. The parents worked together effectively to help the girl gain weight, but on the day of our last scheduled family therapy session, the mother announced that she had tried to kill herself the night before. I realized that I had failed to assess accurately the level of the mother's unhappiness and the weakness of the connection between the parents.

The marriage did not survive. During the separation and divorce, the mother had several more suicidal crises and admitted herself to an eating disorders unit twice. Meanwhile, I worked to promote the girl's growth and development while providing emotional support to the mother. Eventually, the mother met a man for whom she developed strong feelings, and she eventually stabilized as that relationship deepened.

Should I have addressed the marital issues in this family earlier in treatment? A strong argument against doing so is that addressing the marital issues too early in treatment might undermine the message that the parents must do whatever is necessary to join together to save their daughter from anorexia. If marital issues surface early in treatment, it is best to tell the parents that they will be addressed later, after their daughter has begun to eat normally and regain weight. They are encouraged to put their differences aside for the moment, and instead focus attention on helping the girl gain weight. On the other hand, I erred in this case by not paying more attention to the mother's profound unhappiness and her need for a substitute support system as the girl improved and moved out of the family. Thus, as soon as there is evidence that the parents' efforts to help the girl gain weight have been successful, it is important to assess the strength of the emotional bond between the parents. In the case of divorced parents, it is essential that the mother have a sufficiently strong adult support system to replace the girl, and this role should not be relegated to another child.

SUMMARY

In this chapter, I have proposed the following steps for treating families with eating disorders:

- Arrange for a physician to monitor the girl's weight and medical status.

- Negotiate a treatment contract that includes an expanded view of the problem beyond an exclusive focus on food and weight and calls attention to the repetitive patterns of interaction among family members that have enabled the symptom to continue.

- Encourage parental collaboration to help the girl to gain weight by giving the parents the task to decide on a weight goal for the girl and strategies for helping her to meet the goal.

- Facilitate shifts in family interactional patterns by forging strong relationships with each family member and then using these relationships to encourage changes in the ways the family members relate to one another.

- Handle relapses by keeping the focus on family relationships.

- As the symptom remits and the girl begins to eat more normally, work to support the unblocked developmental process of each family member.

- Support the transformation in the family by taking a less central role and gradually disengaging as the family members struggle to resolve their difficulties.

6

Depression and Suicide

When Peter Brandon called me about his daughter, Jenny, I could tell from the resignation in his voice that he had just about given up hope. He had been referred to me by a colleague who was seeing Jenny individually but believed that the individual therapy was not getting anywhere and suggested family therapy. Jenny had been to four other therapists, and she was hospitalized after she tried to slash her wrists. While hospitalized, Jenny had tried to hang herself. She had been on many different medications, including two different antidepressants, a mood stabilizer, an antipsychotic, and an anxiolytic, all with little success. Eventually, the staff told the parents that Jenny might be in the early stages of schizophrenia. Although Jenny had apparently exhibited no overt psychotic symptoms such as delusions or hallucinations, the hospital staff could find no other explanation for her erratic behavior.

Peter, Jenny's 52-year-old father and an executive in a major insurance company, was devastated by this news, since his own mother, now deceased, had been diagnosed with paranoid schizophrenia over 40 years earlier. Peter and his wife, Clare, a registered nurse, had raised a son who was now married and living away from home. When Jenny told her parents that she had been depressed for many months prior to her suicide attempt, they were stunned. They never even suspected that their happy, outgoing daughter was experiencing such unbearable emotional pain.

The prevalence of depression and suicidality significantly increases at puberty (Compas, Ey, & Grant, 1993; Lewinsohn, Rohde, & Seeley, 1996). Some studies have reported that as many as one-third of adolescents experience periods of depressed mood, and between one-third to one-half of these meet the criteria for a diagnosis of major depressive disorder at some time during their adolescence (Compas et al., 1993; Petersen et al., 1993).

Why is depression so common during adolescence? Some authors claim that adolescents are susceptible to depression because of the developmental changes that take place during this phase of life. Hormonal factors might play a role, though it is believed that the effect of hormones on mood is small compared to the much stronger influence of environmental stressors (Buchanan et al., 1992). The physical changes that accompany puberty lead some adolescents, particularly girls, to feel inadequate about their appearance (Allgood-Merten, Lewinsohn, & Hops, 1990; Petersen, Sarigiani, & Kennedy, 1991). The new capacity for formal operational thought makes it possible for adolescents to reflect on themselves in ways that were previously not possible (Elkind, 1967), thus contributing to brooding and self-denigration. Family conflict, which is a major precipitating factor in adolescent depression (Cole & McPherson, 1993; Lewinsohn et al., 1996), becomes more common during the teenage years. Increased cultural pressures toward independence can push many youngsters into roles for which they are not ready, thus promoting disengagement from parents and other potentially supportive adults (Silverstein & Rashbaum, 1994).

Changes in society also play a role in adolescent depression. Many adolescents live in families who are experiencing severe financial stress. Corporate downsizing has led to unemployment and associated financial crisis among middle-aged parents. The increased size of the youth cohort means more competition for slots at the best colleges. Exposure to violence is commonplace for youngsters in inner-city neighborhoods, and many adolescents who live in these environments have experienced loss of a family member or friend to violence. Adolescents are exposed almost daily to violence in the media and in video games.

THE ROLE OF GENDER IN ADOLESCENT DEPRESSION

Among adults, it is widely recognized that depression is more common among women than among men (Culbertson, 1997). It is during adolescence that this gender difference first emerges. Prior to adolescence, depression is more common among boys than among girls, but by age 14, this gender ratio shifts (Petersen et al., 1993).

Many explanations for the gender difference in depression have been proposed. Early adolescence is a more stressful time for girls than for boys. Girls begin developing earlier and are therefore more likely than boys to experience several transitions simultaneously, such as entering middle school at the same time they are going through the first stages of pubertal development (Simmons et al., 1987). Girls and boys also employ different methods of coping with stress. Girls are more likely to react to stress by internalizing their feelings, whereas boys are more likely to distract themselves or turn their feelings outward (Cramer, 1979). Even when exposed to the same degree of stress, girls are more likely than boys to react by becoming depressed (Nolen-Hoeksema, 1987).

Some adolescents engage in a pattern of behavior known as *relational aggression,* which includes efforts to harm another person by manipulating relationships, for example, abruptly breaking off a friendship, excluding someone from social gatherings, or spreading rumors to spoil a peer's reputation (Crick, Casas, & Nelson, 2002). This pattern of aggression is more common among girls, and might be a risk factor for depression because girls tend to be more sensitive than boys to disruptions in their interpersonal relationships.

Other writers have also pointed to specific gender-role-related stressors that differentially affect adolescent girls. Alexandra Kaplan (1991) has argued that the socialization pressures on women to inhibit anger and to assume responsibility when relationships fail increase a woman's vulnerability to depression. Girls experience pressure to silence their own voices in order to preserve relationships that are important to them (Brown & Gilligan, 1992; Jack, 1991, 1999). Mary Pipher (1994) has pointed out that many girls miss the open, warm relationship with their parents, which they have felt forced to sacrifice in order to fit in with peers. Girls are discouraged from expressing or even acknowledging anger, and so might have no option but to suppress these feelings and in some cases turn them back against themselves (Miller, 1991).

Although depression and suicide attempts are more common among girls, boys are more likely to die from a suicide attempt, probably because boys are apt to resort to more lethal methods (Berman & Jobes, 1991; Lewinsohn et al., 1996). This disturbing finding requires us to examine the possibility that gender-related pressures are implicated in the etiology of depression and suicide in boys as well.

Olga Silverstein and Beth Rashbaum (1994) have argued that the expectation in our culture for children to leave home at age 18 can put unbearable pressure on a young man. They write, "There's no permission in our culture for them to postpone the leaving-home rite of passage.... For a young man who is determined not to leave, the alternatives are covert maneuvers, such as ... procrastination ... sickness ... or really drastic actions like suicide attempts" (p. 167). The young man who is not ready or willing to accept the culturally prescribed role of a male might begin to view himself as inadequate and unsuited for life (Pleck,

1981, 1995). For some, suicide might seem to be the only escape from this apparently hopeless situation. Conflicts related to gender-role expectations are particularly intense for GLBT adolescents, as the following case illustrates.

Bart had threatened to kill himself with his father's hunting rifle. Now, he sat sullenly next to his mother, Lois, a frail, depressed-looking woman in her 40s. She was seated next to Bart's father, Ed, a balding, overweight businessman in horn-rimmed black glasses. Next to Ed sat Bart's younger brother, whose baseball hat and athletic build reinforced his self-description as a "jock."

At age 16, Bart had not been to school for the past 3 months because of intractable abdominal pain that had not responded to medical treatment. He had undergone what sounded like a torturing round of tests run by one of the foremost gastroenterologists in the region, and still nothing had shown up. Yet, Bart continued to complain of debilitating pain that kept him confined to his home most of the time. He had lost touch with his friends, except for the few who continued to visit him on weekends.

Patient at first, Ed became increasingly irate at Bart as the medical reports seemed to confirm Ed's suspicions that Bart might be malingering. Because Lois still believed that Bart had an undiagnosed illness and agreed with Bart that he couldn't attend school, Ed felt unsupported in his efforts to get Bart to resume a "normal lifestyle." To underscore his point, Ed would harass Bart daily about his appearance and about minor household chores that Bart had failed to carry out to Ed's satisfaction.

Although Lois sympathized with Bart, she restrained herself from intervening during these arguments because she didn't want to undermine Ed, as she used to do when Bart was younger. In couples therapy 3 years earlier, she had learned that her marital difficulties were fueled by her siding with Bart against Ed, so she stopped interfering and left Bart and Ed to resolve their problems on their own. She remained steadfast even when Bart pleaded with her for support, though she inwardly ached to comfort her son and intervene with Ed on the boy's behalf.

When Bart's abdominal pain began, there was a brief reprieve in the battles between Bart and Ed, as attention shifted to trying to find out what was wrong and how to treat it. But, as Bart became more and more withdrawn and lethargic, Ed became increasingly impatient. At times, he couldn't help comparing Bart to his brother, in an attempt to shame Bart into "acting more like a man." It was after one such particularly volatile confrontation that Bart had made his threat to shoot himself.

One of my colleagues suggested that I work to break the "covert coalition" between Bart and Lois by challenging Lois to be more active in her support of Ed's expectations of Bart. Although I understood the rationale behind this suggestion, it didn't sit right with me. How would it help Bart if he were even more overtly abandoned by his mother, the one person in the family who seemed to have sympathy for him? I decided to try a different approach. I noted that Bart never actually said "no" to his father, but instead would plead illness whenever his father made demands of him. Could I help Bart find his voice so that he could verbalize his resistance in words rather than through physical complaints?

I presented to the family the idea that Bart's pain was related to powerful feelings that he apparently was not ready to express in the family sessions. I suggested that I meet alone with Bart to help him "get in touch" with these feelings and to explore the reasons why he held back these feelings. When I met alone with Bart, I told him that he had to stop using pain as an excuse for not doing things his father expected him to do. If he believed that his father's request was reasonable, then he should do what his father asked, and try to ignore his pain. If he didn't believe that his father's request was reasonable, he should simply say so, loud and clear, rather than pleading illness. If he wanted to get over his pain, he would have to take the risk of challenging his father directly.

With my support, Bart did as I suggested. As Bart began to speak up, Lois became more active, sometimes supporting Ed, sometimes mediating, and sometimes supporting Bart. I encouraged Lois and Ed to air their disagreements about parenting in private, so that they could present Bart with a unified front. I also encouraged Lois and Bart to have a relationship that wasn't based on mutual enmity toward Ed. Bart's pain decreased, but it didn't go away. He started to resume some of his activities and he went back to school.

It was at this point that Bart nervously confessed to me in an individual session that he was being harassed at school by a group of boys who taunted him about being gay. "The problem is," Bart said, "I am. I really am gay. And you're the first person I've ever told."

That session began a lengthy process of helping Bart come to terms with his sexuality. He eventually came out to his parents, who were, to my surprise as well as Bart's, supportive. A year later, Bart was back at school, had no abdominal pain, and had begun dating another young man.

ASSESSMENT OF ADOLESCENT DEPRESSION

Typically, depression is characterized by persistent feelings of sadness and decreased energy level, but other symptoms might be present as well. Adolescents who experience *major depression* might also experience sleep disturbances, appetite and weight loss, social withdrawal, crying, and suicidal ideation. If these episodes alternate with periods of elated, expansive, or irritable mood, a diagnosis of *bipolar disorder* or *cyclothymia* might be warranted. Relatively milder but more persistent depressive symptoms characterize the syndrome known as *dysthymia*. In these cases, depressive symptoms might have been present for many years, and might not have been recognized as such by the depressed person or the family. If depressive symptoms that are not serious enough to qualify for major depression arise in response to a significant life event or transition, the term *adjustment disorder with depressed mood* is applied.

Obviously, the most important factor to consider in assessment of depressed adolescents is the risk for a suicide attempt. All adolescents who present with depressive symptoms should be evaluated for suicidal potential. In general, assessment of risk is based on the presence and specificity of a suicidal plan, access to means, and few barriers to carrying out the attempt. Later in this chapter, I discuss ways of working with suicidal adolescents.

Considerable evidence has accumulated for genetic and biological factors in the onset and development of depression (Rende, Slomkowski, Lloyd-Richardson, Stroud, & Niaura, 2006). However, it is important to keep in mind that these factors are not determinative. Many people with a family history of depression do not develop depression, and many cases of depression arise in families where there is no known history of depression. Some evidence suggests that the level of family conflict interacts with genetic factors in influencing whether an adolescent becomes depressed (Rice et al., 2006). Thus, while it is tempting to assume that biological or neurochemical processes preceded and caused the depressive episode, the evidence at this time remains correlational and does not permit a firm conclusion to be drawn about the etiological significance of biological factors. It is equally plausible that the observed physiological changes result from a depressive episode, or that a third factor (e.g., interpersonal stress) led to both the physiological changes and the psychological/emotional symptoms.

TREATMENTS FOR DEPRESSION

Perhaps the most widely researched approach for treating depression is *cognitive-behavioral therapy* (Lewinsohn et al., 1990; Reinecke & Curry, 2008). According to this model, depression arises in response to automatic negative or pessimistic thoughts about oneself, others, or the environment. The person is typically unaware of having these automatic thoughts but they nevertheless lead to depressive symptoms. Once the depressive symptoms take hold, the person is not only more likely to give credence to negative or pessimistic beliefs, but also might behave in ways that help to sustain the symptoms. For example, depressed persons might withdraw from others, and so cut themselves off from potential sources of social reinforcement. The procedures of cognitive therapy are designed to help depressed persons become more aware of their automatic thoughts so that they can be reevaluated and replaced by more realistic thoughts.

Recently, cognitive-behavioral therapists have incorporated approaches based on *mindfulness* into their treatment of depression (Segal et al., 2002). In this approach, the depressed person is trained in meditative techniques with the goal of helping him or her de-identify with his or her negative thinking. Rather than struggling with their negative thoughts, depressed persons are encouraged to accept them but not treat them as accurate representations of reality or reliable guides to decision making or action. Although practitioners of mindfulness do not explicitly draw the analogy, the approach seems to be compatible with the view of the self as multifaceted. Via the experience of mindfulness, individuals become aware of a facet of themselves that can observe themselves engaging in depressive thinking and behavior, and in so doing they can reclaim part of themselves from the grip of depression. Thus granted more access to this depression-free facet of themselves, they are able to discover ways to amplify its voice and its influence on their lives.

Although it is less well-known than cognitive therapy, *interpersonal therapy* is another approach that has been demonstrated via empirical studies to be effective in treating adolescent depression (Mufson, Dorta, Moreau, & Weissman, 2004). The focus of interpersonal therapy is on social functioning, problem solving, and training in skills for resolving interpersonal conflicts and reducing social isolation. Interpersonal therapy for adolescents also assesses for and addresses the presence of unresolved grief and difficulties adapting to the social role changes that are associated with adolescent development.

Although medications are frequently used in the treatment of depression, it is important to keep in mind that the use of medications with adolescents has been controversial. While there is a body of evidence supporting the efficacy of psychopharmacology for the treatment of depression in adults, there is considerably less evidence supporting its efficacy for children or adolescents (e.g., Emslie et al., 2006). There have also been reports of increased suicide attempts among adolescents who had been taking certain kinds of antidepressants (Olfson, Marcus, & Shaffer, 2006), although others have argued that these risks have been exaggerated (Brent, 2007; Simon, 2006).

Many clinicians are familiar with the term *empirically supported therapy*. This term pertains to those forms of treatment that have been subjected to empirical research and found to be effective. There is empirical support for the efficacy of both cognitive-behavioral therapy (CBT) and interpersonal therapy for treating adolescent depression. However, it is important to note that a considerable percentage (as many as 40%) of individuals treated with CBT do not improve (Kennard et al., 2006; Klein, Jacobs, & Reinecke, 2007; March et al., 2004). Also, there is concern that the process by which research participants are selected for empirical tests of treatment efficacy results in a sample that is not representative of the kinds of complex cases often seen in clinical practice. For these reasons, it is premature to suspend the search for other methods of treatment that might supplement or substitute for CBT. Given the importance of family dynamics in the evolution and persistence of adolescent depression, consideration of family oriented treatment methods seems warranted, especially since there is empirical support for the effectiveness of family therapy for treating depression in adolescents (Diamond, Reis, Diamond, Siqueland, & Isaacs, 2002).

THE ROLE OF FAMILY DYNAMICS
IN ADOLESCENT DEPRESSION

Empirical studies have documented the role of family dynamics in adolescent depression (Allen et al., 2006; Asseltine, Gore, & Colton, 1994; Brent, Kolko, Allan, & Brown, 1990; Forehand et al., 1991; Rueter, Scaramella, Wallace, & Conger, 1999; Sheeber, Hops, & Davis, 2001; Sheeber & Sorensen, 1998). Depressed adolescents experience less supportive family environments than nondepressed peers (Sheeber & Sorensen, 1998). Moreover, studies of depressed adolescents have demonstrated increases in depression in response to increased family conflict and decreased family support, but not the other way around (Sheeber et al., 1997). In other words, high conflict and low support in families do not appear to arise in response to adolescent depression, but rather they appear to be risk factors for the development of depression.

In an interesting study that examined the interactions among mothers, fathers, and depressed adolescents, Sheeber, Hops, Andrews, Alpert, and Davis (1998) reported that mothers of depressed adolescents were more likely to engage in "facilitative" behaviors (e.g., approving or affirming statements) in response to depressive behavior on the part of the adolescent. In contrast, fathers were likely to decrease "aggressive" behaviors (e.g., disapproval, irritability) in response to adolescent depressive behavior. This intriguing finding lends support to the idea that adolescent depression might serve the homeostatic function of helping to regulate the behaviors of the parents; that is, increasing caretaking on the part of the mother and decreasing aggression on the part of the father. These parental behaviors, in turn, positively and negatively reinforce the adolescent's depressive behaviors and thus maintain a self-perpetuating cycle.

There is also evidence that positive parent–child relationships can buffer the youth from the harmful effects of other family stressors (Forehand et al., 1991). Cole and McPherson (1993) reported that the effect of marital conflict on adolescent depression was mediated by the quality of the relationship between the child and parents. Tannenbaum and Forehand (1994) reported that a good father–child relationship buffered the youngster from the negative effects of a mother's depressed mood. Petersen et al. (1991) found that a close relationship with parents moderated the negative effects of stressors during early adolescence and decreased the probability of the youngster becoming depressed later on. Kandel and Davies (1982) found low rates of depression among teenagers who were able to maintain positive relationships with parents and peers. Thus, stronger relationships with parents can help to ameliorate depression in adolescents.

COMMON FAMILY PATTERNS ASSOCIATED WITH ADOLESCENT DEPRESSION

Disengagement/Abandonment

For any number of reasons, adolescents might experience abandonment or loss of support from their parents. The parents might be preoccupied with other stressors, such as a new job, aging parents, financial strains, illness, or marital disruption, and thus be less available to provide the support the adolescent needs to negotiate the developmental transitions of this period of life. Grief associated with the loss of parental support can precipitate depression, which in turn can compromise the adolescent's ability to function. Left to cope with the demands of his or her life with diminished parental support, the adolescent might become overwhelmed and experience a sense of helplessness and hopelessness. Consider the following case.

Connie had lost everything that was important to her, but her parents, Tom and Ellen, didn't seem to realize it. They had just moved to Philadelphia from a small city in the Midwest because Tom had been offered a promotion. Connie didn't want to move and on the day of the move had to be dragged, sobbing, by both of her parents onto the plane. They were living in a rented apartment while they were waiting for their new house to be finished. Connie spent most of her time in her room, refusing to talk with her parents except to rebuff them angrily when they attempted to engage her. She had begun attending school, but the counselor had already contacted Ellen because Connie seemed so withdrawn and unhappy. The final straw came when Tom and Ellen told Connie that after 15 years of being an only child, she was going to have a little brother or sister. Upon hearing the news, Connie ran out of the apartment. Three hours later, Tom found her sobbing and wandering aimlessly in an unsavory part of the city.

After a few sessions with the family, I was able to piece together a hypothesis. For one thing, Connie's difficulty with the move helped to distract her parents from their own grief about leaving their friends and family behind. But another dynamic was also operating. Prior to the move, Tom had been despondent about his career prospects. He worked long hours and interacted little with Connie or his wife. As might be expected, Connie and her mother had developed a close bond that typically excluded Tom, who hardly seemed to notice anyway. When Tom got news of his promotion, his mood brightened and, much to Ellen's delight, he became fun to be with again. Meanwhile, Connie was so morose over the move that she had become unpleasant company for her mother.

Neither Tom nor Ellen knew what to do to help Connie. Eventually, they concluded that she'd "get over it" once she became accustomed to the new surroundings, and they decided that the best thing to do was to leave Connie alone. They had long ago given up hope of having another child, and when Ellen learned she was pregnant, she and Tom were thrilled. The news fueled the exhilaration they were feeling toward one another. For Connie, however, it was just one more loss—her home, her friends, her special bond with her mother, and now her status as an only child. She had lost everything that mattered to her, while her parents, caught up in the excitement of a new city, new house, and new baby, hardly seemed to notice.

In cases such as this, some therapists might attribute the adolescent's depression directly to the stress or transition affecting the family. For example, Connie's depression might be interpreted as a grief reaction to the losses associated with the move. Therapists who view the problem in this way might decide to work individually with Connie to help her grieve her losses. However, it is important to recognize that Connie is also grieving the loss of her relationship with her parents, who have been less available to her because they have been distracted by the changes in their own lives. In this view, the impact on the adolescent of the external stressor (e.g., the family's relocation) is mediated by the strength of the parent–child relationship and the ability of the parents to help the child adjust to the stressors. Adolescents who have strong and secure relationships with their parents are more resilient to the effects of external stressors. Thus, rather than encouraging adolescents in this situation to rely on the therapist for support, it is preferable to use the therapy sessions to help the parents to be more available and supportive to the youngster.

It is also important to note that the effect of the adolescent's depression on the parent–child relationship is bidirectional. James Coyne (1976, 1999) has suggested that individuals in close relationships with depressed persons might at first provide increased support, but then begin to avoid the depressed person because they find his or her mood aversive. Deprived of social support, the depressed person's symptoms intensify, thus perpetuating the cycle. In families, the child's depression might elicit rejecting or abandoning behaviors on the part of the parents, which in turn intensifies the child's depression (Robertson & Simons, 1989; Sheeber et al., 1997). Thus, it is important to consider the possibility that parental disengagement might have intensified following the onset of the adolescent's depression, as a result of the parents' feeling discouraged and defeated in their efforts to help alleviate the depression. In these cases, it is important to empathize with the parents' feelings, not blame them for neglecting the youngster, and help them feel more successful in their efforts to help their child.

Overprotectiveness

The natural response to a suffering person is to try to help him or her by alleviating his or her burdens. It is therefore not surprising that some parents go into overdrive to support their depressed adolescent child. Moved by their child's pain, the parents show their care and concern by relieving the child of responsibilities and providing verbal and physical reminders of how much the child is loved. In moderation, responses such as these are appropriate ways to reassure the child that the parents are available and willing to help. Unfortunately, some parents provide too much of a good thing. They are so eager to help the child that the child becomes more and more dependent on them, which, of course, elicits more parental support. As the parents offer more help, the child becomes more helpless, which elicits more help from the parents in a self-perpetuating cycle (cf. Sheeber et al., 1998). The pattern of protectiveness will often be evident in the interactions among the family members in the room. Parents might answer questions for the child and speak as if they know what the child is thinking and feeling. The following example illustrates this pattern.

No one would doubt that Shana was suffering. She shuffled into the room without responding to my greeting, then slumped into a chair with her hair covering her eyes. Her parents, Brenda and Walter, occupied the seats on either side of her. They each put an arm around Shana's shoulders, gazed at her with worried expressions on their faces, and barely acknowledged my presence in the room.

I began the session by addressing Shana: "You look very sad, Shana. You've probably come to me for help, right?" Brenda jumped in with the response: "She's been like this for the past 3 weeks, and even before that she wasn't herself. She just wants to get back to her old self."

I noticed not only that Brenda immediately interceded between me and Shana, but also that she responded in a way that suggested that she was intimately in touch with her daughter's internal state. However, in the interest of joining with the family, I chose not to address this pattern just yet. I acknowledged Brenda's comment with a benevolent smile and a nod, and then addressed Shana again: "Sounds like you've been having a rough time. Can you tell me in your own words how it's been for you the past few weeks?"

This time Walter jumped in: "We've been trying to help, but she seems to be getting worse. Now she spends the whole day in her room and will hardly talk."

Although Walter's response demonstrated the overprotective pattern once again, I heard in his statement an opportunity to address the pattern. I replied, "I know I just asked you a question, Shana, but I'll come back to you in a minute. Walter, that's an interesting observation you just made." Walter looked at me quizzically and I went on: "You and Brenda have been trying to help, but Shana seems to be getting worse."

"That's right," Walter replied, "we've done everything we can think of for her, but it doesn't seem to help. In fact, I think she's worse now than when we first found out that she was depressed."

I noticed Brenda nodding, so I seized this opportunity to engage the parents directly with one another. "It seems that you both agree that Shana is getting worse even though both of you have been trying everything to help her. Could the two of you talk about this? How do you make sense of this puzzle, that the more you help, the worse she gets?"

Brenda and Walter looked at each other, and then Brenda suggested, "Maybe we aren't doing the right thing." Walter replied, "Or maybe we're doing too much, Bren. I wonder if we're really helping Shana by doing so much for her."

"Maybe you're right," Brenda sighed, "I guess that's why we're here. We need to figure out how to help her better."

This provided me with the opportunity I had been waiting for. However, rather than leading the family in a discussion about how to be most helpful to Shana at home, I decided to start with the interactions in the room.

"And I want to do my best to help," I said. "One of the things I noticed a few minutes ago is that you both quickly answered for Shana when I asked her a question. Did either of you notice that?"

"Now that you point it out, I guess we did do that," Brenda responded.

"What message do you think that might be giving Shana?" I asked.

"I guess it could give her the message that we don't think she can answer on her own," Brenda replied. Walter nodded in agreement.

"OK, then, how about if we start over? Could you be careful not to answer a question unless it is posed to you directly? If I ask you a question, Shana, and you don't know the answer or you don't want to answer, that's OK. If you need time to think, we can wait. OK?" Shana did not respond, so I repeated myself, "Is that OK with you, Shana?" This time she nodded.

The session proceeded slowly, but we had made a first step. The parents and I agreed that we would treat Shana as if she were capable of answering on her own without her parents' help.

In changing patterns based on overprotectiveness, it is best to start with simple interactions that are taking place in the room, as this example illustrates. It is necessary to be creative in finding ways to engage the depressed youngster directly, for example, by asking the youngster to sit in a different seat, allowing the youngster to respond to yes/no questions by nodding or shaking her head, or requesting that she write down her e-mail address, telephone number, or the first name of some of her friends. It is essential to block any attempt by the parents to intercede, even if they appear to be motivated by a desire to be helpful.

The discussions then turn to exploring how the family members are interacting at home. The goal is to break the overprotective patterns and to provide the youngster space to make decisions on her own. The adolescent's refusal to engage in certain activities could be framed as a matter of personal freedom, and the parents' solicitousness thus invoked to protect the youngster's autonomy.

For example, at dinnertime Brenda would invite Shana to the table, but when she did not come, she would bring a plate to her room. Hours later, she would return to Shana's room to find the meal uneaten. I suggested to Brenda that she change this pattern by asking Shana whether she would like her to bring a plate to her room. If Shana did not signal a clear "yes," then Brenda would not bring her food. Meanwhile, I encouraged Brenda to prepare tasty and aromatic meals that she believed Shana would enjoy. If Shana chose not to join them, then the rest of the family would continue to have dinner. They should make sure that they did not spend the time "in mourning" for Shana's absence, but rather avoid talking about her and instead tell funny stories about their day.

It is also important to alert the family to ways in which they might unwittingly reinforce the depressive behavior. For example, the rest of the family would try not to make noise in the house because they did not want to disturb Shana. I discouraged this self-imposed restriction, and instead encouraged them to carry on their daily activities "with gusto," with the rationale that the more they could show that they were enjoying their lives, the more Shana would come to view life as potentially enjoyable.

Sheeber et al. (1998) found that mothers often increased their offers of help and support in response to their adolescent's depressive behaviors. To break this pattern, mothers can be discouraged from offering suggestions or advice. Instead, they can be encouraged to acknowledge the adolescent's distress ("You really seem upset about what happened at school today") and then invite the depressed youngster to engage in a process of brainstorming options together ("Let's take turns thinking about ways you could handle this situation").

In the interactional model of depression proposed by James Coyne (1976, 1999), family members are initially drawn to help the depressed person, but eventually they become frustrated and give up because their efforts to help don't seem to alleviate the depression. Deprived of social support, the depressed person becomes worse. In families who are engaged in a pattern of overprotectiveness, this step does not occur. The parents continue to provide support, thinking that they will eventually alleviate enough of their child's stress so that the child will recover. However, it is reasonable to wonder whether these parents are nevertheless feeling frustrated with the child. They might suppress these feelings of frustration because they think they are unjustified, or because they think they would upset the child if they expressed these feelings. But, by hiding or minimizing these feelings, they give the message that feelings of anger and frustration are destructive and should not be expressed.

To break this pattern, family members can be encouraged to talk more openly about their frustration. The parents can also be urged to invite the depressed child to express feelings of frustration or anger directed at them. For example, the parents might observe, "There must be a good reason why you feel as bad as you do, and we wonder whether there are things that we have done or not done that have disappointed you or made you angry. Please tell us about these things." The parents are then encouraged to focus on and amplify the feelings of anger without becoming defensive or attempting to offer justification for them.

Depression and Homeostasis

In some families, a more complicated pattern emerges whereby the adolescent's depression helps to distract the family from acknowledging issues or conflicts that threaten to disrupt their stability. By focusing efforts on helping the depressed youngster, the parents might be able to avoid dealing with other issues, such as marital conflict or another family member's inadequate functioning. Sometimes, the parents might act in ways to reinforce the depression because they are anxious about other aspects of the adolescent transition, fearful of the consequences of increased freedom or autonomy, or reluctant to "let go" of the child.

The case of Tony illustrates how an adolescent's depressive behavior helped to keep other family conflicts from surfacing. I had warned Tony's parents that after he recovered from his depression, they might wish he hadn't. They dismissed this with a laugh. "Don't worry, we can handle it. Just get us our son back."

The family had certainly weathered its share of crises over the years. Tony's older brother, Al, had been severely injured in a motorcycle accident and was confined to a wheelchair. He had recently left home to live in a supervised apartment and seemed to be doing well. Twelve years earlier, Tony's parents, Paul and Lena, lost their infant son to crib death. They still commemorated his birthday and Lena still got teary-eyed when the baby's name was mentioned. Their youngest child, now 10, was identified by the family as "learning disabled and having attention-deficit/hyperactivity disorder." The family was in constant financial crisis. Paul ran a small business at home and Lena worked as a recreational aide in a nursing home. Tony had always done well in school and was a star basketball player—until he injured his knee in a game. He had a good relationship with both of his siblings and seemed devoted to his family. The problem was that he had stopped going to school. He sat in his room with the lights dimmed, shuffling around the house, not eating, and refusing to talk.

It seemed almost too obvious to wonder if Tony was mourning his brother Al, but I decided to explore this possibility anyway. Tony acknowledged that he missed his brother but also pointed out that he was relieved that Al was no longer living at home, because he was getting tired of helping to take care of him. If anything, Tony said, he was happy that his brother had finally moved out. The rest of the family echoed these sentiments. I decided I'd have to search elsewhere for a hypothesis. Did Al's leaving home reawaken for the parents the grief they felt when they lost their infant son? Was Tony "helping" them by providing them with a distraction for their grief?

Pursuing this direction was a bit more fruitful. Tony challenged Lena on not having "let go" of the baby. He expressed his frustration at his parents for not putting this tragedy behind them. Tony's mood seemed to brighten a bit when he expressed his anger at his parents. Yet, I didn't really believe that talking about this topic was particularly new for this family. If anything, they had the same kind of conversation every year on the deceased baby's birthday.

What I noticed, however, was the process that emerged when Tony began to verbalize his feelings. Tony first criticized his mother for crying every time the baby was mentioned. Lena wept helplessly and Paul reprimanded Tony for hurting his mother's feelings. Tony then lampooned his father, challenging him for "letting" his mother carry on the way she did. This activated Lena, who then angrily began defending herself to Tony. Eventually, Tony gave up, hinting that "Maybe you'd be better off without me." As Tony retreated back into his shell, both parents then rushed to reassure Tony that they loved him and would never want to lose him.

The third time I saw this sequence enacted, it finally hit me. I asked Lena to restrain herself from intervening while Tony confronted his father. Although I had to remind her several times, she eventually got the message. Tony challenged his father, first about his passivity and eventually about the condition of the home, which was in serious disrepair because of years of neglect.

"What kind of man are you anyway?" Tony screamed at his father as Paul sat speechless and tearful.

Trying to activate Paul, I said provocatively, "Are you going to let your son talk to you that way without answering?"

Lena started to intervene, but she restrained herself after I gestured to her to keep silent. With tears in his eyes, Paul looked at me. "What is there to say? He's right. He's right. What kind of man am I?" Paul sobbed.

Lena spoke up, now angry at me, "This is what we've always been afraid could happen. What are we going to do if Pauly can't work? How are we going to live?"

Unrelenting, Tony now challenged his mother: "That's what you always do. You're always protecting him. You let him get away with everything. No one is ever supposed to upset Dad. Dad is too sensitive. Bull! If I've got to pull myself together to get to school, feeling the way I do, then he can pull himself together and start acting like a father."

Paul came to life. "OK, Mr. Know-it-all. You want me to be a father, I'll be a father. Tomorrow you're going to school if I have to drag you out of bed and drop you off there in your underwear."

I wasn't really surprised when Tony only halfheartedly rebuffed his father's threat. The next day, Tony went to school. Soon, he began to go out with his friends and push all of his parents' limits. He seemed to be functioning again, but there were many more tears and confrontations in family sessions, as Tony unleashed torrents of resentment that he had been storing up, unexpressed, for years.

As long as Tony was depressed, then the other conflicts in the family could be kept at bay. The parents did not have to deal with their grief over their other son's injury. Lena's fear over Paul's fragility could be averted by her concern for her son. Although Tony's depression kept his anger at his parents from surfacing, it also immobilized him and prevented the conflicts that provoked the anger from being addressed and resolved. Not unexpectedly, the family had to deal with the torrent of his feelings when he began to function more competently. However, by dealing openly and directly with these feelings the family could address the causes of the resentment and begin rebuilding their relationships with one another.

HELPING SUICIDAL ADOLESCENTS

Not all depressed adolescents attempt suicide, but suicide is strongly linked to depression. In one large national sample of over 4,000 adolescents, those who had experienced depression were 44 times more likely to have experienced suicidal ideation and 6.6 times more likely to have made a suicide attempt compared to those who had never experienced depression (Waldrop et al., 2007). The same study found that suicidal ideation was associated with female gender, family alcohol and drug problems, exposure to violence, and posttraumatic stress disorder.

Suicidal ideation is more common among adolescents than among adults or younger children. Between one-third and one-half of adolescents in community samples report having experienced suicidal ideation, and between 6% and 13% of adolescents report that they have attempted suicide at least once in their lives (Dubow, Kausch, Blum, Reed, & Bush, 1989; Garland & Zigler, 1993; Lewinsohn et al., 1996). Suicide is the third leading cause of death among 15- to 24-year-olds, and the suicide rate has increased more dramatically among adolescents than in the population at large (Garland & Zigler, 1993; Lewinsohn et al., 1996). Contrary to what many adults believe, the vast majority of adolescent suicide attempts are premeditated and are not impulsive reactions to frustration (Lewinsohn et al., 1996).

Family conflict, discord, and rigidity have been linked to adolescent suicide attempts (Brent et al., 1998; Carris, Sheeber, & Howe, 1998; DeWilde, Kienhorst, Diekstra, & Wolters, 1993; Hollis, 1996). Joseph Richman (1979) pointed to disturbances in the family structure, including role conflicts, blurring of boundaries, coalitions, and secretiveness as contributing factors to adolescent suicide. Susan Harter (1990) proposed that suicide might result if an adolescent feels that he or she has disappointed parents whose support is conditional on meeting their high expectations. Krieder and Motto (1974) noted the association between adolescent suicide and "parent–child role reversal," whereby the adolescent is placed in the position of assuming a caretaking role for a helpless or dependent parent. Charles Fishman (1988) described the suicidal adolescent as "a stranger in paradox," torn between "contradictory directives [that] emanate from a split between the parental figures" (p. 161). Fishman also described the families of suicidal adolescents as "prematurely disengaged," in that the family has misjudged the emotional age of the youngster and has withdrawn the support that the adolescent needs. Cynthia Pfeffer (1981) noted that conflicts between parents might be displaced onto the child, who might feel that he or she is not doing enough to prevent the parents' unhappiness. Parents might even communicate that the child is a burden to the family and the family would be better off without him or her. A suicide threat might be the child's desperate attempt to call attention to a problem that the rest of the family has been ignoring.

The most common motives for attempting suicide are to die, escape, or obtain relief (Boergers, Spirito, & Donaldson, 1998). Suicide is a response to hopelessness, that is, the experience that there is no other way out from a situation that is unbearable. Suicidal adolescents feel profoundly alone, and often believe that others would be better off if they were dead. Unwilling or unable to turn to others for support, self-destruction becomes the remaining available option.

When treating suicidal adolescents, the key question is *Why?* The answer to this question must be sought in the relationships in the adolescent's life: *Why did the youngster feel that he or she had no other option but to attempt suicide? Why could he or she not go to the parents for support?* By exploring these questions, rifts in the family relationships can be uncovered and wounds can be exposed, thus permitting an opportunity to promote repair and healing. The following sections provide a recommended strategy for working with suicidal adolescents and also discuss some of the common pitfalls that might be encountered.

Ensuring Safety

When an adolescent is potentially suicidal, protection takes precedence over all other goals. Measures must be taken to prevent the youngster from acting on self-destructive impulses. This does not mean, however, that treatment is delayed. To the contrary, it is possible to use the crisis around the prospect of suicide as a way of beginning the process of change in the family.

One way to provide a protective environment for the suicidal child is to organize a family "suicide watch." This means that the family, under the supervision of the parents, arranges for the adolescent to be personally supervised by a responsible party 24 hours per day until the youngster is no longer suicidal. The institution of a suicide watch can be a powerful message to the child that the parents can and will take care of him or her. At the same time, effective implementation of the watch will require the parents to work together collaboratively to make sure that they don't "burn out" before the crisis is over. The therapist must be willing to hold additional sessions and must be available by telephone to coach the family as needed.

Sometimes, a therapist feels that a family might not be capable of conducting a suicide watch. Perhaps the parents cannot be relied upon to provide effective supervision because of problems of their own (e.g., severe depression, drug abuse). Perhaps the parents are underreacting to the adolescent's suicidality or do not believe that the youngster is "really" suicidal.

Even if the family is not capable of carrying out a responsible suicide watch, it is important to take steps to keep the family as centrally involved as possible. Reinforcements should be recruited first from the extended family or neighborhood. In some communities, specially trained crisis teams can be sent into the home to help the parents supervise the suicidal youth. The key principle is to arrange support that keeps the parents involved and does not supplant the parents as the primary caregivers for the child.

Sometimes hospitalization is necessary and, despite its drawbacks, might be the only alternative. If the therapist has a relationship with a psychiatrist with admitting and attending privileges who supports the therapist's treatment goals, it might be possible for the therapist to arrange to work collaboratively with the hospital staff and keep the parents centrally involved. If the therapist does not have this kind of relationship with the attending physician or hospital staff, the therapist can continue to meet with the parents during the hospitalization as a way of keeping them directly involved in planning how the family will reorganize in preparation for the adolescent's discharge.

Removing the Obstacles to Dialogue

Following a suicide attempt some adolescents deny an intent to die or claim that they no longer wish to die. This might occur because the suicide attempt has had the effect of eliciting a desired response from the parents—either the parents have demonstrated concern for the child or parents have rallied in response to the crisis and no longer appear so distressed by their own problems. At other times, the adolescent feels enormous shame following a suicide attempt. In still other cases, the suicide attempt did not have the intended effect on the family: Rather than rallying to support the child, the family angrily rejects and criticizes the youngster. In yet other cases, the rigidity of the family structure is such that the factors that precipitated the suicide attempt cannot be discussed. To continue to appear suicidal runs the risk of being ostracized from the family because of the danger of calling attention to these "forbidden" topics.

The following procedure, adapted from one originally proposed by John Sargent (1987b), is a recommended template for promoting dialogue in families with suicidal adolescents:

- *Step 1.* The therapist connects with the parents by acknowledging their concern for the child, emphasizing the parents' strengths and the positive aspects of their relationship with the child.

- *Step 2.* Using the relationship with the parents as the springboard, the therapist encourages the parents to take a hierarchical position by telling the adolescent that suicide is forbidden. The parents must make it clear that they value the relationship with the child above all else, so suicide is forbidden precisely because it is a decisive threat to this relationship. The parents should be discouraged from communicating that they forbid suicide because it harms the parents or shames the adolescent. The parents must emphasize that preserving the relationship with the child is their top priority.

- *Step 3.* The parents then express in a calm, caring manner a desire to understand why the adolescent attempted suicide. The parents communicate to the child that they acknowledge that the child must have been experiencing tremendous pain and felt that suicide was the only option at the time. The parents express regret that the adolescent chose not to come to them for help and ask the child to explain the reasons why he or she felt that he or she could not come to them. The entry to this topic is through the questions "Why did you choose to hurt yourself rather than come to us for help? Why did you not come to us first?" It is important that the parents communicate this message in a way that does not accuse or blame the adolescent, but rather recognizes that the child turned to suicide as a last resort. The parents must reassure the child by saying, "Nothing you could tell us could be so bad that killing yourself is the only answer. Tell us what led you to this point so that we can help you. Our relationship is strong enough to handle it." In this way, the parents remove the adolescent from the "Tell me/Don't tell me" bind.

- *Step 4.* After the parents have communicated their sincere desire to listen, then they must give the child a chance to explain why he or she tried to commit suicide. The reasons must go beyond external factors, such as rejection by peers, pressures to perform at school, or grief over the loss of a relationship. The focus of the conversation must be on *the child's relationship with the parents*. While external factors might have played a role, the emphasis should not be placed on these factors. Rather, the conversation should focus on the reasons why the child felt that he or she could not utilize the parents as a resource to help deal with these stressors, but instead sank into hopelessness that culminated in a suicide attempt. The emphasis should be placed not on the external stressors that presumably caused the suicide attempt, bur rather on the child's fear that the parents would not or could not be available to help him or her cope with these stressors. The parents must probe for the reasons why the child did not feel that he or she could come to them, and they must invite the child to tell them what they did (or did not do) that discouraged him or her from doing so.

It is important for this step to follow and not precede Step 3. After Step 3 has taken place, the adolescent's disclosure occurs in a context where the parents have already expressed a desire to listen, have acknowledged failures to listen in the past (deliberate or not), and have reassured the child that they are ready to listen now.

Once the adolescent begins the disclosure to the parent, the therapist must see to it that the parents listen. The adolescent must do most of the talking at this stage. The therapist should intervene as little as possible to facilitate the dialogue and to discourage the parents from responding too quickly.

Many parents are quick to defend themselves when they feel criticized by their child. This defense can lead to pointless bickering or to the adolescent shutting down. At other times, parents are too quick to offer reassurance or comfort, thus communicating the message that they have heard enough and can't handle hearing any more. The parents must be helped to listen nondefensively, to restrain themselves from offering comfort prematurely, and to apologize if they cut off the dialogue with self-defense.

• *Step 5*. After the adolescent has explained why he or she attempted suicide, the parents must make it clear that they have heard what the youngster has said. Parents who react by saying, "I've heard this before," might confirm the child's hopelessness about the relationship. The parents should be encouraged to respond in a way that indicates that they have heard something they had not heard before, or have heard it in a new way, or have gained greater awareness of what the child needs from them. The parents must make it clear that what the adolescent has disclosed to them is important and will be taken seriously. The therapist should encourage the parents and adolescent to identify a specific, concrete way in which the youngster's concern could be addressed. A behavioral change on the part of the parents communicates clearly that they are committed to improving the relationship with the child.

I want to emphasize this point: It is important that the therapist go beyond eliciting verbal reassurance of support from the parents. *It is essential that the parents find specific and concrete ways of demonstrating that they are willing and able to take care of the adolescent.* The therapist should encourage the child and the parents to identify specific behaviors that would demonstrate that the parents are seriously committed to helping the youngster.

• *Step 6.* After the rifts in the relationship have been uncovered and addressed, after the parents have acknowledged their contributions to these rifts, and after the parents have agreed to take concrete steps to repair the relationship, then the parents should ask the child for a commitment not to attempt suicide again. The child must explicitly agree to come to the parents if suicidal feelings were to return, and to give them an opportunity to help him or her deal with these feelings. The parents must again reassure the youngster that their relationship is strong enough to sustain anything that the child might disclose.

Remove the Child from the Parentified Role

Along with helping the parents to provide support for the child, the therapist must also encourage the parents to take care of their own needs. The adolescent will notice if the parents are not taking care of themselves. The parents must acknowledge the adolescent's concern for them and demonstrate that they are taking concrete steps to take care of themselves.

Parents who try to pretend that they are "OK" will only make the problem worse. The adolescent will recognize that the parent is indeed "not OK," and the parent's dishonesty will contribute to the atmosphere of mistrust in the family. In an effort to protect the child from worrying about them, parents might try to hide their own distress. In fact, the child might become even more vigilant if the parents are not honest about how they feel. The message that is most likely to foster the adolescent's growth is:

> "I'm not feeling very good right now, but I recognize that. I plan to do something to help myself, and there's no reason for you to worry or to feel that you have to take care of me. If you think that I'm not taking good enough care of myself, please tell me as soon as you notice it. But you aren't responsible for taking care of me."

In some cases, either because the adolescent is particularly empathic toward the parent or because the parent is in severe need, it is advisable to identify specific ways in which the child can help the parent (similar to an approach recommended by Madanes, 1984, p. 163ff.). For example, the adolescent could assume specific and delimited responsibilities in the home, or commit to spending time with the parent each week. This suggestion does not contradict the idea that the adolescent must be removed from the parentified role. Rather, it facilitates the strengthening of trust in the family because it recognizes that the child indeed has something of value to give to the parent. By identifying a specific way in which the adolescent can help the parent, the child can derive self-esteem from having given something valuable to the parent while being relieved of full responsibility for the parent's welfare.

Pitfalls and Complications

Therapist Gets Angry at the Parent

When an adolescent attempts suicide, the sympathies of most therapists are with the youngster. Parental flaws emerge in sharp relief, and even the best of therapists are tempted to see the parents as villains and the child as victim. This reaction is even more likely if the parents indeed have done something to betray the relationship with the adolescent and fail to acknowledge this betrayal. The child might be trying to tell the parents how they have hurt him or her, while the parents simply refuse to own up to it.

Expressing anger at the parents can confirm their belief that they are a noxious influence on their child, and thus lead the parents to distance themselves from the child even more in an effort to protect the youngster from their harmful influence. The therapist's anger at the parents might prompt the adolescent to protect the parents from the therapist. The child simply shuts down again and minimizes the significance of the suicide attempt in order to shield the parents from the therapist's anger.

Communicating uncertainty about the parents' ability to help and protect the child will discourage the child from confiding in them. Adolescents will take the risk of confiding in their parents only if they believe that the parents will listen and not judge them. In order to listen to the child, the parents will need to feel more secure in their relationship with the therapist and feel that the therapist believes in their competence. Anger at the parents hardly contributes to the climate of safety they need. Rather, it is important to reach out to them, empathize with their position, and express confidence in their ability to help the child.

Parent Underreacts to the Suicidality

In some cases, parents minimize the seriousness of a suicide attempt, or claim that they did not believe that the adolescent "really" wanted to die.

Communicating this message can be tantamount to telling the youngster that he or she is not being taken seriously, and that the parents' offer to listen was not sincere.

In these circumstances, it is best to interpret the parents' underreaction as a defense against the anxiety generated by the suicide attempt, as a sign that the loss of the child is too painful for them even to contemplate. By acknowledging the parents' love for the child, the therapist can provide enough of a "holding environment" (Winnicott, 1965) to allow the parents to tolerate the idea that their child might actually have succeeded in killing him- or herself.

To generate intensity, the therapist might lead the family through a guided fantasy of imagining the child's funeral, seeing the child in the coffin, hearing the eulogy, then leaving the cemetery (similar to the technique "Contaminating the Suicidal Fantasy" described in Sherman and Fredman, 1986, p. 207ff.). The narrative is drawn out in great detail so that the parents can actually imagine details of the situation and how they would feel. This fantasy will often elicit from the parents an outpouring of emotion and show the child how much they really care.

This exercise is most useful when the therapist suspects that mixed in with their love for the child are unconscious desires to be rid of him or her. By emphasizing one side of the ambivalence, the parents' defenses against their hostility are activated and the tender feelings might come to the fore, allowing the therapist to connect with this loving aspect of the parents and bring it into the relationship with the child.

Parent Expresses Anger

Sometimes, parents will express anger at the adolescent for having made a suicide attempt. Often, their anger reflects their terror and helplessness, but children might interpret the parents' reaction as confirmation that they don't care about them.

The therapist should reframe the parents' anger as an expression of their concern rather than rejection of the child. It is necessary to block the dialogue between the parents and the child temporarily, and instead speak directly to the parents. The parents should be encouraged to verbalize their feelings about the suicide attempt while the therapist listens nonjudgmentally. The child can be asked to leave the room if necessary, but adolescents often benefit from watching the therapist express concern for the parents, since it removes the child from that position.

The parents' concern for the child should be emphasized, even if the primary way this concern is being expressed is through anger. In many cases, the parents are angry at the adolescent because of things the youngster had done long before the suicide attempt. In these cases, it is important to acknowledge the validity of the parents' anger while at the same time explore with the family how the situation got so bad that the child resorted to a suicide attempt.

Sometimes, the parents are angry because the suicide attempt added one more burden onto an oppressive load of responsibilities. In these cases, the parents' anger is appropriate but it is misdirected at the adolescent. For example, when a single mother expresses anger at a child for attempting suicide, the anger is more appropriately directed toward the child's absent father, who has victimized both the mother and the youngster by his absence. In these cases, it is important to acknowledge how overwhelmed the parent feels, but also help him or her to recognize that other factors besides the adolescent's behavior have contributed to him or her feeling overwhelmed.

Parents in these situations might be envious of the attention that the adolescent is receiving as a result of the suicide attempt. The parents might express their envy by declaring that the suicide attempt was merely a way of "getting attention." Rather than challenging this perception head on, it is better to invite the parents to consider why the child might have felt that such an extreme way of getting attention was necessary. Often, what the parents are really saying is that they themselves want more attention. The therapist needs to be the one to provide this attention, so that the child is not placed in the position of competing with the parents or denying his or her own needs to make room for the parents' needs.

Adolescent Refuses to Talk

In some cases, despite genuine efforts on the part of the parents to listen, the child refuses to disclose the reasons for the suicide attempt. The appropriate response to this impasse depends on the dynamics that the therapist observes.

Sometimes, the parents ask the child halfheartedly what led to the suicide attempt. The adolescent senses the parents' lack of conviction and accurately identifies this as a "Tell me/Don't tell me" bind. The parents are communicating to the adolescent that they are not confident that they can help him or her. The youngster picks up this message, and so remains silent, feeling even more acutely abandoned as a result.

In these cases, it is beneficial to ask the child if he or she is worried that the parents might not understand or might become upset. It is important to acknowledge that the adolescent might have had valid reasons for coming to this conclusion in the past, but also point out that now the parents seem ready and able to provide the needed support. Therapists should communicate unequivocally their own belief in the parents' competence, and then explore how the parents could convince the adolescent that they are stronger now and ready to hear what the child has to say to them.

If the parents appear to be showing genuine concern but the adolescent is still not opening up, then a modification of this approach is appropriate. Perhaps the child is attempting to keep the parents engaged, and silence is the only way to do so. The adolescent might have had earlier experiences of being abandoned by the parents once a crisis had passed.

The therapist might offer support to the parents by trying to engage the adolescent directly. It is important to do so in a way that does not upstage the parents. Therapists might first ask the parents for permission to intercede, and always refer to "we" when talking about themselves to the adolescent, indicating that the therapist and the parents are part of the same team.

If the child still refuses to talk in the parents' presence, the therapist might suggest a private meeting with the youngster, but in this case the goal must be to reintroduce the parents to the conversation as soon as possible. Another approach might be for the therapist to begin the dialogue by talking for the youngster, perhaps relating reasons "other kids" have given for attempting suicide. The therapist could adopt a strategy of passive refusal, for example, saying to the adolescent, "I'm interpreting your silence as a sign that I'm right," or "Speak up and stop me if I say something that isn't true." Needless to say, persistent silence on the part of the child indicates that the suicidal risk has not abated and the protective measures should continue.

Adolescent Minimizes the Problem

As a variation of the aforementioned complication, the adolescent talks but minimizes the problem that led to the suicide attempt. The youngster professes that he or she "doesn't know" why he or she did it, or mentions a seemingly trivial disappointment as the cause and declares, "I don't feel like killing myself anymore," without a clear reason why the feelings have changed so abruptly.

One reason this might occur is that adolescents often lack the vocabulary to express the intensity of despair they were feeling at the time. Perhaps the child felt ignored in the past unless the issue raised was of a magnitude deemed significant by the parents. Now the adolescent might be "testing the waters" by raising a seemingly trivial issue. The therapist might explore with the youngster what this seemingly trivial issue represented, and then expand the focus of concern to a more general issue.

If the therapist suspects that the adolescent is minimizing the problem because he or she does not believe that the parents could handle the "real" problem, the therapist could suggest that the adolescent "test" the parents by bringing up something that he or she thinks might upset the parents but that "might not" be true, simply to see if the parents could handle it. Alternatively, the therapist could ask the parents to close their eyes and imagine the worst thing their child could tell them. The therapist should linger on this moment and request that the parents imagine this disclosure in vivid detail, and then imagine that they have successfully responded in a way that demonstrated their commitment to supporting their child. The next step is very important. After the parents have indicated that they have successfully imagined the "worst possible thing" their child might tell them, the therapist should say:

> "There is a saying that no matter how bad things are, they could always be worse. Now I'd like you to imagine that your child is telling you something that is even worse than what you imagined the first time, [pause] and now I'd like you to imagine that you are handling it."

The results can be quite dramatic. In one case, a girl who had insisted that there was "nothing wrong" burst into tears and threw herself into her father's arms after watching her father struggle through this exercise. She then proceeded to tell her religiously conservative father that she had been sexually active with her boyfriend and was convinced that she was pregnant.

Let's now return to the case introduced at the beginning of this chapter. This case illustrates many of the principles I have just reviewed. Noteworthy are the ways in which gender issues manifested in this family and how I utilized my relationship with each parent to create a more secure holding environment for the adolescent girl.

CASE EXAMPLE: THE CRYING FATHER

In the first session with Jenny and her parents, I observed a familiar interchange. Clare turned toward Jenny and asked, "Don't you want to know about yourself? Don't you want to find out what's making you so depressed?"

Jenny, not surprisingly, answered in the negative: Perhaps the knowledge was too frightening or dangerous to her or to her family, so she elected to remain blind to a part of herself, even if this part of her had to be silenced through suicide.

Clare pressed on: "Don't you like yourself?"

"No, I don't," Jenny replied.

"Why not? So many other people like you," Clare pleaded.

Though Clare was clearly attempting to express support by pointing out to Jenny that she is indeed likable, she was also giving Jenny the message that one's evaluation of oneself comes from outside, not inside, and that one is really not competent to assess oneself. Also embedded in her statement is the "Tell me/Don't tell me" bind—after asking Jenny why she doesn't like herself, Clare doesn't wait for a reply. Rather, she reassures Jenny that other people like her, thus implying that she has no good reason not to like herself, and that the basis for judging oneself is pleasing other people. Meanwhile, Peter sits on the sidelines, commenting briefly but offering little—the familiar pattern of the seemingly overinvolved mother and peripheral father.

Later in the session, Clare remarked to me, "I think Jenny and I are too close." Neither Peter nor Jenny challenged this idea. When I asked Peter what he thought, he answered, "Well, maybe Clare is right. Maybe Jenny is just trying to tell us that she isn't a little girl any more and she doesn't want to be around us all the time."

I asked Jenny for her opinion. "I don't know," she replied. "I just can't talk to my parents."

I asked her why she felt she could not talk with them, and she answered, "I guess I'm afraid of hurting them."

Clare, struggling to understand, asked incredulously, "So, you're hurting yourself so that you don't have to hurt us?"

This interchange suggests that Clare has bought into the belief that she is hurting her daughter by being too close to her. Attempting to give Jenny the space that she thinks she needs, Clare backs off, but this only intensifies the abandonment the girl is already experiencing. Meanwhile, Jenny and Peter both imply agreement by not challenging Clare's statement. Peter, already peripheral, offers the interpretation that it is Jenny who wants more "space" because she doesn't seem to want to be around them. Presumably, he is referring to "space" from Clare, since he and Jenny apparently don't have much of a relationship.

Jenny offers a different perspective: She points out that the problem is not "too much" relationship, but the absence of one: "I can't talk to my parents." In this respect, Jenny is similar to most adolescent girls, who want to stay close to their parents even as they become more independent and individuated (Kaplan, Klein, & Gleason, 1991).

Interestingly, though, Jenny does not blame her parents for the absence of dialogue between them. Rather, she blames herself—she is afraid of hurting them. Silence is her only option, because to speak what is on her mind risks hurting her parents, and ultimately herself, because the relationship between them will suffer. Young women often find themselves in this bind. They must suppress their feelings and their own voices rather than the baggy sweat suits she used to wear to our early sessions. Rose appeared more confident and began to display an engaging sense of humor. Although Bill attended sessions infrequently, he maintained regular contact with Rose and Tina.

Rather than dismissing conflicts, as they had in the past, the family members persisted until they arrived at more satisfying solutions. For example, during a session with Tina and Rose, Tina burst into tears as she related an incident in which her father yelled at her over the telephone after she told him that she was reconsidering her decision to attend college. As Rose listened, I noted that she restrained herself from protectively soothing Tina or taking this opportunity to attack Bill. Instead, Rose willingly responded to my suggestion that, after listening to Tina's hurt and angry feelings, she encourage Tina to phone Bill to discuss the incident directly with him. A week later, Bill accompanied Rose and Tina to a session and expressed his surprise at Tina's "mature" response to their argument. Tina had phoned Bill, told him she didn't like it when he shouted at her, and asked him to meet her over the weekend so they could discuss her college plans more calmly.

The key at this stage of treatment is for therapists to calibrate carefully their degree of involvement in the family discussions. By now, the family members have developed their abilities to resolve conflicts on their own, and the therapist should remain peripheral, entering only to give the family members a gentle nudge in the right direction. It is important not to overreact to emotional upset in the family and jump in too quickly to soothe hurt feelings or minimize conflicts. Doing so can stunt the family's capacity for growth by distracting them from the conflicts that have been unaddressed or avoided in the past.

I continued to meet weekly with Tina and Rose. Tina visited her father, stepmother, and stepbrother every other weekend. Bill attended family sessions about once a month. He seemed content with his relationship with Tina and Rose, and they seemed satisfied with their relationship with him. Tina continued to gain weight, and finally stabilized at a weight that was well within the normal range for her age and build.

In one of our early sessions, Tina had asked me when she would know that she was "over anorexia." I had responded, "When you have your period. That will mean that you are finally ready to face young adulthood." One day, 6 months after our first session, Tina proudly announced that she had her first period in almost 2 years. Recalling our earlier conversation, Tina declared that she was "not an anorectic anymore" and was ready to face the challenges of "being grown up." Tina and Rose agreed with my suggestion that the focus of our sessions shift to helping them recognize and negotiate the pitfalls associated with young adulthood.

PETER: So, what are we going to do?

Peter has little to offer; he expects Clare to have the answers. But when Clare does propose a solution, Peter criticizes it. Finally, Clare admits, "I don't have the answers." But she doesn't challenge the idea that she *should* have the answers, or that Peter is not offering any himself, or that he should take responsibility to get to know Jenny on his own rather than using Clare as an intermediary. As Betty Carter (1988) has pointed out, "Finding direct involvement with his daughter frustrating and upsetting, father turns the job over to mother and then complains about the way she does it" (p. 113).

The pattern was more complicated, as I later learned. Peter's job took him away from home on extended trips several times a year. During his absences, Clare functioned essentially as a single parent. When Peter returned, Clare would step aside to give him an opportunity to be a parent, which reinforced the idea that it was Peter who was really in charge ("Wait until Dad comes home"). Rather than parenting as a team, Peter and Clare took turns acting as single parents. While this might not have been Clare's intention (perhaps she was simply trying to take a break from full-time parenting), the pattern spoke for itself. From Jenny's perspective, it meant that her relationship with each parent was mediated by the other parent: Her closeness with her mother depended on father's physical presence or absence; her relationship with her father existed only when mother stepped aside. I would need to help Jenny develop a person-to-person relationship with each parent, one that was not mediated by the other parent.

I recommended that Peter and Jenny spend time together, a suggestion they dutifully followed. But the interactions between them remained bland. Although Jenny and her mother argued more, there was more passion in their relationship, more connection, and ultimately more investment by both parties. Peter and Jenny were cordial, but scarcely intimate, and it was clear that simply prescribing time alone together would not stimulate more intimacy between them.

I wondered if Peter's experiences with his schizophrenic mother had frightened him away from Jenny, who had been labeled "preschizophrenic" by the staff at the psychiatric hospital. It would not be the first time that a diagnosis ostensibly given to help an adolescent results in more emotional distance between the child and parents. Peter told me that his father had died when he was only 13, and after his father's death, his mother's male psychiatrist told Peter that it was his responsibility to take care of his mother. I wondered if Peter felt resentment toward his parents for having abandoned him, leaving him essentially orphaned throughout his adolescence and saddled with the impossible responsibility of taking care of his own psychotic mother. However, when I tried to pursue Peter to talk about his inner pain, he pushed me away, dismissing me with reassurance that he had "gotten over" his grief.

We appeared to be at an impasse, but then, as it often does, a crisis arose that provided another opportunity for initiating change. Late one night, I received an urgent message from Clare. Jenny had been rushed to the emergency room after taking 50 acetaminophen tablets. Peter was out of town, couldn't be reached, and wasn't scheduled to return for 3 more days. Jenny had been admitted to the hospital, but the doctors had told Clare that she would be all right and could probably go home the next day. I scheduled an appointment with them late the next afternoon, so that Clare and Jenny could come to my office directly from the hospital.

The story Jenny told was almost unbelievable. She and her mother had just finished eating dinner together. Jenny went up to her room while Clare started the dishes. Hardly 10 minutes later, Jenny came into the kitchen and told her mother that she had taken the pills. Jenny offered no objection as Clare ushered her into the car and drove her to the emergency room.

I began the session by asking Clare to talk with Jenny about the reasons she tried to kill herself.

JENNY: I honestly don't know. I just saw the pills there and I took them.

CLARE: Did it have anything to do with what we were talking about at dinner?

JENNY: I don't even remember what we were talking about at dinner.

CLARE: That's just it, hon, we weren't talking about much of anything, just everyday stuff.

JENNY: I know, Mom. I don't know why it happened.

CLARE: Were you hearing voices?

JENNY: No.

CLARE: Were you planning it all along?

JENNY: (*a bit more annoyed now*) No, Mom. I told you, I don't know why I did it! It just popped into my head.

CLARE: (*getting exasperated*) But I was right in the other room. Why couldn't you come to me?

JENNY: (*sighing*) I told you, I don't know. I just don't know.

I felt sympathy for both Jenny and Clare. I could imagine the guilt Clare felt, since this happened on "her watch," and only minutes after she and Jenny had parted. On the phone the night before, Clare had frantically asked, "Does this mean that I can't leave her alone even for a few minutes?" Although Jenny herself was mystified about her state of mind at the time she took the pills, Clare still felt responsible.

I felt sympathy for Jenny, too. I believed that she really didn't know why she had taken the pills. To her credit, although she knew that she could rescue her mother from her helplessness by fabricating a reason that seemed to satisfy us, Jenny didn't give in to this temptation. But it was poignantly obvious just how much Jenny had lost access to her own voice. Less than 24 hours ago she had taken a near-lethal overdose with no warning and now could offer no explanation.

It crossed my mind that Jenny might have attempted suicide in response to command hallucinations or while in a dissociated state, but I chose to emphasize a different aspect of the problem. It was clear that pleading with Jenny to explain why she took the pills was only pushing her farther away, because our request for a reason presumed that Jenny had knowledge about herself that she really didn't have. The only thing that linked us all was our profound helplessness before a powerful force that none of us understood or could even name. If I were going to be of any help at all, I would have to admit that we were all in the same boat.

I recognized the paradox: By working so hard to save Jenny, we were giving her the message that she was unacceptable as she was. We had been inducted into the cycle of control, as the suicide attempt most poignantly brought to the fore. My relationship with Jenny was predicated on helping her to change (though into what was not entirely clear). Her parents, too, insisted they would "do anything for her," which only underscored how desperately they wanted her to change. Meanwhile, Jenny remained lost. She didn't know herself either, but we were working so hard to help her become who we thought she wanted to be that we inadvertently perpetuated her isolation.

But we were not prepared to allow her to die, even if she believed she wanted to. The bottom line was that we wanted a relationship with Jenny, and that meant she had to stay alive. If living was unbearable for her, then we would do what we could to help share the burden and make it possible for her to go on. But we would never agree that suicide was the only answer. We would keep trying to connect with her even if she wanted to give up.

Stuck as we were in this impasse, I realized the futility of demanding that Jenny tell us why she had attempted to kill herself, an act so extreme that it was really not possible to justify. Jenny knew that she could never adequately explain what she had done, and would not play along. Why should she fabricate a reason only to have it shot down by us as insufficient justification for having attempted to kill herself? She was in a bind:

Give us a reason, and we'll contradict it; don't give us a reason, and we will continue to pursue you ever more frantically until you give us one. The only way out was to let go of our need to understand and to remove the requirement that she placate us by satisfying our need for a reason.

I realized that I needed to help Clare focus back on herself rather than on Jenny. This would be difficult, since Clare's heart ached for Jenny. But pressing Jenny for "reasons" was only pushing Jenny farther away. To break this cycle, I decided to focus on Clare's feelings about what had happened. I asked Clare to tell Jenny how she felt about her suicide attempt. Although I was risking the possibility that Clare might express anger, I thought that my relationship with her was strong enough to allow me to reframe anger as an expression of her anxiety over losing Jenny.

I needn't have worried, because upon hearing my question, Clare paused, and then began to weep.

"How do I feel?" she asked, incredulously. "Devastated. Absolutely devastated."

Jenny looked as if she was going to speak up, but I indicated that she should let her mother go on and not interrupt her.

After a tearful few minutes, Clare said, "No matter how big she gets, she's still that little girl I loved. I wish I could take the pain away from her when she feels that way. I've never felt pain like hers. I can only imagine how agonizing it must feel."

Jenny was now listening intently. Clare wept some more, then went on. "If she had died, I think I would cry until the end of time. I just couldn't be consoled. I would go on, I would live my life, but there would always be this big empty space because Jenny wasn't there anymore."

Clare sobbed. Jenny, also in tears, put her arm around her. After a few minutes had passed, I asked Jenny if she had any reaction to what her mother had said.

Jenny, drying her eyes with a tissue supplied by Clare, spoke as her eyes watered again, "I never knew she cared so much. 'I'd cry until the end of time.' That's, that's like, all the tears in the world wouldn't be enough." Jenny looked at her mother, "I never meant to hurt you, Mom."

Clare held her as Jenny burst into tears again.

"I know, honey," Clare said, "I know. I just wish I knew what to do when that feeling comes over you, sweetie."

I wanted to build on this moment. Clare didn't know what to do to keep Jenny from trying to hurt herself again, and I didn't know either. But Clare knew a lot about being a mother. I wanted to capitalize on the strength of her relationship with Jenny, using Clare's wisdom as the springboard.

"Clare," I asked, "What did you do when Jenny was little and she was sick, but you couldn't do anything but wait until the fever broke?"

Clare looked at Jenny with tears in her eyes, then back at me, "I did what any mother would do. I'd sit with her, I'd hold her hand, I'd tell her that it would be all right, and that I'd stay with her until she felt better."

I restrained myself from speaking, though I smiled and nodded. I waited for Clare to make the connection for herself. A glimmer of insight appeared in her eyes, "So maybe all I can do now is wait, and hold her hand until the feeling passes."

Out of the mother–daughter relationship, strength had emerged, and a discovery that freed Clare from the responsibility that the need to control brings with it. The answer, like many profound truths, was startlingly simple. In surrendering to her helplessness, Clare realized that she was not responsible for changing Jenny's feelings. The pain that afflicted Jenny, like a childhood fever, was temporarily in control. All Clare could do was to hold Jenny's hand, lending Jenny her own strength to fight the emotional fever that had her in its grip. This Clare knew how to do, and she didn't need me or Peter to tell her how to do it. All she needed to do was to be with Jenny, hold her hand, and stay with her until the feeling passed. Jenny also appeared to relax at this realization. No longer was she caught in the bind of having to help her mother by giving her mother a promise she could not keep—that she would not try to harm herself again. But she could surrender herself to her mother's soothing presence while they waited together for the suicidal feeling to pass.

Some suicidal adolescents, like Jenny, back away from their parents out of a misguided sense of love, duty, and responsibility. The adolescent realizes that she hurts her parents when she hurts herself. She knows that they want nothing more than for her to stop harming herself. But the suicidal adolescent is in a bind. If she goes to her parents for help, they go into overdrive trying to reassure her and, in the process, unwittingly discount her feelings. She can't bear to see her parents hurt, so she avoids them, retreating into even more intense isolation, but at least secure in the knowledge that she is not hurting anyone but herself.

If the parents, like Clare, can embrace their own powerlessness, admit that they cannot prevent their child from feeling emotional pain, no matter how much they wish they could, then they can truly be a resource for the adolescent. They must let go of their need to control and protect, and instead focus on their emotional attachment to the youngster. The child can rest in their arms, secure in the knowledge that she needn't produce anything in order to stay cradled there. The parents need not find a way to prevent the child from feeling bad. All they need to do is listen, to be there, to hold her hand until the feeling passes.

The question now was how to bridge from this pivotal event to the next session, when Peter returned. Sometimes, a mother will display competence in a father's absence, only to appear less competent when the father is present. Would Clare revert to her old self when Peter returned? Would she be angry at Peter and hold him responsible for Jenny's suicide attempt? Would she clutch more tightly to Jenny, or would she be able to move away enough to allow Peter in, without letting go of Jenny's hand completely?

I knew that Clare would have liked me to bring Peter up to speed, but I believed that it would enhance Clare's sense of her own competence if she could do it herself. I began the session by telling Peter that we had met the day before, and that I believed that Clare had made a very important discovery that I hoped she could share with him now. Clare then took over and explained to Peter what she had discovered the day before. Peter listened, and I could see that he was struggling to understand. For Peter, as for many men in our culture, helping often means doing something concrete, taking a definite action. Simply sitting together and holding hands did not seem to him as if he was doing his duty as a parent.

After listening to Clare, Peter immediately turned to Jenny: "So is that all you need from us, to hold your hand?"

I inwardly winced: Referring to this simple act of connection as "all" that Jenny needed seemed to devalue it. But Jenny had evidently not picked up on this implication. She replied, "Yeah, that's all. If I knew that I didn't have to talk, that I could just tell you that I was feeling bad, and that you'd stay with me, I think I'd feel better."

Peter was not satisfied: "But why can't you talk to us, Jenny? Why can't you tell us what is making you feel so bad?"

I could see a shadow come across Jenny's face again: "I told you Dad, I don't know. Maybe I just don't want to hurt you."

Peter, more agitated now: "But why do you care about hurting me? Don't care how I feel. Just tell me whatever you need to say."

Jenny just sighed this time. Peter went on: "You've got to help me, honey. I need to hear from you what I'm doing to make you feel this way."

Here is the double bind, explicitly stated. Peter has contradicted himself—don't care how I feel, but help me. In addition, the focus was now off Jenny and onto Peter. The issue was no longer what Jenny needed at that moment, but on what Jenny must give Peter so that Peter could feel better, namely, an explanation that Peter could understand.

But I also sympathized with Peter's frustration. I knew he wanted to do what was best for Jenny, and if that meant that he would have to hear very hurtful things about himself, so be it. What he could not tolerate was the feeling of helplessness. Clare could sit and hold Jenny's hand, but Peter, like most men, needed to do something specific in order to feel worthwhile. He needed to call the doctor, go out to buy medicine, heat up chicken soup, or carry the portable television up to Jenny's room. He needed to do something concrete, something active, to feel that he was helping.

As a man, I could empathize with Peter's position. Often, we men are put in the position of feeling that we must be instrumental if we are to feel good about ourselves. But, in Peter's case, I sensed that something else was also going on. He was frightened of the emotions associated with helplessness and surrender. The seeming irrationality of Jenny's behavior reawakened the ghost of his mother, and offering to share Jenny's burden had too much potential to open up his wounds. But these wounds had to be opened if he was going to relate to Jenny person to person and not as a container of his own projected fears. I realized that it was now time to pursue Peter. He must confront his own demons if he was going to understand Jenny. But I knew that I had to proceed gently, lest I become the rejecting parent or his mother's psychiatrist who told him to suppress his feelings for her sake.

MICUCCI: (*to Peter*) I want to know about your sadness.

PETER: (*looking at me as if I had spoken in a language he didn't understand*) What do you mean?

MICUCCI: I can see the sadness in your eyes. I can hear it in your voice. I want to know about it.

PETER: I don't know what you are talking about.

MICUCCI: Just tell me how it feels right now.

PETER: I feel like there's a pounding jackhammer in my chest.

MICUCCI: So you're feeling anxious?

PETER: I guess.

MICUCCI: Do you know what's making you feel anxious?

PETER: I don't know. I guess it started when you asked me about being sad. Like, maybe you see into me and I don't like that.

MICUCCI: See into you?

PETER: Yeah, like maybe you know me better than I want you to.

MICUCCI: And do you know why that would make you feel so scared?

PETER: I guess it scares me to be so close. I just feel better when I can keep a bit of a wall up, I guess.

Like many men, Peter was threatened by intimacy with another man, what Stephen Bergman (1995) has called "male relational dread." I understood that, and I didn't want to push so hard that I scared him away. On the other hand, if I was going to help this family, I would have to push Peter farther than he had gone before. I wanted him to get in touch with his emotional side, and learn that he could not only tolerate it, but could also be enriched by it.

MICUCCI: OK, Peter, I understand. Can you let me in just a little? If it gets too uncomfortable, you can always put up the wall again.

PETER: (*hesitantly*) Sure, but I don't know what you want.

Many men are so unaccustomed to intimacy with another man that they are not sure what it means. They are a bit suspicious and wonder what they might discover about themselves if they allow another man to get close.

MICUCCI: All I want is to understand that sadness in your voice and in your eyes.

PETER: (*sighing, letting go just a bit*) I don't know. I'm so confused. Clare looks like she knows what to do for Jenny. The two of them look so close together. I guess I just feel out of it, like a third wheel.

Here was Peter's isolation. Clare looked as if she was about to speak, perhaps to reassure Peter, but I gestured to her to remain silent for now.

MICUCCI: So you're feeling left out. Alone?

PETER: Yeah, alone, helpless, like they don't need me.

MICUCCI: You'd like to feel needed.

PETER: Sure, I'd like to. But then, what do they need me for? I don't have any answers for them. I don't know what to do (*tears welling in his eyes*).

MICUCCI: It's OK, Peter. I can imagine how bad that must feel for you.

PETER: It's like when that doctor told me I had to take care of my mom. I didn't know what to do. I was only a kid. What was I supposed to do?

The tears came. Clare looked at me for a sign, and I gestured that it would be all right for her to move over to Peter and put her arm around him. Jenny didn't wait for a sign from me. She went to Peter's other side and put her head on his shoulder.

One theory to explain what had happened in this family is that Peter had projected the threatening and disowned parts of himself onto Jenny. By doing so, it helped Peter feel that this split-off part of himself was more controllable because it was someone else—Jenny—who was losing control, not he. The cost, however, was that Peter then lost access to the parts of himself that could feel, that could let go, that could surrender, and as a result, the rational, intellectualized parts of him hypertrophied. If Peter could reclaim even some of these disowned parts of himself, he would have a better opportunity to know Jenny for who she was, and so have a more genuine and intimate relationship with her.

In subsequent sessions, we talked about Peter's loneliness and how Clare and Jenny had misinterpreted it as lack of interest in them. Jenny told her father that she often felt intimidated by him. I could see that Peter winced on hearing this: He didn't want to be seen in this way by his daughter, yet he could understand how it had happened. As the discussion unfolded, the family members both figuratively and literally held each other's hands. They listened to each other's pain, to fragments of thoughts and ideas that came up but didn't necessarily connect in a meaningful sequence, and in so doing, Jenny, Peter, and Clare became both more connected and differentiated. They could see each other as individuals rather than as projections of their disowned feelings.

Eventually, the parents, on their own, solved the dilemma of "what to do when Jenny wants to hurt herself." They decided that they would simply ask her on a regular basis how she was feeling and remind her of their presence and support. If she were feeling bad, they would keep her company and hold her hand. She did not have to produce an explanation or even an elaboration. They would just be there for her until the feeling passed, keeping her company, lending her their strength, and, in the process, they all realized that they felt stronger.

SUMMARY

Although biological and environmental factors play a role in some cases of depression, in this chapter I have emphasized the role of family dynamics and relationships. Underlying depression and suicidality in adolescence are isolation and disconnection from supporting and validating relationships. Thus, a key theme in treatment must be reconnecting the adolescent with the parents so that the parents can become a more supportive resource to the child. I presented the following procedure for working with depressed and/or suicidal adolescents:

- Ensure the adolescent's safety by helping the parents take whatever measures are necessary to prevent a suicide attempt.
- Open up dialogue. Often, the "Tell me/Don't tell me" bind is

powerful in these families. Some depressed and suicidal youngsters feel responsible for their parents' welfare and worry about upsetting their parents. Some fear rejection were they to share their true feelings with their parents. Others are reluctant to trust the parents because of past experiences of abandonment. In addition to showing empathy and concern for the adolescent, it is important to provide support to the parents to enable them to listen to the child without becoming defensive, angry, or dismissive. Parents must help the adolescent answer the following key question: *Why did you choose to hurt yourself rather than come to us for help first?*

• Help the parents find specific, concrete ways of demonstrating that they have heard the adolescent's concerns and are committed to addressing them.

7

Anxiety

It has been said that we live in an age of anxiety. As one patient put it, "The world is getting scarier and scarier." With the threat of terrorism, global warming, economic collapse, and toxins in the environment, it is not surprising that many people feel anxious. However, most people are able to cope with these anxieties and go on living in spite of them.

Some people, however, are immobilized by anxiety. They live in a constant state of tension or worry. Some experience unexpected and apparently random attacks of intense anxiety or panic. Others develop avoidance strategies to keep the anxiety at bay. As a result, they live restricted lives, often considerably compromising their functioning by doing so. Some develop elaborate compulsive rituals that are designed to ward off intense anxiety, but the rituals themselves become the focus of the person's life and prevent him or her from engaging in other activities.

Frequently, the other people in the sufferer's life become embroiled in the anxiety and the efforts to avoid it. This is particularly true when a child or adolescent experiences anxiety. Members of the family, especially the parents, become involved in the problem. As is true in most cases of the problems discussed in this book, the family's efforts to resolve the problem often have the unintended effect of exacerbating the problem. Attempts to reassure the anxious youngster are either ineffective or reinforce the child's helplessness by cultivating dependence on the parent for emotional support. The parents' efforts to relieve the child's stress (which they presume causes the anxiety) by reducing expectations of the child or accommodating to the child's fears have the unintended effect of reinforcing the fears and the child's helplessness.

ANXIETY AND THE FAMILY

In order to understand the role of family dynamics in anxiety it is necessary to identify the particular manner in which children or adolescents signal to the parents that they are experiencing anxiety. In other words, it is important to attend to the adolescent's behavioral expressions of anxiety. It is via these behavioral expressions that the family members become aware of the anxiety, and thus these behaviors are the logical place to begin an exploration of the interpersonal cycles surrounding the anxiety. It is important to inquire what is going on in the family at the times when the adolescent's anxiety becomes noticeable, and also to track carefully the family interactional patterns during the session when the child displays signs of anxiety. Questions to consider include:

- What immediately preceded the first noticeable manifestations of the adolescent's anxiety?
- Who is the first to notice that the adolescent is anxious? Which family members seem most and least sensitive to the adolescent's anxiety?
- How did the family members respond to the emergence of the symptoms?
- How did the symptomatic adolescent respond to the responses of the other family members?

The patterns might be more complex than they first appear. It is important to be astute, not only to the overt behaviors, but also to the more covert or subtle responses of the family members, as is illustrated in the following example:

During a session an adolescent begins talking about her fears of ridicule at school. As she does so, signs of anxiety become noticeable. After a few minutes, her mother moves closer to her and puts her arm around her shoulder. The mother's response seems to imply that she is attuned to her daughter's anxiety. We might even speculate that the mother's readiness to offer support encourages the girl to depend on the mother for support. However, the attentive observer might have noticed that another interaction preceded the mother's apparently supportive response. As the girl began to relate her fears of ridicule, the mother looked at the father, who avoided her eye contact and turned his face away from both the girl and the mother. The mother then turned to the girl and put her arm around her.

Ignoring the intervening response of the father, and the mother's reaction to it, could lead to the erroneous conclusion that the mother's response to the girl might be reinforcing her anxiety, or that the girl's anxiety is the only way that she can elicit a desired supportive reaction from her mother. On the other hand, when the father's contribution is considered, another hypothesis is plausible: The girl's expression of anxiety triggers the mother to seek the father's support. When this support is not forthcoming, the mother turns to the girl, thus supplying the comfort that she thinks the girl needs, and also obtaining from the girl the closeness that she could not get from the father.

What happens next is also relevant: The girl and her mother have a conversation about the girl's fears, and as they do so they become physically closer. Mother moves away from the father, who now turns toward that dyad but does not participate. At one point, he tries to enter the conversation but is ignored. He then turns away and looks at the floor again, not protesting or persisting.

Being astute to these subtleties can lead us to consider other hypotheses worth exploring further: The girl's expressions of anxiety invite her mother to comfort her, and in so doing divert attention away from the conflict between the mother and father over the mother's perception of the father's unavailability. The girl's anxiety and consequent avoidant behavior also keeps her from engaging in activities outside the home and thus keeps her from separating too quickly from the family. One could also speculate that the father does not intervene in the cycle because alleviation of the girl's anxiety could result in her moving out of the family, and thus moving out of the triangle with his wife, which could exacerbate overt conflict between the parents. As the mother apparently comforts the girl, the mother also receives comfort from the closeness that she is not receiving from her husband. Also supporting the idea that the family has established a comfortable homeostasis are the observations that neither the mother nor the girl responds to the father when he tries to intervene and the father does not insist on being involved.

If we were to miss the father's contribution to the cycle, then we might be tempted to block the mother's support for the girl, thinking that her apparently supportive response might be encouraging or reinforcing the girl's helplessness. As a result, the girl might become more anxious. If the girl's anxiety were to intensify to a level that could threaten the family's homeostasis, then the father might join the mother in comforting the girl, and in so doing bring the system back to the original homeostatic level.

The therapist who notices the father's contribution, however, has other options to intervene. The therapist could invite the father to join the mother in comforting the girl, or encourage the mother to talk with the father about her own concerns while she remains in physical contact with the girl. The therapist could also talk directly to the girl herself, thus taking over the role of support that the mother was providing. Perhaps another sibling could be introduced into the session. The therapist could encourage the sibling to offer support to the girl, or redirect the mother's attention to the sibling while the father took responsibility for helping the anxious girl.

It is important to emphasize that the foregoing analysis does not intend to imply that the parents are the "cause" of the girl's anxiety. Rather, as is the case with all formulations based on systems thinking, the girl's expression of anxiety elicits particular responses from the parents, and these responses elicit, encourage, or fail to discourage more expressions of anxiety on the part of the girl. Furthermore, this formulation assumes that the expressions of anxiety (and presumably the girl's subjective experience of anxiety) help to maintain a particular pattern of family interactions, which stabilizes the family by distracting attention from other problems (e.g., the marital problem).

Empirical Support for the Role of the Family in Child and Adolescent Anxiety

Empirical studies of families with anxious children and adolescents support the claim that particular types of family interactions are correlated with symptoms of anxiety in children and adolescents. The idea that parental behaviors might encourage a child's avoidance behaviors was supported by an observational study by Dadds, Marrett, and Rapee (1996), who reported that parents of anxious children were more likely to support avoidance behaviors, while parents of nonanxious children were more likely to agree with and listen to the child's own ideas about ways to cope with the problem. The association between child anxiety and overprotectiveness was supported in a study by Bogels, van Oosten, Muris, and Smulders (2001), who reported that a child's social anxiety was associated with maternal overprotectiveness. McFarlane (1987) found that children's response to a fire disaster was moderated by their mother's response: Mothers who were more anxious and overprotective after the disaster were more likely to have children who exhibited posttraumatic symptoms. Rapee (1997) noted a connection between maternal control and child anxiety, and argued that parental overprotectiveness communicates to the child that danger is continually present and also restricts the child's opportunities to develop successful coping mechanisms. In a similar vein, Krohne and Hock (1991) found that mothers of highly anxious girls were more likely to intervene in the child's attempts at independent problem solving and tended to retain control over the problem-solving situation rather than relinquish it to the child, thus inhibiting the child's opportunity to learn effective problem-solving skills. Interestingly, exactly the opposite pattern was found for boys, implying that maternal rejection and failure to intervene supportively might be associated with anxiety in boys.

Although parents of anxious children might be overprotective and intrusive, they are not necessarily perceived as warm or engaged by the child. Hale, Engels, and Meeus (2006) reported that adolescents with symptoms of generalized anxiety perceived their parents as alienated and rejecting. Wolfradt, Hempel, and Miles (2003) found that anxiety among adolescents was associated with an authoritarian parenting style and lower parental warmth. Barrett, Fox, and Farrell (2005) reported that parents of anxious children showed more control, less paternal warmth, and less maternal reinforcement of coping behavior than parents of nonanxious children.

Taken together, these studies imply that families with anxious children are not only overprotective, but intrusive. Although their efforts to help might be well-intentioned, they interfere with the youngster's own efforts to self-regulate and solve problems independently. Moreover, the child does not experience the parents' intrusiveness as positive. Instead, the adolescent might become overly sensitive to signs of parental rejection or displeasure, which increases the youngster's anxiety. Weak interpersonal boundaries in the family make the anxiety contagious. When the adolescent becomes anxious, the parents become anxious, and what appear to be their efforts to alleviate the child's anxiety in fact are efforts to alleviate their own anxiety. As the parents' frustration increases, they begin to communicate this frustration to the child, who becomes even more worried about disappointing the parents. As discussed below, the ultimate fear is the fear of abandonment. As the adolescent becomes more and more worried about the parents' anxiety and disappointment, he or she becomes more and more terrified at the prospect that the parents (who have cultivated dependency on them via their "supportive" efforts to help the youngster) will abandon him or her.

COGNITIVE FACTORS IN ADOLESCENT ANXIETY

Much attention has been directed to the role of cognitive factors in adolescent anxiety. Anxious adolescents tend to exhibit certain biases in the way they perceive the world. For example, they tend to overestimate the probability and cost of negative events (Rheingold, Herbert, & Franklin, 2003). Several studies have found that CBT, which emphasizes the discovery and alteration of these cognitive biases, is an effective treatment for anxiety disorders in children and adolescents (Cartwright-Hatton et al., 2004).

Claims that CBT is an "empirically supported therapy" for the treatment of anxiety has led many therapists to assume that it is the best or the only effective treatment for anxiety disorders. However, CBT is not effective in all cases. In a review of 10 randomized controlled trials, Cartwright-Hatton et al. (2004) reported that CBT was effective for 56.5% of the treated cases. Although this rate exceeded the rate of 34.8% of non-treated controls, over 40% of children and adolescents treated with CBT continued to be symptomatic. Furthermore, in a study of adolescents who had received CBT for anxiety during childhood, many reported ongoing anxiety and about 30% had symptoms so severe that they required additional treatment for anxiety (Manassis, Avery, Butalia, & Mendlowitz, 2004). There are promising reports that including parents in treatment can improve the success rate of CBT for child and adolescent anxiety by directly addressing parental behaviors that could be maintaining the child's anxiety (Barrett, Dadds, & Rapee, 1996; Bogels & Siqueland, 2006; Ginsburg & Schlossberg, 2002). Training parents in the application of CBT techniques for their children might seem like an effective strategy, but it can also encourage parental overprotectiveness, as exemplified in the following case.

Adam had many worries, and would often be distracted from his homework by ruminations about things that had happened during the day at school, not having handled situations the "right" way, or fears about the future. His parents had divorced when he was a young child, and he also worried that he might be "scarred for life" because of the divorce. He had a close relationship with his mother, and would frequently seek her out for support when he felt particularly anxious. Before consulting me for family therapy, Adam had been treated by a therapist who followed a CBT protocol. Mother had been included in the therapy, and coached on things to say to Adam to remind him that he was engaging in irrational patterns of thinking or not appraising situations realistically. Mother used these techniques when Adam would come to her for aid, and they appeared to be effective. Adam would come to his mother and report his worries. She would interrupt what she was doing, sit down with him to write out his dysfunctional cognitions, and help him substitute more appropriate ways of thinking. After these sessions, which would typically last 20–30 minutes, Adam would feel better and return to his homework. Recently, however, these sessions were becoming more frequent. They would occur on a daily basis, and sometimes Adam would come back to his mother later in the evening after what was apparently a successful session of cognitive restructuring.

I inferred from this pattern that the role taken by Adam's mother was perpetuating an overprotective relationship and excessive dependency on her, almost as if she were an extension of his own rational mind. Without her, Adam could not engage in the CBT analysis on his own. Moreover, his father was rarely consulted during these episodes of anxiety, even though Adam visited him at least once a week and he had a cordial working relationship with Adam's mother.

I intervened in the following way: I suggested that Adam continue to come to his mother whenever he felt anxious, but before engaging in a conversation with him about his fears, the mother should encourage Adam to contact his father to get his father's perspective. After talking with his father (or if his father was not available), Adam could then talk with his mother if he wished. However, his mother was to take a different role than she had taken in the past. Rather than employing CBT techniques with Adam, his mother was simply to listen nonjudgmentally to Adam's fears, reflect back his feelings, and refrain from offering suggestions. Instead, she was to remind Adam that he had learned techniques for managing his anxiety and that she was confident that he would find a way to do so without her direct assistance. Meanwhile, she would hold him accountable for his schoolwork, and give consequences if she received reports that he was not completing assignments.

The first few times the family tried this new approach, Adam appeared to get more anxious and agitated when his mother did not immediately respond to his request to help him get rid of his fears. But both parents persisted in this approach (it helped that I had warned them about Adam's reaction). When Adam got agitated, his mother suggested that he call his father. If Adam refused to call his father or if his father was not available, his mother would simply acknowledge how anxious Adam was, communicate empathy and sympathy, and remind him that she was confident of his ability to use the techniques he was taught to help him manage his own anxiety. Eventually, Adam stopped going to his mother. He began to call his father on his own, without having to be reminded by his mother. Eventually, he decided that he wasn't really getting much benefit from asking his parents for help, so he decided to handle his anxious feelings on his own.

ANXIETY AND ABANDONMENT

Fear of abandonment is a common fear shared by all family members of an anxious child or adolescent. All family members fear being abandoned and left alone to cope with unbearable adversity without the support of others on whom one has come to depend. The child fears loss of the parents, the parents fear that they can't count on one another, and they fear losing the child to madness.

Families of anxious children and adolescents might appear to be close and supportive, but closeness comes at a price: restriction of free-

dom, parentification, loss of identity, or the injunction against expressing feelings of anger or disapproval, which then can become internalized
and experienced as anxiety. Their apparently close attachment to one
another is fraught with insecurity. The child, dependent on the parents to
help regulate his or her anxiety, becomes hypersensitive to signs of parental unavailability, distress, or disapproval. The parents become hypervigilant to signs of distress in the child so that they can intervene quickly
to prevent the anxiety from escalating. They sacrifice their relationship
with each other in order to provide the attention they believe their child
needs.

As the parental relationship weakens, the parents feel more isolated
from each other and so more likely to seek closeness with the child to
compensate for what is missing in the marital relationship. The adolescent is apt to interpret the parents' anxiety as evidence that the parents
believe that what the adolescent fears is indeed a significant threat. This
interpretation is reinforced by the fact that parents will often give the
youngster mixed messages: On the one hand, they will reassure the child
that "there's nothing to fear," while on the other hand they accommodate
to the child's anxiety by reducing expectations or tolerating avoidance
behaviors, thus giving credence to the adolescent's fears. Feeling increasingly helpless to deal with the child's anxiety, the parents' own anxiety
increases. As the parents' distress mounts, the adolescent becomes more
anxious about losing the parents or irrevocably alienating them.

Because abandonment anxiety is often a theme for the entire family,
it is not surprising that anxious children have anxious parents. When
the child is anxious, the parents are anxious. The parents' responses to
the anxious youngster are not only motivated by a desire to alleviate the
child's anxiety, but also motivated by a need to alleviate their own anxiety. Since the anxiety has permeated the family, treatment in these cases
can be long and difficult. The following case illustrates this process.

I received an anxious call from Evelyn, the mother of 13-year-old
Caleb. About 6 months prior to the call, Caleb had begun to experience anxiety at bedtime, and would be unable to sleep unless one of
his parents stayed with him in his room until he fell asleep. Eventually,
these fears progressed into an elaborate ritual that Caleb felt compelled
to perform before he would allow himself to get into bed. After making
sure that all of the articles in his room were carefully arranged in their
"proper" place, he would then recite a series of prayers, often having to
start over again from the beginning if he believed that he had missed a
particular phrase or if he had "allowed" his mind to wander while pray-
ing. These rituals took over an hour to complete, and within the past 2
weeks Caleb had been pressuring his parents to participate in the rituals
as well. If they refused, or if they demanded that he stop and get to bed

immediately, Caleb would become frighteningly agitated, cry uncontrollably, and beg his parents to allow him to proceed. Since these outbursts would not only be unpleasant for the parents but also take more time than the rituals themselves, the parents would relent. However, they were becoming more and more anxious as the amount of time required to complete the rituals was increasing.

At the first session, Caleb refused to sit down in a chair, claiming that he preferred to stand because he might catch "a germ" from the chair in my office. I asked him to explain what might happen if he caught a germ. He claimed that he might get sick and die, or he might pass on the germ to another family member who might get sick and die. I asked him about his nighttime rituals, and he said that he could not sleep unless he had completed them because he was convinced that either he or one of his parents would die if he fell asleep before completing the ritual. If both he and his parents were to die, he was afraid that his parents would go to heaven and he would go to hell, so he had to recite an elaborate series of prayers that would ensure that he would not go to hell if he died.

Caleb's father, George, worked the night shift, and Evelyn reported that Caleb's symptoms were worse when George was at work and not as bad on those nights when he was at home. George said that he was prepared to take a leave of absence from his job so that he would be home at night for Caleb, but I encouraged him not to take that step "just yet" until I had a chance to get to know them a little better and see if there might not be another solution. George admitted that he had similar fears as a child, although he had not felt compelled to engage in compulsive rituals. He did, however, admit that for many years he had felt the urge to pray several times a day lest some harm come to his wife or children.

Although Evelyn and George were willing at first to accommodate to Caleb's rituals, they were beginning to lose their patience and get frustrated. I asked them why they thought that Caleb's symptoms were less intense when George was at home. I expected that they would say that George was firmer with Caleb and so Caleb was discouraged from engaging in elaborate rituals when he was present. I did not get the answer I expected. Caleb's symptoms were less intense when his father was at home because George readily agreed to "help" Caleb with his rituals and would then allow Caleb to sleep in the parental bed with him while Evelyn slept in Caleb's room. Caleb said that he felt more comfortable sleeping in the bed with his father because then his father would notice if he was about to die in his sleep and would be able to prevent him from dying by waking him up.

It was obvious that Caleb's parents were never sleeping together in the same bed. Either George worked nights (and slept during the day) or on his days off he would sleep with Caleb rather than with his wife. I wondered if George might be engaging in sexual activity with Caleb, but this was not the case: It was Caleb who pressured his father to allow him to sleep with him, and Caleb denied that he had ever been touched inappropriately by an adult when I asked him about this in private. It was clear, however, that this sleeping arrangement would become a regular nighttime pattern if George followed through on his plans to take a leave of absence from his job. I wondered how the parental marriage would survive such an arrangement, but I also wondered whether the arrangement helped to ensure the survival of the marriage by keeping the parents at a comfortable distance from one another. Of the three of them, Evelyn was least happy with the sleeping arrangements. On the other hand, she was not willing to risk "a meltdown" from Caleb if she did not go along with his demands. It appeared to me that this arrangement helped everyone be less anxious: Obviously, Caleb was less anxious, but the parents were less anxious too, because they felt that they were helping their son and preventing him from having "a breakdown."

Although I had developed a sketch of the relevant family dynamics, it was not so obvious how to intervene to help this boy and his parents. If I instructed the parents not to participate in or encourage Caleb's rituals, then Caleb could develop even more elaborate rituals or his anxiety might escalate to the point that the parents would feel they had no choice but to accommodate to his demands. If this happened, I would quickly lose credibility with the family. On the other hand, it was clear that continuation of the current pattern was not going to work either. Over the past few months, despite parental compliance with Caleb's rituals, they had become more elaborate and time-consuming.

I asked the parents if they believed that Caleb's fears were founded or unfounded. George asserted that Caleb's fears that he or his parents might die were "probably" unfounded. Everyone in the family was healthy, and there "seemed" to be little chance of a 13-year-old boy or a 40-something parent dying unexpectedly in their sleep. Evelyn didn't speak, but nodded her head as George spoke. I detected equivocation in this answer, and it is possible that Caleb detected it as well. In an attempt to elicit a stronger conviction from the parents that Caleb's fears were excessive, I asked them: "Are you absolutely convinced that Caleb's fears are unfounded? Do you have any doubt in your mind that he might have a good reason to be afraid?"

Not unexpectedly, Evelyn was more convinced than was George that Caleb's fears were unfounded. George said that he did not think that it was "likely that anyone would die in their sleep" but he understood why Caleb might worry about it because "sometimes people do die in their sleep." I directed the parents to talk together and reach a consensus.

in order to prevent the loss of a relationship (Brown & Gilligan, 1992; Jack, 1991, 1999). Jenny is in a no-win situation. If she silences herself, she contributes to her own isolation. If she speaks, she risks hurting her parents and damaging her relationship with them, which in turn will intensify her isolation. Therapy must help Jenny and her parents find a way out of this bind. The way out is to help them open up the dialogue without sacrificing their relationships.

Throughout this session, Peter remained aloof. I knew that he cared about Jenny—in fact, it was he who first contacted me for help. But the pattern in the family session underscored his peripheral position. He remained on the sidelines, entering only to contradict Clare or to speak for Jenny when the tension threatened to escalate between Jenny and her mother. Perhaps he was trying to reconnect with Jenny and communicate that he did indeed want a relationship with her. Unfortunately, he was doing so in a way that robbed Jenny of her own voice and undermined his relationship with his wife.

I also noted that Clare was willing to accept responsibility for part of the problem ("I think Jenny and I are too close"), while Peter stated the problem more impersonally, framed in a way that relieved him of blame ("Jenny doesn't want to be around us"). Peter was using his peripheral position to exonerate himself: How can I be responsible for this problem if I've really not been around very much?

Later, to explore further the relationship between the parents and to see how I might capitalize on their strengths, I asked Peter and Clare to talk together about how they thought they could be helpful to Jenny.

PETER: (*to Clare*) So what do you think we should do?

CLARE: Well, I think we should keep on doing what we are doing. We're trying to listen to her, trying to find out how she would like us to change, and …

PETER: (*cutting her off*) Yeah, but that doesn't seem to be getting us anywhere. She still won't talk. I think we're back at square one, almost.

CLARE: Well, I don't. I think Jenny is really interested in finding out what's bothering her.

PETER: But what *is* bothering her? We keep asking and asking and she doesn't tell us.

CLARE: I think she is telling us. She's telling us that she's afraid to hurt us.

PETER: And we tell her not to be afraid. So where does that leave us?

CLARE: (*with a sigh*) Peter, I don't have the answers.

Before we could proceed, both of them had to be absolutely sure that Caleb's fears had no basis in reality. This conversation between the parents took the better part of two sessions, but eventually Evelyn prevailed. The turning point occurred when George said, "You're right, Ev. No one is going to die. He's worried about something that just isn't going to happen. Period."

I then asked the parents the following question: "Since you both believe that Caleb's fears have no grounding in reality, how do you think you could act in ways that are consistent with your belief?"

Evelyn quickly made the connection that giving in to Caleb's fears was giving him a mixed message. If they really believed that there was no basis for his fears, then they should not participate in his rituals or alter their family routines in order to ward off an outcome that they didn't think was going to happen anyway. George was able to change his schedule to a day shift temporarily so that he and Evelyn could work together to help Caleb deal more effectively with his anxiety. George agreed that he would no longer spend the night in Caleb's room and he would not allow Caleb to sleep in the parental bedroom. Each night before bedtime, Caleb would be permitted to talk with them for no more than 10 minutes about his fears. They would listen sympathetically, offer reassurance and express confidence that he would be able to beat his fears, but they would not try to convince him or argue with him. If Caleb became agitated or aggressive during these conversations, then the parents were simply to walk away and refuse to talk with Caleb any more that night. They were not to interfere with Caleb's rituals, but he could not disturb the other family members and he was expected to be up on time for school the next day.

But they did have another fear, and we all agreed that this feared outcome was much more likely to occur: that Caleb would become increasingly anxious if they did not comply with his rituals. I took their concern seriously and asked them to spell out exactly what they feared could happen. George said that he feared that Caleb might "go crazy" and never recover, thus expressing his own fear of losing Caleb. I asked him to talk with Evelyn about this concern. Evelyn responded with her own fears: Although she did not think it was very likely that Caleb would "go crazy," she could not say for sure that it would not happen. I assured them that this outcome would not occur. Caleb might get very anxious and *appear* to be losing control, but my experience told me that he would eventually recover. If nothing else, he would get exhausted. To help reassure the parents, I gave them my cell phone number and told them they could call me if they became so frightened that they felt they could no longer tolerate it. I emphasized that they shouldn't share the number with Caleb, and that I would not accept a call from him. The number was to be used only by the parents and only if they felt that the impulse to participate in Caleb's compulsions was becoming irresistible.

It wasn't pretty. I got several phone calls, and we had to increase the frequency of our meetings. One night Caleb had gotten so upset that he began to throw up. While I felt sorry for him and realized he was suffering, I also noted to myself that by running to the bathroom to throw up Caleb had interrupted his rituals. Following a few minutes of what was clearly uncomfortable retching, Caleb was so exhausted that he fell asleep immediately, albeit on top of his blanket with his clothes still on.

Meanwhile, I met alone with Caleb to explore the basis for his anxiety. I listened attentively to his fears, and did not try to argue with him or convince him that he was wrong. I asked questions to help him articulate the fears and the expected feared outcomes. As a result of these conversations over several sessions, I learned:

• Caleb sometimes used his fears as an excuse to avoid doing something he didn't want to do. For example, his aunt had invited him out to lunch, and he did not want to go. Rather than telling his aunt that he didn't want to go (because he didn't want to "hurt her feelings") he said that he was afraid to go because he might pick up a germ at the restaurant.

• Caleb worried about displeasing his parents. As I expected, he feared that if he displeased them enough they would stop loving him and they would leave him. I noted that this fear actually provided Caleb with an incentive to comply with his parents' expectations that he limit the time spent on his rituals and be up on time for school the next morning. He said that it gave him "strength" to resist the compulsions because he didn't want to upset or displease his parents.

• Caleb admitted that he was sometimes very angry at his father, but he was afraid of expressing his anger because his father had a temper. With Caleb's permission, we brought this issue into a family session. I challenged George to help Caleb express his anger at him in a way that George felt was tolerable and appropriate.

• Caleb admitted that he was getting "tired" of his compulsions. He was beginning to feel that they were taking up too much of his time and kept him from doing some things he wanted to do, like spend the night at a friend's house.

Caleb was also very interested when I offered to help him learn ways of coping with his anxiety. Some of the techniques we used were:

- Practicing progressive relaxation and the use of relaxing imagery.

- Identifying and challenging (in writing) the dysfunctional thoughts that precipitated his anxiety.

- Externalizing the anxiety and finding ways to foil it. Caleb called his anxiety "The Bully." We talked about ways in which he had learned to outfox "The Bully" and argue against its demanding and demeaning messages.

- Substituting less conspicuous and less time-consuming compulsions for his elaborate and time-consuming rituals. We developed a shorter series of prayers he could say in 2 minutes rather than the lengthy prayers that required over 30 minutes. We practiced meditation as a substitute for vocal prayer. We substituted clenching his fist for touching and rearranging the articles in his room.

- We played the "game" of "What if?" I challenged Caleb to think about what could happen if his fears were to come true. If he died, what would he tell God to convince Him to send him to heaven rather than hell? If his parents died, how would he cope? Where would he live and what would he do? How did he think other children coped when they lost their parents? By encouraging him to talk openly about these fears while I maintained a calm presence, I hoped to defuse their power over Caleb. These discussions were anxiety-provoking for Caleb, so we deferred them until Caleb had become more secure in practicing self-soothing techniques.

In family sessions, I encouraged Caleb to talk with his parents about the fear that they might abandon him, either because they might die or because he might do something "bad" that would cause them to leave him. The parents repeatedly reassured Caleb that they would never abandon him, but it was clear that this wasn't working. The more they tried to reassure him, the more examples of "What if?" Caleb concocted. Their reassurance was inviting Caleb to think of more and more ways that he could possibly lose their love.

Instead, I encouraged the parents to listen to Caleb and express empathy for his feelings without trying to convince him to think or feel differently. They were permitted to state that they did not think or feel the same way, but that did not mean that Caleb was compelled to think or feel the way they did. If either parent became anxious during these conversations, I encouraged the other parent to offer physical support in the form of squeezing the anxious parent's hand or putting an arm around the anxious parent's shoulder.

Over the next few months, Caleb's anxiety gradually (very gradually) subsided. Some weeks were better than others. I encouraged the family to consider the "good weeks" as harbingers of great progress, while "bad weeks" were simply expected and understandable setbacks that should not be accorded great significance. I used every opportunity to spend session time on "normal" adolescent issues. I helped Caleb negotiate for more privileges and strategized with him how to handle annoying peers. Eventually, I noticed that these discussions were taking more of our session time, and less time was being spent talking about fears of death or dying. After 8 months we reduced the frequency of our sessions to biweekly, then monthly, and finally 18 months after our first session we agreed that our work was done. By then, Caleb was in 10th grade and doing well. I next heard from the family 2 years later: They sent me a picture of Caleb in his graduation cap and gown, along with a note informing me that Caleb would be going to college in the fall and living on his own in a dormitory. Although he still had brief episodes of anxiety, they were not frequent and they did not prevent him from having an active social life.

FREEING THE FAMILY FROM THE GRIP OF ANXIETY: A DETAILED CASE EXAMPLE

The following case demonstrates how anxiety in an adolescent is linked to interactive processes in the family and how intervening in these processes can provide a new direction for the adolescent and the parents. By presenting this case in detail, I hope to illustrate how themes emerge and develop during sessions, and how the therapist can link together and emphasize different themes to keep the session moving forward.

Danielle is a 16-year-old sophomore at a public high school. Her mother, Abigail, contacted me because she was worried about Danielle, whose school performance had slipped and who appeared unhappy and "moody" at home. Danielle was Abigail and Ray's only child.

At my request, both parents and Danielle attended the first session. I started the session by asking each family member to describe their perception of the problem.

MICUCCI: Can you tell me why you are here today?

ABIGAIL: We've been concerned for a certain amount of time, maybe 6 months, that Danielle doesn't seem to be focusing. She's not doing as well as she used to do in school. She doesn't sleep. She's more moody than I'd expect from a 16-year-old girl. My husband and I talked about it and we thought that before it got worse we should talk to a professional to find out what's going on and how we can help her.

MICUCCI: So you're concerned because Danielle has changed?

ABIGAIL: Yes, and I think she's not as happy as she used to be.

MICUCCI: She's not as happy as she used to be?

ABIGAIL: Yes, she doesn't sleep, she has a poor appetite, she seems to be nervous and worried, and I don't know what to do to help her.

MICUCCI: OK. How about you, Ray? What's your point of view?

RAY: Well, we've seen a drop in grades. Danielle has said that she is anxious and worries a lot. I wonder if we are putting too much pressure on her. I don't want her to be unhappy.

MICUCCI: So both of you are seeing something in Danielle that concerns you?

RAY: Yes, she seems sad, nervous.

MICUCCI: OK, sad and nervous. Danielle, what do you think about these things that your parents have said?

DANIELLE: I think that sometimes they are overprotective. Yes, I don't get a lot of sleep, but I have a lot of work. If they want me to get good grades, then I have to skip on sleep, but I don't think it is a big deal.

MICUCCI: So you think your parents are concerned unnecessarily?

DANIELLE: Sometimes, yeah. I know I've been anxious lately, but I don't think it is such a big deal.

MICUCCI: And what have you been anxious about?

DANIELLE: I don't know, grades, college, sports, just regular stuff like that. I have a lot on my plate, but I don't think it is anything that they should be worried about.

From these descriptions, I inferred the following:

- Abigail has been appointed the spokesperson in the family. She is the one who speaks first and presents her concerns about Danielle.
- Ray has concerns that are similar to those of Abigail, but he is also concerned that he and Abigail might be putting too much pressure on Danielle.
- Danielle dismisses her parents' concerns and instead claims that they are "overprotective."
- Abigail frames the problem as existing inside Danielle. Ray introduces a relational dimension by wondering if Danielle is reacting to parental pressures.

I pursued these themes by asking Danielle to elaborate and carefully tracking what she says.

MICUCCI: So you think your parents might be overly concerned, but you do feel anxious sometimes?

DANIELLE: Yeah, sometimes I guess. But I think they are just looking for things to worry about. Like, the other day, I came home from school and said that I was going to lie down, and she was like, "What's wrong? Why do you have to lie down? Didn't you get enough sleep last night?"

MICUCCI: Is that what you mean by overprotective?

DANIELLE: Yeah. I love them, they do take care of me, but it's tough being the only child.

MICUCCI: It's tough being an only child. What's hard about it for you?

DANIELLE: You're the center of attention. OK, I do like being the center of attention. But sometimes it's just too much.

MICUCCI: Sometimes the attention is too much?

DANIELLE: Yeah, I just want to be like the other kids.

MICUCCI: Have you noticed whether the attention you've been getting from your parents has increased or decreased?

DANIELLE: Definitely increased. Maybe since starting high school. They started asking a lot more questions, where I was going, what I was doing, how much sleep I got, whether I did my homework, stuff like that. It just felt like more babying, and I don't need so much babying.

In the preceding segment, Danielle elaborated on the theme of overprotection and implies that the family may be struggling with age-appropriate issues of independence and differentiation. To keep the process in motion, I then asked the parents to comment on what they heard Danielle saying.

MICUCCI: (to parents) What do you think about what Danielle has been saying?

RAY: Well, I'm not sure what came first. About a year ago the bouts of crying started and grades started to go down.

ABIGAIL: She wants to go to college, and her grades have to be good.

RAY: We don't want to put pressure on her, we want to support her, but now that she's in high school the grades count more.

MICUCCI: OK, you want to be supportive. What about Danielle's comment that she thinks you two have been overprotective?

RAY: Well, it's ... (*Looks at Abigail.*)

MICUCCI: Ray, I noticed you looked at Abigail when I asked that question.

RAY: Well, we talk about this. I think I probably tend to back off more than she does. I think she might worry a little too much, and she thinks I don't worry enough.

ABIGAIL: I don't think you can worry too much. I'm not trying to say that you don't worry enough, but I'm just saying that in this day and age a parent can't worry too much.

I had to redirect the parents to focus on the relational theme ("What about Danielle's comment that she thinks you two have been overprotective?"), then I commented on a nonverbal behavior that could reveal a more subtle aspect of the parental relationship ("I noticed you looked at Abigail when I asked that question"). In response, Ray differentiated his position from that of Abigail. In claiming that Abigail "worries too much," Ray implied that he is less concerned than she and that Abigail's anxiety is excessive. This statement also highlighted a potential coalition between Ray and Danielle, as both were minimizing Abigail's concerns as a reflection of excessive worry.

Rather than highlighting the conflict at this point, I chose to invite Abigail to elaborate on her worries. My goals in the next segment were to strengthen my relationship with Abigail, to avoid becoming inducted into the father–daughter coalition, and to learn more about the nature of Abigail's concerns that could point toward a more complex and complete understanding of the dynamics in the family.

MICUCCI: (*to Abigail*) What are you worried about?

ABIGAIL: I'm worried that in 10 years Danielle won't have lived up to her potential. I'm worried that she's affecting her health by not eating right and not getting enough sleep. I'm worried that she takes on so many things, activities, and sports, and I worry that she will be a jack-of-all-trades and master of none.

MICUCCI: So one thing you're worried about is that the future will turn out badly.

ABIGAIL: Yes.

MICUCCI: That in 10 years she might be very unhappy.

ABIGAIL: Yes, and disappointed.

MICUCCI: And disappointed.

ABIGAIL: Yes, this is the time in a person's life, a young person's life, when the choices she makes really are going to matter. I know some kids her age don't eat right and don't sleep well, but I think it is too much.

MICUCCI: You're worried about her sleeping and eating, and earlier you said that you thought she was anxious.

ABIGAIL: I think she's a really anxious kid, and I think the anxiety is what is causing her to lose her appetite and not sleep well. It's more than I think ...

MICUCCI: ... should be happening.

ABIGAIL: Exactly, thank you.

By ending Abigail's sentence for her, I expressed my understanding and empathy for her position and suggested that it needed to be taken seriously, rather than dismissed as done by Ray and Danielle. In the next segment, I attempted to promote more interaction among the family members, in hopes that I might understand some of the interactional patterns that might be related to the problem.

MICUCCI: So, Danielle, what do you think, do you think you've been more anxious lately?

DANIELLE: Yeah, like I said before, I do have a lot on my plate. And I do think I worry more about things than some of my friends, but I don't agree with my mom that I should be planning out the rest of my life when I'm 16.

MICUCCI: So you and your mom disagree about this?

DANIELLE: Very much so. We agree on a lot of things, but ...

ABIGAIL: Danielle, I never said you had to decide on your future at age 16, but I said that you had to plan for your future.

DANIELLE: I don't know what I want for my future.

ABIGAIL: That's what a plan means, not ...

RAY: Well, Danielle, I think what your mom means ...

MICUCCI: Ray, could you just let the two of them talk about this a little bit, and I'll get to you in a minute?

RAY: Sure.

DANIELLE: But why do I have to be so worried about the future? Can't I just live my life right now?

ABIGAIL: But you can't just forget about the future.

DANIELLE: Who said I was forgetting about the future? You always turn my words around.

ABIGAIL: I do not turn your words around. You need some kind of plan, not written in stone, but a plan that will help you …

DANIELLE: But I don't know what I want.

ABIGAIL: So you need to consider different options.

DANIELLE: I *am* considering options!

ABIGAIL: You've got to explore different paths, but I don't think you're doing that.

MICUCCI: Let me stop you there. Ray, what are you seeing? What do you observe going on here?

Rather than commenting directly on a pattern that has emerged in the session, I will often ask another family member to comment in order to elicit the family member's perspective and to help family members become better observers of their own interactions.

RAY: Well, this is the way they communicate.

MICUCCI: You've seen this before.

RAY: Yeah, they argue a lot and I don't think they listen to one another.

MICUCCI: And it looked to me like you wanted to jump in.

RAY: Well, I see both of their points.

MICUCCI: You see both of their points.

RAY: These are two powerful, intelligent women, and I love them both. But they butt heads. And sometimes I think that I wind up being the intermediary.

MICUCCI: But I noticed that you volunteered for that role, too.

RAY: I know, I did try to jump in.

MICUCCI: What was your reason for doing that?

RAY: There have been some shouting matches, and I didn't want that to happen here. I don't like to see them upset with one another.

MICUCCI: Who do you think gets more upset about the arguing, Danielle or Abigail?

RAY: I think it disturbs Abigail more. I think she worries a lot right now.

MICUCCI: Do you think your jumping in might have been a way to protect Abigail from getting too upset?

RAY: I haven't thought of it that way, but I guess that's it. I don't want Abigail to get upset, and I'd like her to worry less.

MICUCCI: You'd like her to worry less?

RAY: I respect her a lot, but I think she's worrying too much.

ABIGAIL: I think Ray has the same issues with Danielle that I have. He just doesn't call it worrying. But I do think he is worried.

MICUCCI: So you feel that the two of you are on the same page?

ABIGAIL: Very much so.

MICUCCI: Ray, I'm wondering if Danielle has ever talked with you about what she's anxious about.

RAY: Maybe a little bit, not much.

MICUCCI: I wonder if it would be good to do that right now. Danielle, could you tell your dad what it is that worries you the most?

Ray acknowledged that he tries to mediate between Danielle and Abigail in order to prevent the conflict between them from escalating, and he also admitted that he is trying to keep Abigail from getting upset. He tries to differentiate himself from his wife by claiming that he worries less than she does. This seems to exempt him from responsibility for the problem, and now shifts the locus of the anxiety away from Danielle and onto Abigail. While Abigail appears to be an overly protective, anxious parent, she is also closer to Danielle than is Ray and so knows more about her daughter's struggles than Ray does. Rather than seeing Abigail's perspective as biased toward exaggerating her daughter's problems, I chose to pursue the possibility that Ray has not been involved enough to understand how anxious Danielle has been. From Ray's perspective, Abigail is worrying "too much" because he is not aware of how anxious Danielle is and what is provoking this anxiety. So, rather than putting the focus on the parental relationship and encouraging them to resolve the differences between them, I decided to put the focus on the relationship between Danielle and Ray by providing an opportunity for Danielle to talk directly with her father about her worries.

RAY: What are you worried about, Danielle?

DANIELLE: I do worry about my future. Mom doesn't think that I care but I do.

MICUCCI: Can you tell your dad more about your worries?

DANIELLE: I worry if I'm going to be successful, whether I'll have a good future, and I feel that maybe you two wouldn't be so proud of me if I didn't do well.

RAY: What makes you think that about us?

DANIELLE: Well, when I got a C on my report card you freaked out.

RAY: But you didn't do any work in that class.

Before the discussion veered off into an argument between Danielle and Ray, I intervened to redirect the focus to Danielle's worries.

MICUCCI: Can you tell your dad more about your worries that he and your mom might not be proud of you?

DANIELLE: I do worry about that. I worry that I might not make you proud of me and then you'd be unhappy.

MICUCCI: You worry about making your parents unhappy.

RAY: Danielle, you don't need to worry about that …

MICUCCI: Ray, why don't you just listen right now, and help Danielle explain to you how she is feeling?

DANIELLE: Like, Dad, I know you don't like my boyfriend, and I worry what might happen if I wanted to marry him.

RAY: (*Rolls his eyes, but doesn't speak.*)

MICUCCI: What might happen?

DANIELLE: I worry that they wouldn't be proud of me, that they would not get along, and I'd be stuck in the middle.

MICUCCI: And then what?

DANIELLE: And then I might have to choose between them. And I worry about my boyfriend, and I worry that the relationship might not work out.

MICUCCI: Tell your dad how that would make you feel.

DANIELLE: Really sad. And I worry a lot about letting my teammates down. Like I missed that goal in that game last week, and I felt awful, really depressed, because they were counting on me and I let them down.

MICUCCI: (*to Ray*) Ray, do you hear a theme here? Danielle seems to worry a lot about letting people down.

RAY: Yes, I do hear her saying that.

MICUCCI: And if you let people down, then what?

DANIELLE: Then they wouldn't like me.

MICUCCI: They wouldn't like you. That's what you worry about.

Danielle proceeded to talk about this theme, and I assisted by interjecting questions to keep the conversation on topic. Ray listened intently and nodded at appropriate intervals. Abigail was also listening, but holding back from intervening so that Danielle and Ray could talk directly with one another. I then asked the parents to comment on what they had been hearing.

MICUCCI: So, Ray, what do you think about what Danielle has been saying?

RAY: I knew that she was worried, but I guess I didn't know how much.

MICUCCI: I wonder why Danielle hasn't talked with you about this before.

DANIELLE: Because they always rush in with suggestions and solutions, like, "You've got to figure this out right now." That makes me more upset.

MICUCCI: What would be helpful?

DANIELLE: If they just listened.

ABIGAIL: She's right about that. I do try to come up with solutions.

MICUCCI: What I hear her saying is that what would be helpful for her is for you to listen and not rush to come up with solutions. Do you think you'd be able to do that?

ABIGAIL: I can try, but I think it would be hard.

MICUCCI: I wonder if what drives your desire to offer solutions is that you get anxious about what Danielle is telling you. You try to put salve on the wounds, so to speak, rather than let the wound heal naturally on its own.

ABIGAIL: (*after a brief silence*) That would never have entered my mind to let it heal naturally on its own, but that's a different way to look at it, and I will.

MICUCCI: But what about your worries, your anxieties?

ABIGAIL: I guess I would just have to handle them.

MICUCCI: How could Ray help you?

ABIGAIL: If he wouldn't tell me that I was being crazy to worry so much.

MICUCCI: It would help if Ray would listen to you, just like it would help if you could listen to Danielle.

ABIGAIL: Yes, that would help.

MICUCCI: Ray, do you think you could do that?

RAY: I would certainly try.

Here I expanded the theme to include Abigail's anxiety, but this time in a new context. Rather than labeling Abigail as an overly worried or overly protective parent, I used her anxiety to help to link her and Ray together. The family needed to become a better container for anxiety, and this means that they needed to be able to tolerate hearing that someone is distressed without feeling compelled to find a solution. The urgency to find a solution doesn't help, but rather makes the other person more anxious. Ray's attempts to reassure Abigail are intended to be helpful, but they have the effect of making Abigail feel more isolated and more anxious, and thus less able to listen to Danielle without feeling compelled to find a solution. My suggestion was intended to help Ray validate Abigail's feelings and provide support by listening, without trying to convince her that her fears were excessive or unfounded.

MICUCCI: I'd like to make a suggestion. Would that be OK with you? (*Parents nod.*) During this coming week, I'd like you, Ray and Abigail, to go out alone together, somewhere where you can talk and not be disturbed. And I'd like you, Ray, to invite Abigail to tell you all of her worries about Danielle. I'd like you to listen, and not try to talk her out of her worries or offer solutions.

RAY: You're telling me not to try to solve them.

MICUCCI: Not try to talk her out of them.

RAY: Not try to talk her out of them, right.

MICUCCI: After she's told them to you, after you've made sure she's said all that she wants to say, then you are free to comment. But only after she is finished.

RAY: OK. Kind of bite my tongue.

MICUCCI: Right, until she's finished telling you all of her worries.

RAY: Got it. We'll try that.

We scheduled an appointment for the following week and ended the session. When the family returned the following week, none of them looked happy. Both Abigail and Danielle looked like they had been crying, and Ray had a somber expression on his face. While I recognized that the family members were suffering, I did want to follow up on the task I had given Ray and Abigail the week before. If I did not do this, I risked giving the family the message that the tasks I asked them to do were really not important.

MICUCCI: Hello, how are you?

RAY: We had a bump in the road.

MICUCCI: I'm interested in hearing more about that, but before we get into that, I had asked the two of you to take some time together and I was wondering how it went.

RAY: Well, because of what happened it kind of put our plans on hold. We weren't really able to get to that.

MICUCCI: Oh, that's too bad.

ABIGAIL: Ray and I haven't been able to concentrate on ourselves or each other. Danielle's been crying all week and hasn't left her room. She isn't even going to school.

RAY: But I do think we have been a little more conscious of how we talk to one another. I noticed that I was trying to listen more and not jump in.

The parents had absorbed the first message—that they should listen more without rushing to solutions—but not the second—that Abigail needed to take her worries to Ray and Ray needed to listen and validate them. I decided to table this issue for now, and instead inquire about what had gone wrong this week.

MICUCCI: So, let's get to what's been preoccupying you this week. Can you fill me in?

DANIELLE: Tuesday night my boyfriend broke up with me.

MICUCCI: That must have been a big disappointment.

DANIELLE: And I know why he broke up with me. At first I thought it was because I wasn't good enough for him, but then he told me it was because I wouldn't have sex with him. It was devastating.

MICUCCI: Were you able to talk to your parents about this?

DANIELLE: A little. I told my mom the reason, but not my dad.

MICUCCI: Do you think your parents understood how upset you were?

DANIELLE: Yeah, I think so. And he's been spreading rumors about me, you know, that I did sleep with him.

MICUCCI: That must hurt.

DANIELLE: Yeah, now everyone thinks I'm a slut.

MICUCCI: So you've been feeling really, really bad and staying in your room?

DANIELLE: Yeah, I just don't want to leave.

MICUCCI: What do you think would happen if you did leave your room?

Danielle's sequestering herself in her room has potentially serious implications, not the least of which is the possibility that her avoidance behavior could develop into full-blown agoraphobia. I decided to focus on this aspect of her experience and find out more about her anticipated fears.

DANIELLE: I don't know. I just don't want to face anyone.

MICUCCI: What would that be like for you?

DANIELLE: I'm afraid I'd get all emotional in front of people and I don't like that. And I'm afraid that I wouldn't be able to work as hard as I normally do in school and on the team.

MICUCCI: Then what would happen?

DANIELLE: I'd let my teammates down.

MICUCCI: And what would happen if you did?

DANIELLE: They might not like me any more, and I'd be even more unhappy.

MICUCCI: So you worry that your friends might leave you?

DANIELLE: Yeah.

MICUCCI: Like your boyfriend did. If you do something they don't like, they might leave you, and then you'd be all alone.

DANIELLE: Yeah, I do worry about that.

We were back to the theme of abandonment that first surfaced in the last session. At the root of symptoms of anxiety is the dread that one will be abandoned and left alone to cope with one's fears without support. Now that we had touched on this theme, I wanted to expand on it.

MICUCCI: (*to parents*) Did Danielle share these worries with you this week?

ABIGAIL: Not really. When she got off the phone with him she was hysterical and all she could say is that her life was over and it would never be the same. She never said to me the things that she just said to you. All she could say was how devastated she was. That was all I heard.

MICUCCI: And how did that make you feel?

ABIGAIL: Sick. I got physically sick. And weak. Because my child was hurting and I couldn't do anything to make her feel better.

This presented an opportunity to return to the task that I had assigned at the end of the last session.

MICUCCI: Do you think Ray understood how upset you were?

ABIGAIL: Somewhat, I don't know. He just seemed angry at the boy. It was almost like, "I knew this kid was bad news." It was like he was blaming Danielle for being with the kid.

RAY: I am proud of Danielle for doing the right thing. I know how boys can be.

DANIELLE: He was really mad when he found out about the birth control.

MICUCCI: The birth control?

ABIGAIL: I had gotten birth control for Danielle. I hadn't told Ray about it because I knew how he would be.

MICUCCI: How would he be?

ABIGAIL: He wouldn't understand. He'd be against it.

RAY: You don't know that. I'm a reasonable guy. I know how life works. I don't understand why I was left out of this.

MICUCCI: Let's find out. Abigail, could you tell Ray why you felt you couldn't discuss the birth control with him?

ABIGAIL: Ray, I wasn't sure that you wouldn't flip out. You've gone on and on the past few months about how you disliked this boy. You've been very verbal about it. And frankly, I didn't want to add any more fuel to the fire. I had to be proactive and I didn't want a confrontation with you. I didn't want to keep it from you, but I felt that I did not have an alternative.

Abigail's decision to get birth control for Danielle without first consulting Ray exemplifies the structure that was apparent in the previous session. Abigail and Danielle have a bond that sometimes excludes Ray. This has the effect of depriving Danielle of the support and guidance of one of her parents, and also deprives Abigail of the support of her husband. Ray contributes to this pattern by not challenging it and by reacting with anger rather than listening.

MICUCCI: Ray, what's your reaction to what Abigail has said?

RAY: It's hard to hear it, but I can see her point. I was really against Danielle seeing this kid. I knew what kind of kid he was.

ABIGAIL: See, there you go, Ray. You knew what kind of kid he was, so you had made up your mind and there was no talking to you about it.

RAY: Yeah, I see what you mean. (to therapist) I grew up with two brothers. I didn't have any sisters.

MICUCCI: So maybe you know boys but you don't know girls so well?

RAY: Yeah, that seems real clear.

MICUCCI: But now you have an opportunity to learn. By listening.

RAY: Right.

ABIGAIL: Ray, I know I should have discussed the birth control thing with you, and I'm sorry, but I didn't feel like I had a choice.

RAY: I understand that now.

The parents seemed to have reached a resolution of sorts on this issue, and I wanted to return to the theme of abandonment that had emerged earlier in the session.

MICUCCI: OK, can we go back to something that came up earlier? A few minutes ago Danielle said that she worries about being left all alone. Abigail and Ray, could you talk with Danielle about this feeling?

ABIGAIL: I guess I'd like to know how long you've been feeling this way.

DANIELLE: A long time, I guess. I always worry about people not liking me.

ABIGAIL: Why might people not like you?

DANIELLE: I don't like making other people angry. I have to watch what I say and do because I don't want to make them mad. I'm always thinking about this.

RAY: So what can we do to help you not feel this way?

Ray jumps in with an offer to "fix" the problem. As we saw in the last session, the parents' rush to find solutions aborts the conversation about feelings. However, I didn't want to exclude Ray from the conversation so I decided to let it go for now.

DANIELLE: I just wish you guys could back off a little and let me be around my friends more. I wish you guys could just trust me.

ABIGAIL: It's not that we don't trust you, Danielle, it's that we don't trust other people. This is 2009, and I know what can happen out there.

In this family where anxiety rules, Abigail asserts her perception that the world is a dangerous place.

DANIELLE: But I'm 16, Mom. I think I can handle myself.

ABIGAIL: But I thought you were overwhelmed with everything you had to do. Now you want more time with your friends? I don't get it.

DANIELLE: I have so many activities because you wanted me to get involved. I'd like to have a life, eventually. I mean a life outside my soccer friends and my lacrosse friends.

ABIGAIL: OK, so maybe we should sit down and look at your activities and prioritize them.

RAY: (*to Abigail*) Are we starting to fix now?

ABIGAIL: Yeah, maybe.

RAY: Maybe we should let her come up with a proposal and we'll consider it, and maybe offer a counterproposal.

DANIELLE: Like extend my curfew on weekends.

RAY: (*to therapist*) Should we talk about this now?

MICUCCI: No, I think you can take this up at home. I'd like to move on and look at another issue here. Danielle, I know you've been feeling really bad the last few days, but I think we should talk about getting back to school. How could your parents help with that? Could you tell them right now?

The negotiation for age-appropriate privileges is certainly important, but it takes second priority to helping Danielle return to normal functioning.

DANIELLE: Just be there when I need someone to talk to. Don't try to fix things, just listen. That's all I need.

ABIGAIL: I can do that Danielle, I mean, we can do that, but I worry about you. I worry that you might make some bad decisions that will affect the rest of your life.

This is a theme that has emerged before. Abigail's anxiety about Danielle's future prevented her from being able to listen to Danielle without rushing to offer solutions. I decided to pursue this theme now.

MICUCCI: Abigail, what if that happened? How would you feel?

ABIGAIL: Devastated.

MICUCCI: Devastated?

ABIGAIL: Yeah, I would feel sorry for her that she wasted a good portion of her life, that she wouldn't be able to pick up the pieces, that she'd never accomplish what she wants to accomplish.

RAY: She would think it was her fault.

ABIGAIL: I think most mothers would.

MICUCCI: So you would feel very bad, you'd feel worried, you'd feel guilty.

ABIGAIL: At that point, she would be 26, and it's a lot harder to fix the problem when you're 26 than when you're 16.

MICUCCI: And if this came about, how long do you think you'd feel bad?

ABIGAIL: Forever.

MICUCCI: Forever?

ABIGAIL: Yeah, forever, or at least until I could see some progress, that she was back on track and feeling better.

MICUCCI: So you would continue to feel bad as long as Danielle felt bad or until Danielle did something to change the situation?

ABIGAIL: I would continue to feel as badly as I feel until something changed.

MICUCCI: So, if Danielle didn't change the situation, or if she even made things worse, you would just feel worse and worse?

ABIGAIL: I know I shouldn't, but I would.

MICUCCI: Do you think there would be anything you could do to deal with those feelings?

I'm pursuing the theme of enmeshment here. I'm introducing the idea that Abigail might be able to differentiate her feelings from Danielle's, and in so doing she would be in a better position to support her daughter.

ABIGAIL: Well, I could talk with Ray, and I think we'd come to the point that it's her life, and she can do what she wants with it. But I could not imagine myself saying that at this point.

MICUCCI: Your choices would be either saying that to yourself or feeling horrible?

ABIGAIL: I guess I would just have to accept the situation. It would be extremely difficult.

MICUCCI: But you would go to Ray?

ABIGAIL: Yes, I would go to Ray.

MICUCCI: And rely on his support, and do what you can to feel better?

ABIGAIL: Hopefully. Hopefully, I would feel better.

MICUCCI: You know, I think it would be very helpful to your daughter if that "hopefully" could become a "definitely." And here's why I think that. Danielle is frightened about many things, but mostly about being abandoned. We could try to soothe her and say, "Oh, you won't be abandoned. Your friends will stick by you." But we really don't know. No one can absolutely guarantee that bad things won't happen.

ABIGAIL: That's right.

MICUCCI: So what does that leave us with? The only thing we have is our confidence that we will be able to handle anything that might come up. Together, we can handle *anything*. Say to Danielle, "We have absolute confidence in you that you can handle this thing and we will be there for you."

RAY: We would try our best, hopefully.

MICUCCI: We would *definitely* do our best. We would *definitely* be there for you.

ABIGAIL: We would definitely be there for you.

MICUCCI: And it applies to you, too, Abigail. If Danielle made some bad decisions, you would definitely handle it. You might cry for a while, you might be unhappy for a while, but as a strong woman you know you can handle anything.

ABIGAIL: I never looked at it like that.

MICUCCI: But you are a strong woman.

ABIGAIL: Yes, I am.

MICUCCI: The root of all fear is the fear that I'm not going to be able to handle it and I'll be all alone. But once you believe that you can handle anything, fears lose their power over you.

ABIGAIL: That's true.

MICUCCI: So, if Danielle comes to you and tells you that she is worried about something, or upset about something, rather than telling her that what she is worried about won't happen, or that it's not a big deal if it does, wouldn't it be better to listen and convey to her your confidence that she could handle it? To give her the message, "If this thing happens, we have the utmost confidence that you will be able to handle it. And if you need us, we are here."

ABIGAIL: That would be good.

The antidote to anxiety and dread is confidence. Sometimes, we have to "fake it until we make it," but belief in our own competence is more reliable than empty reassurances that feared outcomes will not come to pass. I also want to emphasize here that Abigail can be of most help to her daughter if she modeled confidence and communicated to Danielle that she believed in her capacity to handle adversity. I now wanted to explore Danielle's reactions to this conversation.

MICUCCI: Danielle, if your parents said that to you, how would you feel?

DANIELLE: It would give me a confidence boost, that they have confidence in me.

MICUCCI: We can never be guaranteed that bad things won't happen, but we can believe in ourselves that we can handle them if they do.

ABIGAIL: To be perfectly honest, I never would have thought to handle it like that. I would never have thought of saying that.

RAY: But it is not foreign to us.

MICUCCI: Maybe you've already done it sometimes without realizing it.

RAY: Exactly.

MICUCCI: So, Danielle, what about going back to school?

DANIELLE: I have to go back.

MICUCCI: The longer you stay away, the harder it might get.

DANIELLE: I know that. I will be hard, though.

MICUCCI: Maybe not as hard as you think. After all, you're a strong person and you've probably handled harder things in the past. And if you need support, your parents are there to believe in you.

DANIELLE: OK, I see that.

MICUCCI: And then, maybe you could negotiate for more privileges, because then they will see you having more confidence in yourself and will believe you can handle them.

I ended by returning to an earlier theme: Danielle's desire for more freedom to be herself and make her own mistakes. I link this desire with the theme of confidence, that by demonstrating to her parents that she is able to handle difficult situations she will encourage them to give her more freedom.

In this case, what was presented as the daughter's symptom was linked to a family pattern characterized by an enmeshed mother–daughter relationship that both promoted and was sustained by a distant, disapproving father. Rather than directly challenging the mother's presumed overprotectiveness, I validated her feelings and encouraged her husband to do the same. Rather than encouraging the parents' efforts to reassure Danielle and soothe her anxieties by finding solutions for her, I instead encouraged them to support her confidence in her ability to handle difficult situations when they arose.

Danielle's fear of abandonment doesn't really have an "answer." No one can guarantee that she will not be rejected and that people will not disappoint her or disapprove of her. The rejection by her boyfriend brought this message home. The more the parents tried to run interference for her by arranging her life so that she wouldn't feel bad, the less confident Danielle became that she could handle difficult situations on her own. As we discovered in the second session, Abigail's motive for being so "helpful" was to prevent her own fears from coming true: that Danielle might have a "bad life" and this would prove that she was a bad parent. These fears all needed to be uncovered, and the family relationships reorganized so that the family members would be more resilient. This meant that Abigail needed to differentiate herself from Danielle, and rely on Ray's support to do so. It also meant that Ray needed to listen and validate feelings without rushing to find a solution. Finally, it meant that Danielle needed to feel that her parents had confidence in her, which could happen only if they "backed off" and allowed her to struggle with her own problems while they listened to her empathically and communicated their belief in her competence.

SUMMARY

In this chapter I presented several case examples illustrating how to help families with anxious adolescents. Here are some principles to keep in mind when working with anxious adolescents and their families:

• Symptoms of anxiety, as are all symptoms, are embedded in a cycle of interactions in the family. By identifying and interrupting these interpersonal cycles, the therapist can help to free the family from the constricting influence that anxiety has over all of their lives.

• When an adolescent is anxious, it is often the case that other family members are anxious as well. In some cases, a child's anxiety helps to distract the family members from other problems or conflicts.

• Often, the parents' efforts to help the anxious child are making the problem worse. By trying to help their child by accommodating to the anxiety, they give the child the message that the youngster's fears are justified. These messages contribute to the child's insecurity and intensify the worry that he or she will be left alone to cope with overwhelming terrors. By blocking parental overprotectiveness and giving the family members space to express their true feelings to one another, it is possible to help these families gradually free themselves from the grip of anxiety.

8

Defiant and Disruptive Behavior

As it so often happens, the boy before me belied the description I had received from his mother on the phone only 4 hours earlier. With wavy brown hair stuffed carelessly beneath a baseball cap and an impish smile, 15-year-old Keith greeted me with a firm handshake that reminded me that he had been a leader in the military boarding school he had attended until he was expelled for his behavior 3 months ago. This was not the angry, bitter boy I had expected to see.

Keith's mother, Pam, had called in desperation on the recommendation of a colleague who suggested they see me. He was becoming increasingly disruptive and confrontational in his behavior, culminating recently in an incident in which he threatened his mother with a kitchen knife when she refused to give him $20. Pam was sure that Keith was using drugs, certainly marijuana and possibly hallucinogens, because she had overheard some of Keith's telephone conversations. Keith made no attempt to conceal his drug use, declaring, "Marijuana is not a drug."

Keith respected none of his parents' limits. He defied his 11 P.M. curfew, and several times a week stayed out all night, coming home mid-afternoon the next day in a disheveled state, falling into bed and then sleeping until 10 P.M., only to repeat the pattern. When his parents challenged him, he'd defiantly retort, "Try to stop me. I'm making my own rules now." After being expelled from military school, he enrolled in the local public school but had stopped attending. On three occasions, Pam had discovered money missing from her purse, and she suspected that Keith was stealing from her.

Keith's father, Stu, a shy, soft-spoken man in his mid-40s, had sometimes tried to block the front door to prevent Keith from leav-

217

ing the house, but Keith would push his father aside. These confrontations had grown more violent, as both Stu and Keith stood their ground more decisively. A week before our session, Stu and Keith were wrestling on the floor of the living room while Pam looked on in horror. Unable to take it any more, Pam cried out, "Just let him go, Stu. Let him go." Stu stopped struggling, and Keith ran out of the house. The next day, Pam quit her job so she could stay home all day to supervise Keith. It didn't work. Keith continued his rampage, and Pam was even more frightened now, because she was alone in the house most of day.

"We just don't know her anymore," Helen sighed in response to my question about the problem in the family. She and Tammy's father, John, had been divorced for 5 years but had maintained a good relationship. "For the sake of the kids," John said. Their older daughter was attending college, and their younger daughter, Tammy, age 14, was, in their words, "running wild." She was a good student until she started ninth grade this year, and then "all hell broke loose." Since Tammy developed earlier than most of the other girls, she attracted the attention of older boys. Before long, she was associating with a "bad crowd." Within months, she was pregnant and had an abortion. Now, she was being treated for a sexually transmitted disease.

Tammy didn't deny that she was sexually active, and described herself as "serially monogamous," a rather sophisticated term for a 14-year-old, I noted. When I asked her what she meant, she replied that she never slept with more than one boy at a time, but that she had "hooked up" with five or six different boys over the past 6 months. Each relationship burned with intensity for a few weeks, then fizzled, only to be replaced by the next.

Tammy's grades had fallen from A's and B's to C's and D's. She was skipping school but did attend most of the time. She violated curfew regularly but had never stayed out all night. Though verbally disrespectful to her parents, she had never physically assaulted them or anyone else. The worst incident she and her parents could recall was when she threw a book at the wall in a fit of anger.

Tammy admitted that she had tried marijuana and alcohol but didn't use them on a regular basis because she didn't like them. "I don't know what all the fuss is about," she said, "I don't need that stuff to feel good." She associated with friends who used drugs and alcohol but denied that she was tempted to join them: "It's cool, you know, like they do their thing and I do mine." When I asked her what "her thing" was, she thought for a moment and answered, "Life, man. I just want to enjoy my life. And I am. They [indicating her parents] just need to chill."

Tyrone had been diagnosed with attention-deficit disorder and was taking methylphenidate. Seen for his late afternoon appointment when the medication was wearing off, Tyrone fidgeted in his seat. He typically came to sessions 10 or 15 minutes late, sheepishly apologizing that he had "lost track of time," even though I noticed that he wore a wristwatch.

Tyrone and Lureen, his mother, agreed that they had a good relationship. They spent time together and talked often about Tyrone's plans for the future. He played sports at school and had a part-time job on the weekends. Tyrone denied using drugs, and his mother believed him, because she trusted Tyrone and knew that he had never lied to her.

"He's a good boy," Lureen said, smiling at Tyrone, "but I'm scared. He's so close, now, and I don't want him to fall."

Indeed, Tyrone had accomplished much compared to the other boys in his neighborhood. He was in his senior year at high school and had won a track scholarship to college. But his grades had slipped and he wasn't coming home on time. He and his mom were having more and more arguments, and Tyrone was staying away just to avoid the confrontations. Tyrone had been dating a girl for 6 months and was very attached to her.

"When I'm out with Cindy, I just find it so hard to leave," Tyrone said. "I'm having such a good time that I can't break away. I know I should, but I can't."

Lureen snapped back, "Well if you can't now, what will you do when you get to college? You tell me, Tyrone. If you can't walk the walk now, how are you going to make it in college?" Tyrone sighed and didn't answer.

These vignettes present three different faces of adolescent problem behavior. These cases seem so different from one another, it's easy to miss what they have in common. In each, there is conflict between the parent and the child about what constitutes "appropriate" behavior. The adolescent's misbehavior has seized the attention of the parents, and arguments about the youth's behavior have begun to dominate the family interactions. The parents feel frightened, helpless, angry, and guilty. Their sense of control over their own environment has been shaken, and they cling desperately to what little authority they have left.

There are also important differences among these three families. Keith's family is on the brink of chaos, and there is a high risk that he or another family member could be harmed. Tyrone, and even Tammy, though crossing the limits, still maintain a relationship with their parents, still see their parents as important figures in their lives, and want to stay connected to them. While Keith seems so self-involved that he can't fathom what his parents might be feeling, Tammy and Tyrone seem to be able to empathize, at least partially, with their parents' predicament. Tyrone, on the verge of leaving home, has already accomplished much, but Tammy is still in the dawn of her adolescence and still has 3 years of high school ahead of her; 3 years in which she could drift farther and farther into trouble.

HOW COMMON IS PROBLEM BEHAVIOR DURING ADOLESCENCE?

It's difficult to obtain accurate estimates of the prevalence of problem behaviors among adolescents. Statistics are based either on self-report or arrest records, and both sources are likely to be biased, the former by the veracity of the reporters, the latter by varying community definitions of what constitutes a delinquent act. According to statistics released by the National Center for Juvenile Justice (Snyder & Sickmund, 2006), the arrest rate in 2006 for all juveniles between the ages of 10 and 17 was about 6.6%. The arrest rate for boys (9.2%) is higher than that for girls (3.9%) and the arrest rate for African Americans (12.2%) is more than twice that for Caucasians (5.8%). One factor contributing to this racial difference in prevalence is that police are more likely to arrest a minority youth suspected of an offense than a white youth suspected of a similar offense. Another factor is the correlation between economic poverty and delinquency (Elliott & Ageton, 1980).

When less serious problem behaviors are considered, the rates are even higher. By age 17, 43% of all youth have stolen something worth less than $50, 37% have vandalized property, 33% have been suspended from school at least once, 18% have run away from home, and 8% have belonged to a gang (Snyder & Sickmund, 2006). In all instances, rates are higher for males than for females. Because of a tendency for problem behaviors to cluster together (Jessor & Jessor, 1977), it is important to note that some adolescents are multiple offenders while most engage in none of the more serious forms of problematic behaviors.

National surveys have revealed that over 70% of high school seniors and almost 40% of 8th graders have drunk alcohol (Johnston, O'Malley, Bachman, & Schulenberg, 2008). The same survey reported that nearly 30% of 12th graders and 5% of 8th graders admit to having been drunk at least once in the past month. Over 40% of 12th graders have tried marijuana, about 10% have tried LSD or other hallucinogens, and about 8% have tried cocaine. About 5% of seniors reported daily use of marijuana. Because these statistics are based on self-report, they probably underestimate the actual prevalence of substance use among adolescents. Regional differences in prevalence must also be taken into account.

DEVELOPMENTAL PERSPECTIVES

Contrary to popular belief, hormonal changes are not the primary cause of erratic behavior during adolescence (Buchanan et al., 1992). While hormonal changes associated with puberty have a small influence on behavior and moods during early adolescence (Archibald et al., 2006), environmental factors are far more important than biological factors in influencing adolescent behavior.

Timing of pubertal development appears to be a risk factor for girls but not for boys. Early developing girls are at higher risk for behavior problems, but only if the girls had problems prior to adolescence, or if they associate with older peers (Caspi & Moffitt, 1991; Magnusson, Strattin, & Allen, 1985; Silbereisen, Petersen, Albrecht, & Kracke, 1989). For young adolescents (and older adolescents who are delayed in their development), the "personal fable" of invulnerability leads them to underestimate the risks involved in potentially dangerous activities (Elkind, 1967; see also Chapter 2).

Some adolescents have difficulty appreciating the effects of their actions because of delayed development in perspective-taking abilities (see Selman, 1980, and Chapter 2). By age 14 or 15, most adolescents can appreciate the perspective of another person, but some teenagers are unable to hold in mind at the same time their own perspective and the perspective of another person, a necessary step in arriving at a solution that meets the needs of both parties.

In terms of Kohlberg's stages of moral development, most adolescents are at Stage 3, where earning the approval of others constitutes the basis for making moral decisions. If adolescents associate mainly with deviant peers, then their decisions are likely to be based on what they think will earn the approval of these peers. Youngsters who have not yet reached Stage 3 are motivated primarily by concrete rewards (Stage 2) or avoidance of "getting caught" (Stage 1).

According to Kegan's theory (see Chapter 2), most adolescents are at the "interpersonal" stage of development (i.e., they have not yet fully differentiated themselves from the reference group of peers). Thus, many adolescents have difficulty distinguishing their own values from those of the peer group. As an additional complication, rule-breaking (so-called "deviant") peers are likely to comprise the primary reference group for adolescents who exhibit problem behavior.

FACTORS RELATED TO ADOLESCENT DEFIANCE

Some adolescents who engage in defiant behavior have limited capacity for impulse control associated with other complicating factors such as attention-deficit disorder, learning disabilities, or serious psychiatric problems such as psychosis, bipolar disorder, or substance abuse. While a thorough assessment for the presence of any of these factors is always indicated, in this chapter I emphasize the role that relationships with parents and peers play in the development and maintenance of defiance among adolescents.

Peer Relationships and Defiant Behavior

One finding that consistently emerges in the literature is that adolescents who associate with peers who are engaged in defiant behavior are likely to engage in similar behaviors themselves (Ary et al., 1999; Aseltine, 1995; Dishion & Loeber, 1985; Heinze et al., 2004). One factor that appears to influence the adolescent's choice of associates is the degree to which the adolescent is attached to societal institutions such as school, home, church, or place of employment (Hirschi, 1969). Adolescents who are involved in a variety of activities are less likely to gravitate toward deviant peers. An adolescent who does reasonably well academically, seems to have decent relationships with teachers, is involved in some extracurricular activities, has a job, or regularly attends religious services is less likely to be attracted to (or be attractive to) a deviant peer group. If an adolescent's school experience has been frustrating and humiliating, the adolescent might repudiate the importance of school in his or her life. This can snowball into repudiation of all activities associated with school, such as organized sports or clubs. Once adolescents have earned a reputation for being irresponsible, it is harder to redeem themselves and harder for them to compete with the more successful youngsters for the limited job opportunities for teenagers. These kids will have plenty of time on their hands to find the other disenchanted youth in their community.

In considering the role of the peer group in promoting defiant behavior, it is important to understand that the relationship between peer-group norms and the behavior of individual group members is bidirectional: Peer-group norms do influence individual behavior, but it is also true that "birds of a feather flock together" (Brown, 1990). Adolescents gravitate toward so-called "deviant" peers, who then reinforce each other's rule-breaking behavior. True, there are some adolescents who have such low self-worth and are so famished for approval that they will do almost anything to get accepted. But this case is the exception rather than the rule. Most of the time, troublesome kids find each other and then egg each other on (Dishion, Patterson, Stoolmiller, & Skinner, 1991).

The Importance of Relationships with Parents

While it is true that association with deviant peers is linked to problem behavior, the adolescent's relationship with parents also plays an important role. Research has demonstrated a link between association with rule-breaking peers and ineffective parental monitoring and discipline (Dishion, Capaldi, Spracklen, & Li, 1995; Snyder, Dishion, & Patterson, 1986). Furthermore, adolescents who associate with rule-breaking peers are less likely to engage in similar behavior themselves if their parents effectively monitor them (Farrell & White, 1998; Galambos et al., 2003; Vitaro et al., 2000; Wood et al., 2004).

But parental monitoring and discipline are not the only factors that are important in preventing defiant behavior among adolescents. The strength of the adolescent's attachment to his or her parents has also been shown to be an important factor. Studies have demonstrated that weak attachments to parents are associated with problem behavior among adolescents (Allen et al., 1998, 2002; Arbona & Power, 2003; Eamon & Mulder, 2005; Farrell & White, 1998; Marcus & Betzer, 1996; Paschall, Ennett, & Flewelling, 1996; Smith & Krohn, 1995). Moreover, relationships with parents and peers interact in influencing the frequency and severity of an adolescent's involvement in problem behavior. Adolescents who have a strong relationship with their parents are less likely to associate with deviant peers (Brown et al., 1993; Freeman & Brown, 2001). Moreover, a strong relationship with parents attenuates the link between having "deviant" associates and engaging in problem behavior (Dorius et al., 2004; Farrell & White, 1998; Vitaro et al., 2000; Wood et al., 2004).

In other words, adolescents who have a strong relationship with their parents are less likely to gravitate toward deviant peers. Among those who do associate with deviant peers, having a strong bond with parents reduces the chances of engaging in problem behavior.

Longitudinal studies have discovered a reciprocal relationship between defiant behavior and the gradual erosion of the parent–adolescent relationship (Buist et al., 2004; Laird, Pettit, Bates, & Dodge, 2003; Scaramella, Conger, Spoth, & Simons, 2002). The more the adolescent acts out, the more helpless and angry the parents feel. Parents begin to feel they have no influence or importance to the child, and so may abdicate their parental role, or become so focused on controlling the youth that they lose sight of other aspects of their relationship. The more the adolescent acts out, the less the parents like him or her, the more they treat him or her not with kindness and affection, but with redoubled attempts at control, which elicits more defiant behavior. The defiant behavior weakens relationships that already have a weak link.

Thus, in families with defiant adolescents, the symptomatic cycle operates in the following way (see Figure 8.1):

1. Defiant behavior first arises in the context of weakened attachments to parents and/or ineffective parenting.
2. As the defiance intensifies, the bond between the adolescent and parents is weakened further. The adolescent may gravitate

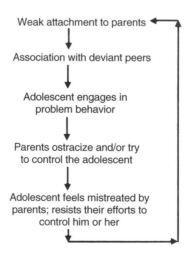

FIGURE 8.1. The symptomatic cycle in adolescent problem behavior.

toward deviant peers as a "substitute family." These deviant peers encourage and reinforce more defiance.

3. In response, the parents, who feel that they have little influence on the child, may abdicate their parental role, distance themselves from the youth, or instead become focused on controlling the adolescent using ineffective punitive methods.

4. These parental responses lead to further estrangement in the family, push the youngster even more in the direction of deviant peers, and result in more anger and defiance, thus continuing the cycle.

Helping families who are caught in this cycle requires the therapist to address both the loss of parental authority as well as the weakened relationship between the adolescent and the parents. Therapists must resist the pull to join the parents in trying to tame an "out of control" kid. Rather, the therapist must balance efforts to strengthen the parental hierarchy with efforts to repair the dislocated relationships in the family. The therapist must shift back and forth between supporting the parents and supporting the adolescent, between strengthening the hierarchy and encouraging age-appropriate autonomy (Micucci, 1995, 2006). How these ingredients are blended depends on the severity of the problem.

ASSESSING THE SEVERITY OF THE PROBLEM

Problem behaviors in adolescence often cluster together, so that involvement in one tends to predict involvement in another (Jessor & Jessor, 1977). However, I find it useful to think of problem behavior as falling on a continuum from mild to moderate to severe that depends on the variety and frequency of the behavior and the potential for harm to self or others (see Table 8.1).

When the problem is *mild*, the adolescent might "test limits" by violating rules or showing verbal disrespect to the parents. However, there are also many instances of compliant and prosocial behavior, with no incidents of violence against property or people. A youngster, such as Tyrone, who comes in after his curfew, talks back to his parents, or refuses to clean his room, would be classified as exhibiting "mild" problem behavior.

When the problem is *moderate*, the adolescent will show a more persistent pattern of defiance in a number of areas. These kids might be regular users of alcohol or drugs, or, like Tammy, might be engaging in promiscuous sexual activity. School performance is often marginal, and there are likely to be frequent arguments with family members, often involving

TABLE 8.1. Assessing the Severity of Adolescent Problem Behavior

Mild problem behavior

- Adolescent tests limits by violating rules or showing verbal disrespect to parents
- Many instances of compliant and prosocial behavior
- No violence against property or people

Moderate problem behavior

- More persistent pattern of defiance
- Might be regular users of alcohol or drugs
- Might be engaging in promiscuous sexual activity
- Marginal school performance
- Frequent arguments with family members, involving cursing, threats, fits of temper
- No violence to anyone in the home
- Legal involvement, if any, has been minimal

Severe problem behavior

- Possibility of serious danger either to the adolescent or to other family members
- Running away or staying out overnight
- Daily use of drugs and/or multiple drug use
- Problems with the law
- Theft from the family
- Physical violence
- Truancy, failure, and/or serious behavior problems at school

cursing, threats, and fits of temper. However, they have never assaulted anyone in the family, and legal involvement, if any, has been minimal. Adolescents who are failing at school, known to be using marijuana on a regular basis, regularly defy curfews, and curse at their parents would be classified as exhibiting "moderate" problem behavior.

Severe problems pose the risk of serious and imminent danger either to the adolescent or to the family. There might be a pattern of running away, staying out all night, repeated and/or multiple drug use, problems with the law, theft from the family, or physical violence. If these kids are attending school at all, they are likely to be truant, failing, and defiant. The case of Keith, which opened this chapter, exemplifies severe problem behavior.

Whether to emphasize interventions to strengthen the parental hierarchy or interventions to repair the ruptured relationships in the family depends on the severity of the problem. When the adolescent's defiant behavior is mild or moderate in severity, relatively more emphasis should be placed on strengthening family relationships. If attention in these cases is given to shoring up the parental hierarchy, these interventions should be embedded in a larger context of repairing relationship ruptures and strengthening the adolescent's bond to the family. Parents should not be encouraged to view therapy as a means of helping them tame or control an "unruly" adolescent. Rather, efforts to support the parents' authority should be firmly grounded in their care and concern for the child. Parents should be encouraged to replace erratic or reactive modes of response with carefully planned consequences that are delivered in a caring, benevolent manner, motivated by their desire to protect the adolescent, themselves, and other family members, and not by a desire to punish the child.

To focus attention on the relationship between the adolescent and the parents, it is important to use the language of feelings and emotions. The therapist should explore with the adolescent and the family how it came to be that the parents' feelings and wishes have become unimportant to the adolescent. This issue must be addressed explicitly and the parents must be helped to listen to the answer. Key questions that are important to explore include:

> "Since you have made it clear that your child's behavior gravely distresses you, why does your child seem to care so little for your feelings?"
> "Why doesn't he or she do what you ask simply because he or she doesn't want to upset you?"
> "How did it come about that your child stopped wanting to please you and instead decided that what you want is no longer important?"

For example, Harry was frustrated because his 14-year-old son, Bryce, had started smoking and refused to do his household chores. He threatened the boy with a variety of consequences, but none of them seemed to work. Harry wanted me to "talk some sense" into the boy. Instead, I asked, "Why does Bryce seem to care so little for your feelings? Why doesn't he do what you ask simply because he doesn't want to upset you?"

Questions such as this frequently take parents by surprise because many of them have given up on the prospect of a relationship with their child that is based on mutual care and concern. Since they don't think the kid cares how they feel, they never mention to the child how sad their behavior is making them feel and instead they simply resort to power struggles. My question was designed to break this unproductive pattern. By focusing attention on the quality of the relationship between Harry and Bryce, I hoped to encourage them to begin talking with one another about their feelings, and thus change the nature of their interactions from one characterized by conflict and control to one characterized by care and concern.

As a result of my question, Harry and Bryce talked about their relationship. Bryce revealed that he believed that Harry didn't like him anymore, and grudgingly admitted that he missed the good times they spent together when Bryce was younger. "Why should I do anything for someone who hates me?" Bryce asked. Harry was surprised to hear that his son believed that he hated him, but agreed that their relationship had seriously deteriorated over the past few years. I encouraged Harry to talk with Bryce about his care and concern for the boy, and why Bryce's smoking and refusal to help out around the house made Harry sad. As the bond between father and son began to repair, Bryce became more amenable to his father's influence, and more willing to accept his father's guidance and restrictions as manifestations of the care and concern his father had for him.

In each of the sections below, I discuss specific ways in which these principles might be applied to families who are struggling with angry and defiant adolescents. The theme remains the same: Although work must proceed on two fronts simultaneously—supporting parental authority and repairing ruptured relationships—the emphasis should generally be on the latter, except when the adolescent's defiance is so severe that either the adolescent or other family members are in immediate danger.

INTERVENTIONS WHEN THE PROBLEM IS MILD

The emergence of mild problem behavior in an adolescent otherwise developing normally often signals that the family is experiencing difficulty making a developmental transition. Mild episodes of defiance are to be expected during early adolescence, as the youngster begins to assert autonomy and challenge limits. Families who have difficulties at this stage might be struggling with the developmental transitions involved in becoming parents of adolescents, who no longer willingly comply with parental expectations. Providing guidance on adolescent development and effective parenting strategies can help these families.

In some cases, difficulty adapting to commonplace adolescent defiance could signal that the family might be experiencing stress in another area of their lives, which might be impeding the necessary structural changes. For example, a weak marital bond might be weakened further by the normal demands of having an adolescent child. The developmental transitions associated with midlife (Steinberg & Steinberg, 1994), the demands of caring for aging or infirm parents, changes in job status, or health crises could all be creating demands on the family that manifest in a struggle over relatively minor episodes of adolescent defiance. In these cases, it is important to place the adolescent's defiance in context, and not focus exclusively on this issue. Rather, the focus of therapy should expand to include attention to other stressors affecting the family.

The case of Louis first introduced in Chapter 3 illustrates these principles. The parents sought therapy for their son because they were frustrated with his curfew violations and falling grades. At my request, the parents accompanied Louis to the first session. In Chapter 4, I discussed how I structured this first session, and arrived at a definition of the problem that focused on the relationships among the family members rather than solely on Louis's noncompliance. In subsequent sessions, it became clear that problems in the marital relationship were undermining the parents' ability to respond effectively to Louis's defiant behavior.

The symptomatic cycle in this family is illustrated in Figure 8.2. Mickey's job required him to be "on the road" traveling between Monday morning and Friday evening. During the week, Judy was responsible for managing the household and dealing with Louis. Judy was lonely and sought out Louis's company. Louis, however, experienced his moth-

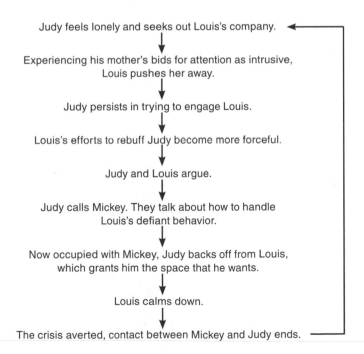

FIGURE 8.2. The symptomatic cycle in Louis's family.

er's bids for his attention as intrusions on his independence, and would respond by defiantly pushing her away. This would lead to an argument between Judy and Louis. Judy would then call Mickey, who, after first berating her for not being more effective, would help her calm down and think about possible responses to Louis. Since Judy was now occupied with Mickey, Louis was freed from his mother's intrusive attention. Louis was then able to calm down and the conflict between him and Judy dissipated.

It was clear from this pattern that Louis's defiance could not be understood apart from the dynamic in this family. While Louis was certainly defiant and at times oppositional, it was also the case that Judy's pushing him for more closeness than he could tolerate provoked a defiant response. When Judy backed off, Louis calmed down. But what helped Judy to back off was contact with Mickey, which alleviated her loneliness and allowed her to step back from Louis. In order to help this family, the relationship between Mickey and Judy needed to be addressed.

The first few sessions had focused almost entirely on the relationship between Mickey and Louis. Through these conversations, Mickey came to see a different side of Louis, and began to realize that Louis was not as unreasonable as he thought he was. They were able to talk over some of their arguments and Louis seemed willing to compromise on his parents' rules and expectations. Following these conversations, Louis's behavior on the weekends when Mickey was at home started to improve. However, the weekday arguments between Louis and Judy continued. This was not surprising, given the symptomatic cycle described above.

The next intervention focused on the relationship between Mickey and Judy. I asked them to talk with each other about ways in which they could be more supportive of each other during Mickey's weekly travels. I then suggested the possibility that Judy might accompany Mickey on some of these trips. The parents were initially reluctant to consider this idea, fearful that Louis would take advantage of their absence to "run wild." However, the foundation laid by the conversations between Mickey and Louis provided an opportunity for them to talk about "ground rules" that would be followed while Judy was away. Another incentive for Louis, I pointed out, was that it was an opportunity for him to demonstrate to his parents that he was capable of more independence and could be trusted. The parents eventually agreed that Judy would meet Mickey mid-week and then drive back home with him on Friday night. Louis agreed to behave, and as a demonstration of his trustworthiness, offered to meet with me alone during his parents' absence. This was the beginning of work to help strengthen the parental bond, which allowed Louis the room to make his own mistakes and removed the pressure from him to be Judy's companion while Mickey was away.

Mild Defiance in Older Adolescents

When an older adolescent suddenly develops a pattern of mild defiant behavior, it is likely that the issue involves the developmental transition from living in the parental home to living more independently. These cases often reflect an adolescent's attempt to manage anxiety associated with increased demands for independence, and the parents' anxiety over letting go.

The key to successful intervention in these cases of mild defiant behavior is to facilitate more effective conflict resolution by the family. Unlike cases of more serious defiance, which are discussed later in this chapter, the focus should not be on strengthening the parental hierarchy. While it might indeed be the case that parents are not consistent or united in their response to the problem behavior, what is more significant is the fact that the family is struggling with a developmental transition. Thus, it is important to expand the focus beyond the presenting problem of the adolescent's defiance. By encouraging direct discussion of the adolescent's and parents' worries about the transition, the therapist can facilitate the identification of more appropriate solutions. Youngsters can be encouraged to talk with their parents about their feelings about growing up, their plans for the future, and worries about the years ahead. Concentrate on what the family is doing right, direct attention away from the problem behavior, and put the kid's behavior in the context of the developmental transitions that the family is facing (see Table 8.2).

In Tyrone's case, for example, I expanded the dialogue beyond the issue of Tyrone's curfew violations. His difficulty saying "good-bye" to his girlfriend at the end of the evening was framed as a metaphor for the developmental transition that was about to take place in this family:

TABLE 8.2. Interventions for Mild Problem Behavior

Key = Facilitate more effective conflict resolution by the family.

- Focus should not be on strengthening parental hierarchy.
- Concentrate on:
  - Strengthening relationships.
  - Improving dialogue.
  - Improving conflict resolution.
  - Helping parents provide age-appropriate guidance.
- Build on what the family is doing right.
- Put the problem behavior in the context of the developmental transitions the family is facing.
- Expand the dialogue beyond the immediate problem issue.

Tyrone was leaving for college and saying "good-bye" to his mother, his home, and his neighborhood. As we explored the implications of this metaphor, Tyrone began to understand that leaving his girlfriend's house in time to make his curfew would be good practice for the bigger "good-bye" he was to face in a few months. Lureen realized that berating Tyrone for his lateness or imposing more severe consequences didn't really help. While these measures might encourage more compliance from Tyrone around curfew, it would actually undermine what she really wanted, namely, that Tyrone would come to monitor and regulate his own behavior. She realized that the issue was, in fact, "leave taking" in general, and not obedience to rules. With my encouragement, she decided to leave the hour of curfew up to Tyrone. However, before he left the house, he would commit himself to coming home at a specific time. Thus, both goals were served: Tyrone would recognize that leave taking was inevitable, and he would also be responsible for regulating himself to meet a commitment he had made rather than simply capitulating to his mother's limits. Meanwhile, I encouraged Tyrone to challenge himself to grow by forcing himself to leave his girlfriend's house on time and then writing down his feelings in a journal after he returned home.

INTERVENTIONS FOR MODERATELY SEVERE DEFIANCE

When the problem has escalated to the point of repeated defiance, open hostility toward the family, or a persistent pattern of potentially dangerous behavior (e.g., frequent drug use), more decisive interventions are required. At this point, the family interactions more often than not revolve around struggles with each other about the adolescent's behavior. External systems, such as the school or the police, might now be involved, and the parents might be in direct conflict with each other and with the external systems about what to do about the adolescent. The youngster is likely to feel misunderstood and alienated, and might redouble efforts to assert independence in ways that invite only more efforts at control from adults.

When problem behavior has progressed to this level, it is often the case that attempts to control the adolescent have eclipsed the parents' efforts to maintain or strengthen their emotional attachment with their child. In contrast to the milder cases discussed in the previous section, which pose no physical danger to anyone and where family members retain positive relationships with each other, in cases of moderately severe problematic behavior the family interactions are dominated by the problem. Anger and frustration pervade the family. The more ineffective the parents are in reining in the adolescent, the more their authority erodes in a repeating cycle. The involvement of other systems (e.g., school, legal authorities) reinforces the parents' feelings of failure. While the therapist cannot discount the degree of frustration experienced by the parents, it is imperative to keep in mind that the adolescent is also experiencing intense feelings of alienation and abandonment.

The central principle of intervention at this level is to redirect the parents' efforts away from control toward rebuilding their relationship with the adolescent (see Table 8.3). This is not an easy task, since the youth's behavior invites controlling responses from the parents. The parents are understandably reluctant to relinquish what they feel is the last vestige of control over a young person who seems determined to self-destruct. They may be convinced that the kid is "out of control" and needs them to impose even firmer controls "for his or her own good." On the other hand, some parents simply give up, abdicate responsibility, and withdraw in defeat. Both strategies are likely to increase the child's alienation from the parents and promote involvement with deviant peers who are in the same boat.

From Control to Relationships

There is a way to reconcile the importance of supporting the parents while also discouraging efforts to dominate the adolescent: Encourage the parents to employ methods of influence that are grounded in their emotional investment in their child rather than methods oriented toward restricting or overpowering the child. For example, consider the case of Harry and Bryce discussed above. Harry was locked in a futile power struggle with Bryce over the boy's apparent defiance of his father's wishes that he not smoke and do his chores. The more Harry berated Bryce, the more Bryce defied his father. The pattern shifted when Harry was encour-

---

TABLE 8.3. Interventions for Moderate Problem Behavior

Key = Redirect the parents' efforts away from control toward rebuilding their relationship with the adolescent.

- Help the parents distinguish between what they can and cannot control.
- Emphasize the parents' emotional investment in the adolescent.
- Encourage both the adolescent and the parents to express feelings of hurt, betrayal, sorrow, or anxiety.
- Facilitate negotiation of rules and consequences that respect the needs of both the adolescent and the parents.

aged to express in a genuine and authentic way the softer feelings that lay buried beneath his anger. These other feelings—hurt, betrayal, sorrow, and anxiety—were rarely, if ever, expressed. But, by calling attention to these feelings, I was able to shift the focus away from issues of control onto issues of emotional attachment, care, and concern. Harry admitted that he indeed could not control what Bryce did, but it was equally true that Bryce's actions had an emotional impact on Harry. By bringing these feelings to the forefront, the discussion shifted away from "What can I do to make Bryce behave?" to "Why does Bryce seem to care so little about the way his actions are making me feel?" This shift opened up an exploration of the ways in which the father–son relationship had deteriorated over the years, and ways that it could be repaired. Sometimes parents are reluctant to share their feelings of hurt with their children for fear of "laying a guilt trip." But guilt can be a powerful motivator for changing behavior, and many times defiant adolescents experience far too little of this important emotion.

It is essential that parents not get the impression that expressing feelings is simply another way to manipulate the adolescent. The feelings the parents express must be genuine, and their disclosure of them must be honest. The primary reason for expressing these feelings is to emphasize that the relationship is still important, at least as far as the parents are concerned. The adolescent might choose to disregard the importance of the relationship, but can't "make" the parents stop caring about him or her. Youngsters who assert their autonomy by claiming that their actions have consequences for them alone come face-to-face with the reality that when one is in a relationship, one's actions always have consequences for other people.

Case Example: "Daddy, Don't Worry about Me."

Let's return to the case of Tammy that was introduced at the beginning of this chapter as an example of "moderate" problem behavior. Tammy's parents had been trying to rein her in by restricting her and ineffectively grounding her when she violated curfew, only to find out that she had sneaked out of the house after they had gone to bed. In the family session, Tammy glared at her parents, as if daring them to start an argument that was almost sure to end in her leaving my office in a fit of high dudgeon. I had seen this pattern in the second family session and didn't want to risk letting it happen again.

John began the third family session by telling me with a mixture of fury and resignation in his voice that the weekend before our session Tammy came home at 2 A.M., 2 hours later than their negotiated curfew.

When he confronted her, she blithely told him that she was "hanging out" with her most recent boyfriend, a 22-year-old, unemployed high school dropout, whom her parents had expressly forbidden her to see. Interrupting her parents' account of the events of that night, Tammy interjected with a provocative tone, "Don't worry, we're using condoms. I won't get pregnant again."

John was fuming, but I caught a glimpse of great sorrow on Helen's face. I turned to her and asked if she would share her feelings about what Tammy has been doing. She burst into tears.

"It's breaking my heart," she sobbed. "I can't bear it any more. Every day I wonder if today might be the last time I see her."

Tammy looked incredulous. "Oh, Mom, don't be so dramatic," she sighed.

"No, it's true, honey." Helen continued, "I can't sleep at night for worrying about you. I know there's nothing else I can do to convince you to change. And it hurts me so much I can't think of anything else."

Helen burst into sobs again. I noticed that John was about to shift into anger, and I wanted to prevent what was sure to be another unproductive outburst that would overshadow Helen's poignant self-disclosure.

"John, I can see that you're angry at Tammy for putting you and her mother through this," I said, "but I also sense that you might be having some of the same feelings that Helen just talked about."

"Of course I do," he said. "How couldn't I? Tammy is my daughter. Sure I get angry, but it's just to keep me from crying my eyes out over what this girl is doing to herself."

"Daddy, don't worry about me," Tammy feebly interjected. "I can take care of myself."

"Honey, I do worry about you," John said. "And no matter how many times you tell me not to, I will. I love you and I don't want to lose you."

"You won't lose me," Tammy replied unconvincingly.

"I'm not so sure, honey," John continued. "Just the other day, I read in the paper about that girl they found in the river. They said she was probably raped. I couldn't even finish the article, because all I could think of was that it could have been you."

Tammy tried to bait her parents with remarks that seemed designed to pull from them an angry or controlling response against which she could react. But I was able to help the parents stay with their own feelings of helplessness, frustration, and anxiety, and to communicate these feelings to Tammy. Eventually, Tammy shifted from defending herself to trying to soothe her parents by attempting to convince them that they had no reason to worry. All she wanted was to be left alone. I encouraged John and Helen to continue to state their position and to let Tammy know in every way they could that they were committed to a relationship with her.

I helped the parents distinguish between what they could and could not control. Short of monitoring Tammy around the clock, they could not control what she did. They could not control how she chose to express her sexuality, and they could not control what gave her pleasure. They had more control over what they permitted in their home, but even in this arena, their control was limited because they were not prepared to evict Tammy from the house if she violated their prohibitions. They had some control over their own feelings, more control over their actions, and thus some control over the kind of relationship they would have with Tammy. The latter also depended on what kind of relationship Tammy wanted with *them*, and what they thought would be best for Tammy. Both parents claimed that they wanted a close relationship with Tammy. Tammy said that she wanted a relationship with her parents, but she did not want them to "force" her to do anything. After some discussion, both parents agreed that it would be best for Tammy if they were available and supportive, and that little would be gained from giving her ultimatums that could lead to her running away from home.

The parents struggled with the question of what to do when Tammy was late and they did not know where she was. They concluded that all they could do was call the police. Tammy bristled at this idea: "How could you call the police on me? I thought you just said that you loved me." Her parents explained that they were calling the police not to get her into trouble (though it might) but because they were worried about her and they didn't know what else to do.

This distinction was an important one. If the parents were calling the police in yet another ploy to control or reform Tammy, then they were playing into the symptomatic cycle. However, if the purpose of calling the police was not to punish Tammy, but rather to allay their worries about her and to carry out what they saw as their duty as parents, then the pattern of mutual reactivity would be broken.

It is necessary to deal directly with the parents' anxiety and frustration when they begin to accept the limits of their control over the adolescent. Parents need help to set reasonable limits and avoid futile power struggles. Ideally, rules and limits should be negotiated between the adolescent and parents, but in some cases the adolescent refuses to enter into negotiations, either because of mistrust in the parents or fear that any concession will lead to loss of autonomy. In these cases, the parents should do their best to develop a system of rules and consequences that seem fair, even if the adolescent initially rejects them.

After the parents have expressed the feelings that are evoked by the adolescent's behavior, then the adolescent is invited to share his or her feelings about the parents' disclosure.

The following is an illustration from Tammy's case:

MICUCCI: Tammy, how does it make you feel to hear your parents say they are worried about losing you?

TAMMY: They shouldn't care so much.

MICUCCI: But how does it make you *feel* to hear that they care about you so much?

TAMMY: Good, I guess.

MICUCCI: Knowing that some of the things you have done have really scared and hurt your parents, how does that make you feel?

TAMMY: Not so good. I really didn't want to upset them. I just wanted to have fun.

JOHN: We want you to have fun, too, honey. But what you were doing was scaring the bejeebers out of me.

HELEN: Me too.

TAMMY: I'm sorry, Mom and Dad. I'm really not bad.

JOHN: We know you are not bad, Tammy. That's why we were so confused about what was going on.

TAMMY: I guess I'm confused, too.

MICUCCI: You're confused about why you were acting the way you were?

TAMMY: Yeah, it seems so pointless now. Maybe I was just looking for someone to care about me, and I didn't think my parents cared as much as they did.

In some cases of moderately severe defiance, such as Tammy, the teen's defiance might be motivated more by self-gratification than by rage or anger at the parents. In these cases, articulation of the parents' care and concern for the child often leads the child to reconsider his or her unwillingness to comply with the parents' wishes. In other cases, such as Bryce, the adolescent's feelings of hurt and anger need to be addressed directly before the adolescent is willing to defer self-gratification out of deference to the parents' feelings. In cases of severe defiance, however, the adolescent may *want* to hurt the parents, in retaliation for what he or she has experienced as rejection or betrayal. In the next section, I discuss how to be helpful in these cases.

INTERVENTIONS FOR SEVERE DEFIANCE

At this level of severity, the adolescent is engaging in a pattern of disruptive and potentially dangerous behaviors. Examples include running away, repeated drug use, serious thefts, or physical violence against other family members. The youngster appears unconcerned about the potential consequences of his or her actions either to him- or herself or to others. If the adolescent comes to therapy, he or she does so only under duress and, when there, participates halfheartedly, if at all. Parents feel helpless and defeated. Often, they are so preoccupied with the adolescent's behavior that they have little energy for anything else. Their lives have become so constricted that they are completely isolated from friends and extended family. They might be afraid of the child and go to great lengths to avoid provoking a conflict, even if it means abdicating their parental authority.

If the adolescent is engaging in severely defiant behavior that is potentially harmful to self or to others, then the first step is to restore order to the household by reducing the impact of the adolescent's behavior on the other family members. While the parents might be powerless to change the adolescent's behavior, they often have more power than they realize to protect themselves and their other children from the adolescent's actions. The challenge is to do so without alienating the adolescent and thus losing any hope of engaging him or her in treatment (see Table 8.4).

In these cases, I recommend the following procedure:

• An initial family session, in which the goal is to focus attention away from the adolescent's defiance and onto the relationships in the family.

• A series of meetings held separately with the parents and with the adolescent. Because these adolescents are often very angry at the parents and might even refuse to attend sessions with them, I believe that more progress can be made by meeting separately with the parents and with the adolescent. In these sessions, work proceeds on two fronts simultaneously. In the sessions with the parents, the goal is to help the parents develop reasonable and enforceable rules and consequences as well as effective ways of protecting themselves and their other children from the symptomatic adolescent's defiance. In the sessions with the adolescent, the goal is to help the adolescent identify and articulate the painful feelings of hurt and betrayal that are presumed to be motivating the rage, anger, and destructive behaviors.

• Finally, the family is reunited for a series of sessions focused on

TABLE 8.4. Interventions for Severe Problem Behavior

Key = Find a balance between strengthening parental authority and rebuilding the relationship between the adolescent and the parents.

- Initial family session in which the definition of the problem is expanded beyond an exclusive focus on the defiant behavior and onto the family relationships.
- Separate parallel sessions with the adolescent and parents.
- In sessions with parents, help them to:
  - Restore order to the household.
  - Wipe the slate clean and acknowledge parental mistakes.
  - Reclaim control over their own lives.
  - Distinguish between *disagreeable* and *destructive* behavior.
  - Choose appropriate consequences.
  - Avoid participating in arguments with the defiant child.
  - Reduce isolation from extended family and community.
  - Explore their beliefs about the problem.
- In individual sessions with the adolescent:
  - Encourage exploration of feelings of hurt, betrayal, or loss that are obscured behind anger and rage.
  - Explore the origin of the ruptures in the adolescent's relationship with the parents.
- Bring the parents and adolescent back together to:
  - Encourage the adolescent to express the feelings of hurt, betrayal, or loss directly to the parents.
  - Help the parents to listen and make a concrete commitment to repair the relationship.
- Find ways to build or strengthen the adolescent's ties to mainstream societal institutions, such as school, work, religious, or service organizations.

acknowledging the relationship breakdowns and taking concrete steps toward forging a more trusting relationship between the adolescent and parents.

The Initial Session

The initial session is conducted in the same way as previously recommended (see Chapter 4). The goal of the initial session is to call attention to the link between the defiant behavior and family relationship patterns.

For example, in the first session with Keith and his parents, I asked them to talk about the incident described at the beginning of this chapter, when Keith and his father got into a physical struggle over Keith's attempts to leave the house. Within minutes, the conversation devolved into mutual shouting, followed by silent "stonewalling" on Keith's part. Pam turned to me: "See, we can't do anything with him. He's just completely out of control."

Although I agreed that Keith seemed to accept no limits on his behavior and might indeed be out of control, I wanted to use this opportunity to call the family's attention to the disintegration of their relationships with each other and how all three of them were suffering as a result. I offered the following comment: "What I observe is a very low level of trust in this family. You, Pam and Stu, don't trust Keith, and you, Keith, don't trust your parents. We must work at restoring your trust in each other."

When offering a frame such as this one, it is important that it be *bidirectional,* that is, one that links the adolescent and parents in a mutual dilemma, in this case, the absence of *mutual* trust. It can then be suggested that an important goal of therapy would be to help restore mutual trust.

To work on this goal, a series of separate meetings with the parents and with the adolescent are proposed. It is important at this point to discuss the issue of confidentiality, especially since adolescents might disclose in an individual session with the therapist information about their behavior that the therapist believes the parents should know. It is important to be very clear about the limits of confidentiality, and to let the adolescent and family know in advance what will and will not be disclosed without the adolescent's permission. The reader is referred to other suggestions regarding confidentiality discussed in Chapter 4.

Engaging Reluctant Adolescents

If the adolescent expresses reluctance to participate in the sessions, the therapist might say in the presence of the parents that he or she understands that there are many sides to every story, and that the therapist sees his or her role as taking no one's side consistently but rather helping the family members to resolve their disagreements with each other. The therapist acknowledges that the decision whether or not to participate is up to the adolescent, but if the adolescent declines to participate, then the therapist is left with no choice but to meet only with the parents. The therapist emphasizes that the adolescent's decision not to participate means that the therapist will not have an opportunity to hear the youngster's side of the story or to help the parents understand it.

The therapist should express genuine interest in getting to know the adolescent, point out something that he or she sincerely likes or admires about the youth, and emphasize that the purpose of the individual sessions is not to "fix" the kid but rather to listen to him or her. The therapist acknowledges that the adolescent probably feels misunderstood or unappreciated by the family members, expresses interest in understanding his or her point of view, and offers hope that he or she might be able to help the family view the youth differently.

If necessary, the therapist might entice the adolescent to participate by offering to do something concrete for him or her or to advocate on his or her behalf. For example, if the adolescent is in legal difficulty, the therapist might offer to try to convince the court to be lenient, saying, for example:

> "I'm prepared to write a recommendation to the court that says they should give you another chance. Most of the time they'll go along with my recommendations. But I need to be convinced that if I stick my neck out for you, I'm not going to get it cut off. Before I write this recommendation, you'll need to convince me that if you're given a second chance, you won't prove me wrong."

If the adolescent rebuffs all of the therapist's offers and simply refuses to participate, the therapist should communicate respect for the youth's decision but explain that he or she will nevertheless try to engage the adolescent periodically while continuing to work with the parents. The therapist, from time to time, might telephone the kid, send unsolicited letters and birthday cards, or perhaps even visit the youngster at home. In meetings with the parents, the therapist attempts to introduce the adolescent's perspective, and invites the parents to consider ways in which they might have damaged their relationship with the child, either deliberately or unwittingly.

Sessions with the Parents

Whether or not the therapist is successful in engaging the adolescent in an alliance, the therapist then proceeds to meet with the parents to discuss ideas for handling the defiant behavior. However, before sharing these ideas, *it is important to obtain the parents' assurance that they will carry out the therapist's suggestions in such a way as to make the youngster think that the parents (not the therapist) had come up with these ideas.*

The therapist explains that this "deception" is necessary if there is going to be any hope of ever engaging the adolescent in treatment. While this intervention might strike some as devious, in fact it strengthens the parental hierarchy by restraining the parents from carrying out any of the therapist's suggestions until they are convinced they could do so in a way that does not implicate the therapist in the adolescent's eyes. Thus, the parents assume more ownership of the interventions, and more responsibility for the outcome.

Restoring Order to the Household

A primary goal is to decrease parental reactivity and to help the parents plan ahead for confrontations they anticipate might arise. When the parents react to the adolescent's behavior, they are ceding control to him or her. The kid sets the tone for the interaction, and by following his or her lead the parents experience more helplessness. The parents might feel that their reactions are justified and necessary to assert control over the youth. However, by allowing the youngster to set the tone, they are colluding in the cycle that saps them of their authority (Keim, 2005). If the kid is friendly and compliant, the parents are happy and responsive to the kid. If he or she is angry and defiant, the parents shout, threaten, or withdraw. In either case, the adolescent, not the parent, is setting the tone for the interaction. Pointing out these patterns can help parents modify their customary responses to the child's defiance.

Wiping the Slate Clean

The therapist suggests that the parents tell the child that they are willing to wipe the slate clean and start all over. Past infractions are forgiven, and they are prepared to begin again. They admit to the adolescent that they have made mistakes in the way they have treated him or her in the past and they apologize. They invite the child to come to therapy so the parents can tell the child how they have failed him or her as parents. They then offer to do something small and concrete for the kid, such as buying him or her a new pair of jeans or preparing a favorite meal.

The parents should be cautioned against taking this step until they are committed to it and prepared to see it through. They should be warned that doing so incompletely would probably make matters worse, so they should refrain from acting until they have dispelled any doubts about their decision. The therapist then explores in detail how their relationship with their child would be different if they were seriously committed to wiping the slate clean. How would they act toward him or her if they had in fact forgiven and forgotten past offenses?

The point here is that by changing the parents' response and, in some cases, even their perception of the adolescent, the symptomatic cycle is broken. The parents are no longer responding in their predictable way, but are instead treating the child as if he or she were not just a "problem child." This change opens up space for other new responses to emerge as well.

Reclaiming Control Over Their Lives

The parents must be redirected away from controlling or "reforming" the adolescent and toward a focus on themselves and their own needs—what they need to do to reclaim control over their *own* lives. The therapist might discuss with the parents how they have suffered from the problem and how their lives have become more and more constricted as a result. It is important to acknowledge that they have lost the feeling of comfort in their own home and encourage them to think about what they need in order to feel secure again. This discussion shifts the emphasis away from controlling or changing the child and onto what the parents can do to restore their own sense of security.

It is essential to help the parents focus on what *they* can do to restore a sense of order, even without the adolescent's cooperation. This enables the parents to see that they can set reasonable limits and stand by them regardless of what the youngster does. Perhaps they need to know that they are safe from violence, so they decide to tell the adolescent (as did Keith's parents) that they will call the police and press charges if he threatens violence. Perhaps they need to know that their property will not be damaged or stolen. After making reasonable precautions to secure their belongings, they tell the child that they will assume he or she stole the item if they discover anything missing, and they will either report him or her to the police or confiscate one of the child's possessions equal in value to the missing item. Perhaps the parents have neglected their relationship with each other and need to arrange to spend some time together. Perhaps they have been neglecting another child while they have been preoccupied with the "problem" adolescent. In any event, it is important to help the parents define what is *essential* for them to reclaim a sense of order and sanity in their own lives.

Distinguishing between Disagreeable and Destructive Behavior

It is often necessary to help parents distinguish between *disagreeable* and *destructive* behavior. Disagreeable behavior includes behavior that is troublesome or obnoxious, but not necessarily destructive or dangerous. Examples include surliness, sloppiness, mild disrespect, or argumentativeness. Destructive behaviors pose the risk of danger, such as threats or acts of violence, stealing, staying out all night, and so on. Many parents who feel powerless over the adolescent's more flagrantly destructive behaviors resort to trying to control the disagreeable behavior. Sometimes these parents think they are being "consistent" by disallowing any type of rule breaking, however slight. In fact, these parents might effusively criticize the adolescent for relatively minor disagreeable behavior while failing to impose effective limits on more serious and potentially dangerous behaviors. This policy serves only to damage the relationship even more, as the parents become hypervigilant to any occasion to criticize the kid and the adolescent begins to feel as if he or she can't do anything right. Parents should be encouraged to ignore the disagreeable behavior as much as possible and to "choose their battles" by focusing on the more flagrant episodes of potentially dangerous or destructive behavior.

Choosing Appropriate Consequences

Any consequences imposed by the parents should be under their control, and should not require the adolescent's cooperation. "Grounding" a defiant adolescent such as Keith invites disaster, as he simply defies the parents by violating the grounding. Parents have more control over resources or privileges they provide to the youngster, such as money, rides, or use of the family car or other family property.

For example, Stu and Pam complained that Keith would receive telephone calls from people they did not know, and they suspected he might be buying or selling drugs, using their telephone as a means of communication. As one of the strategies for restoring a feeling of comfort in their own home, they decided they would invest in a "caller ID" service offered by their local telephone company. This service allowed them not only to monitor incoming calls, but also to block calls from certain numbers. Though Keith was furious when he heard of this decision, he grudgingly accepted his parents' explanation that they had a right to have the "caller ID" service because it was their home and their phone. They also informed Keith that they would no longer pay his cell phone bill and would confiscate any cell phones they found around the house.

Refusing to Participate in Arguments

One of the "resources" parents control is their own participation in an argument. Parents of severely defiant adolescents often complain that they are engaged in constant arguing with their child, and that these arguments sometimes escalate to the point of violence. To break this pattern, parents can simply refuse to participate in an argument. I point out to parents that it "takes two to argue" and that there is no argument if the other party does not join the fray. I encourage them to "stay cool" when their adolescent attempts to engage them in a verbal battle, state their position simply and confidently, and then refuse to respond to any efforts to provoke an unproductive argument.

Reducing Isolation

Families with severely defiant or violent adolescents are often isolated from the extended family or their communities. Perhaps the parents have been so preoccupied with the child's outrageous behavior that they have neglected other relationships in their lives. Perhaps the parents are embarrassed by the kid's behavior and so they have distanced themselves from family and friends. Perhaps the family was always isolated and cut off from extended family and community, and this lifestyle served them well until the adolescent's behavior began to frighten them, so that now they feel intensely alone and disconnected from other sources of support.

Whatever the reason for the family's isolation, the therapist should strive to help the family reconnect with members of the extended family and the community. For example, the therapist might suggest that the parents contact the parents of the adolescent's peers, to talk with them about what they might do together to solve the problem they share. The therapist might encourage the parents to attend (or start) a parent support group in their community, or help the parents list the people they could call to serve as reinforcements if a conflict were to escalate between them and the kid.

Exploring Beliefs about the Problem

It is important to explore the parents' beliefs about the problem, with an eye to discerning how these beliefs have interfered with finding solutions. Sometimes parents see the adolescent as a *troubled* youth, and so believe that it is their responsibility to give plenty of leeway and to provide a sense of security and unconditional love. These well-intentioned parents contribute to their own powerlessness by setting no limits at all on the child's behavior. In these cases, therapists might encounter resistance from the parents when suggesting that they set firmer limits. In other families, the parents are so angry at the adolescent that they see him or her only as a *troublesome* youth. They want to punish the youth for his or her actions and be rid of him or her as quickly as possible. In these cases, the therapist encounters resistance when suggesting that needs for more understanding and nurturance hide behind the adolescent's troublesome behavior.

It is important to address this dualistic thinking that views the youngster as *either* "troubled" *or* "troublesome." The parents need to expand their views to include other aspects of the kid, to see him or her as a more complex individual. The adolescent is *both* a troubled *and* a troublesome youth who needs *both* firmer controls *and* more understanding. It is important to assess where the parents fall on the continuum of seeing the adolescent as troubled or troublesome, and then work to move the parents closer to the middle of the continuum. If the parents are reluctant to set limits or seem willing to take most of the blame for the problem, therapists might suggest that the parents talk to other parents who are in similar situations, they might share stories of other families with whom they have worked, or they might ignite the parents' indignation and outrage at the way the child has been treating them. If the parents emphasize the other side of the coin and are so angry at the kid that they are unable to see him or her as a troubled youth, therapists might point out some of the adolescent's positive qualities, help them recall ways in which the child had demonstrated loyalty to them in the past, invite them to remember earlier times when they felt some connection to the youngster, or emphasize that the adolescent still needs them and that they have much to offer him or her.

Sometimes one parent sees the child as "troubled" and the other sees the child as "troublesome." Not only does this difference of opinion lead to mutual undermining between the parents, but it can also escalate into ugly conflicts between the parents over whose approach is the right one. Some therapists believe that a child's problem behavior is symptomatic of detoured marital conflict between the parents, and so they welcome the surfacing of these conflicts as an opportunity to work on the "real" problem in the family. The problem with this view is that it is linear: It fails to acknowledge that the adolescent's problem behavior is also fueling the conflict between the parents, or might be helping to transform a minor problem in marital conflict resolution into a major impasse.

I recommend utilizing the crisis created by the adolescent's problem behavior as a way to improve parental collaboration. The parents are advised that the top priority is to reduce the level of danger in the household. In order to do so, they will have to put aside any other differences between them and join forces. The parents are told that both of them are right, that the child is both troubled and troublesome, and that each needs to consider the merits of the other's position in order to reduce the polarization between them. Each parent's view might be compared with the view from a single eye, and the integration of both views to "binocular vision." Thus, the parents are encouraged to help each other see the "blind spots" in the view that each favors.

Sessions with the Adolescent

Concurrently with the meetings with the parents, the therapist meets individually with the adolescent. These sessions with the adolescent are guided by the acronym *ARCH* (see Chapter 1). The therapist *accepts* the youngster as he or she is, without feeling compelled to change or "fix" him or her. *Acceptance* does not mean that the therapist approves of the adolescent's behavior. Rather, it means that the therapist accepts that it is completely up to the adolescent whether he or she will grant the therapist any influence over him or her and whether the youth will accept the therapist's offer to help. The therapist treats the adolescent with *respect*, that is, with empathy for his or her predicament rather than as a "problem" child. The therapist attempts to engage the more mature aspects of the adolescent by treating him or her as someone capable of self-reflection, delay of gratification, and compassion for others (even if the adolescent has not been showing these qualities in his or her interactions with the family). The therapist's attitude is characterized by *curiosity*, which is grounded in a willingness to listen to the kid and to help him or her express him- or herself, even if the therapist does not agree with the content of what he or she is saying. Curiosity means that the therapist seeks to understand the kid rather than trying to figure out ways to compel him or her to change. Finally, the therapist is *honest*, giving sincere, thoughtful, and balanced feedback as appropriate, keeping promises and commitments, and refusing to collude with the youngster in lying or deceiving the parents.

The goal is to steer the direction of the conversation onto the adolescent's feelings, especially feelings about the relationship with the parents. While adolescents who engage in milder forms of defiant behavior are able to empathize with their parents' care and concern for them and trust that these feelings are real, adolescents who engage in severely defiant, destructive, or dangerous behavior have such a weakened attachment to the family that they either deliberately want to retaliate or simply don't care that they are hurting the parents. It is important to strive to understand how the relationships became damaged. A way to do so is to invite adolescents to examine their feelings about the parents and explore how their childhood trust in their parents eroded over the years.

Often, anger is the first feeling to emerge. The youth feels angry at the parents for punishing him or her or standing in the way of his or her autonomy or happiness. The discussion should be directed toward the feelings of hurt, betrayal, or loss that are obscured behind the anger and rage. The goal is to help the adolescent become aware of and articulate the "softer" feelings of hurt and sadness that reflect the ruptures in the emotional attachment to the parents. Useful questions might be, "I know you feel angry, but I wonder if you might also be feeling a little bit hurt at what your parents have done?" or "If I were in your place, I think I'd be angry too, but I think I'd also feel sad. What about you?" These questions can lead to recall of specific events that led the adolescent to feel betrayed or abandoned by the parents.

It is important that the therapist not imply that the adolescent's defiant behavior was a justified response to the experience of abandonment or betrayal. Rather, the message that must be emphasized is that the defiance was the adolescent's way of dealing with the *underlying feelings* that resulted from the experience of abandonment or betrayal. The defiance per se is not justified, but the feelings are. In linking the defiance to the adolescent's experience of abandonment or betrayal by the parents, it is important that the mediating feelings be included in the explanation. For example, the adolescent's drug use is not justified as a retaliatory response against rejecting parents, but rather drug use is his or her way of dealing with the painful feelings that resulted from the experience of being rejected or abandoned.

After helping the adolescent articulate these feelings, the next step is to orchestrate a conversation between the adolescent and the parents about these feelings. The intent is to repair the ruptures in the relationship by giving the parents an opportunity to acknowledge that they have let the child down and then express the resolve to repair the relationship.

Family Sessions

Preparing the Parents

Once order has been restored to the household, the emphasis shifts to rebuilding relationships in the family. In later sessions with the parents, the therapist begins to explore ways in which the parents might have (deliberately or unwittingly) abandoned the child in the past, thus evoking feelings of rage and entitlement that erupted into a pattern of destructive behavior.

If the parents are struggling with feelings of resentment toward the child, the therapist might invite them to reflect on the process by which their relationship with their child deteriorated, and help them identify ways in which they might regain access to positive feelings for the child. With the adolescent's permission, the therapist might introduce into the dialogue information obtained from the adolescent about how the child had come to feel hurt, betrayed, or abandoned by the parents. Drawing on the individual meetings with the adolescent, the therapist paints a positive picture of the youngster, one that depicts the child as sad, hurt, or frightened rather than angry and vindictive. The goal is to prepare the parents to listen nondefensively while the adolescent expresses these feelings directly to them.

The parents are reminded prior to the family session that the purpose of the session is to give the adolescent an opportunity to talk directly with them about the feelings disclosed to the therapist in the individual sessions. The therapist prepares the parents for the possibility that they might feel unjustly attacked by the adolescent, and so feel compelled to defend themselves or to "correct" the adolescent's perception of events. The parents are encouraged to listen supportively to whatever the adolescent says to them, even if they don't readily understand or agree. They are reminded that the purpose of this phase of treatment is to help restore positive feelings in the family and to give the parents an opportunity to express care and concern for the child.

Encouraging Dialogue

Others have written about the process of using emotions to strengthen the attachment between adolescents and parents. Susan Johnson (2004) described the process of *softening* by which careful tracking, reflection, and questioning by the therapist can elicit vulnerable feelings from couples who are engaged in hostile interactions. In his work with adolescent substance abusers, Howard Liddle (1999) has demonstrated how interactions between parents and adolescents can be shifted toward expressions of support and nurturance by the parents. Diamond and Stern (2003) have also discussed the process of rebuilding the attachment between parents and adolescents.

These approaches provide guidance for conducting the family sessions and stimulating more productive dialogue between the adolescent and parents. Here's the recommended procedure:

1. At the beginning of the session, the therapist reminds the parents and the adolescent that the purpose of the session is to talk about feelings, not to resolve disagreements or to negotiate rules.
2. The therapist invites the adolescent to share feelings about something the parents did or failed to do that hurt or disappointed him or her. If the adolescent expresses angry feelings, the therapist works to uncover the "softer" feelings of hurt, sadness, or loss that lie beneath these feelings.
3. The therapist intensifies these softer feelings of hurt by paraphrasing and suggesting words that articulate the feelings. For example, the therapist might say, "What I hear you saying is, 'Mom and Dad, you've let me down. I counted on you and you weren't there for me. I felt so lost and alone I couldn't stand it.' "

4. The therapist gradually introduces the parents into the dialogue by asking them to express their own feelings about what their child had just disclosed.

5. Finally, the therapist elicits from the parents a commitment to engage in concrete and specific efforts to demonstrate that they have heard the adolescent and have taken him or her seriously. For example, if a boy expresses sadness over his father's withdrawal from him after a divorce, the father must not only listen supportively to the feelings but also commit to spending more time with his son.

This procedure is illustrated in the example of Keith. He disclosed in an individual session one of the reasons why he was so angry at his parents: He "couldn't forgive them" for having sent him to military school. He tearfully related the brutal hazings he had experienced there, and the rage he felt at the upperclassmen who victimized the younger students. Although he begged his parents to allow him to come home, they refused.

In the next family session, the therapist encouraged the parents to talk about this issue. Pam asked Keith why he had never told them about the abuse he had experienced at school. Laughing sardonically, Keith told about another boy who had reported the hazing to his parents, who then came to the school to confront the administration. The offenders were punished, but the boy who reported them was victimized even more brutally by other students and ostracized by his peers, who feared being associated with him. Eventually, the boy had a "breakdown" and left the school in shame.

Almost in tears, Keith told of the rampant drug use on the campus and the hypocrisy of the administration and faculty, who denied that there was a drug problem at the school. He talked about his initiation into smoking marijuana, and how it helped him feel a sense of calm he couldn't get any other way. "I begged you to take me home," Keith cried, "but you wouldn't listen. You wouldn't even talk with me about it. Now I'm living by my own rules and you can't stop me!"

Stu began to defend his decision to send Keith to military school. I realized that this would quickly lead to an impasse, so I redirected him.

MICUCCI: Stu, how do you feel about what Keith just said about living by his own rules?

STU: It scares me, because I'm afraid of what could happen to him.

MICUCCI: And how do you feel about the way Keith was treated at military school?

STU: It breaks my heart. I ache for him. I wish I had not been so stubborn and I wish I had at least tried to do something to help him.

MICUCCI: Can you tell Keith directly how you feel?

STU: Keith, I am so sorry for what happened to you, and I'm sorry that I put you in that situation. I can understand why you are so mad at me and now don't trust me.

Pam was silently weeping. I turned to her next and asked her to tell Keith how she was feeling.

PAM: I'm feeling so bad that I put my son in that place. I'm so sorry, Keith. We made a bad decision. I hope you can find a way to forgive us.

KEITH: I dunno.

PAM: I understand. It hurt a lot. I'm really interested in hearing more about what happened there and how you were feeling.

The session continued with Keith expressing the terror he felt at the prospect of being victimized, and how he helped himself feel less frightened by focusing on the anger he had for his parents. But beneath the anger was his deep sense of hurt, loss, and betrayal.

After these feelings were expressed and acknowledged, concrete steps needed to be taken to repair the ruptures in the relationship. I encouraged Pam and Stu to keep telling Keith how much they cared about him and how sad they felt that a decision that they had made had caused him so much pain. As a concrete demonstration of their commitment to repairing the relationship, we planned opportunities for Keith to spend time alone with each parent.

Repairing Ruptured Relationships

The relationship between Keith and Stu had never been very close. Stu had kept his distance, worked long hours, and pursued his own interests apart from the family. Some boys, like Keith, might act out aggressively as a way of asserting their image of a masculine ideal, or as a way of engaging a peripheral father (Osherson & Krugman, 1990). Father must help the boy develop a more inclusive image of what it means to be a man by validating his son's masculinity in nonaggressive areas and modeling positive qualities associated with masculinity, such as loyalty and commitment to others. It is valuable to encourage the father and son to engage in a specific activity or project that helps them to work collaboratively rather than competitively. Toward this end, I suggested that Keith and Stu plan a weekend camping trip together, something they had done (and enjoyed) once before, when Keith was 10 years old.

We also explored ways in which Pam could remain an important person in Keith's life. We started with simple things, such as buying him a small article of clothing, or cooking him a meal he liked. Keith started coming home at night for dinner with his parents. As many mothers do, Pam was careful to give Keith "plenty of space." She would allow him to decide how much contact they would have. As Silverstein and Rashbaum (1994) have pointed out, while this strategy might appear respectful of the boy's boundaries, it runs the risk of allowing distance to grow in the mother–son relationship: The boy feels that it is "not manly" to want to be with his mother, and so does not approach her. He reads her reticence to approach him as evidence that she's not interested either.

In family sessions, we talked explicitly about this pattern and explored ways in which Pam might play a more active role in Keith's life. At first, Keith was willing to accept only traditional "mothering" activities such as cooking meals and doing laundry. Pam, a remarkably astute and sensitive woman, was patient. She made him dinner and neatly folded his T-shirts. Eventually, Keith began to help his mother in the garden, and by midsummer, they were redecorating Keith's room together. Stu supported this activity by giving Keith the money to buy the wall paint. And, of course, as Pam and Keith worked, they talked, and their relationship blossomed.

Strengthening Ties to Society

As discussed above, some theories maintain that a primary cause of delinquency is weak ties to societal institutions, such as school, work, or religious organizations. Adolescents who are weakly bonded to family or social institutions gravitate toward similarly alienated peers and become even more disengaged from mainstream institutions. To help reverse this trend, the therapist can encourage adolescents to join a sports team, to do volunteer work, or to return to church. Rather than trying to pull the adolescent away from deviant associates, it is preferable to encourage more diversity in the adolescent's peer network by exposing the youngster to other kids who are engaging in prosocial activities.

For example, rather than concentrating on pulling Keith away from his "bad" friends, we tried to think of ways to help Keith strengthen ties with more mainstream kids. Keith wanted to earn money, so he was encouraged to find a job. He wasn't successful. His parents were willing to pay Keith an hourly wage for doing volunteer work at a soup kitchen. Keith accepted their offer. He began spending more and more time at the soup kitchen, and even started attending a youth group at the church that sponsored the kitchen.

SUMMARY

The main point of this chapter is that defiant and disruptive behaviors are signs of ruptures in the adolescent's relationships with the family. The more the parents try to control the kid, the more the kid resists their control and gravitates toward deviant peers who reinforce problem behavior. The key to successful intervention is to break this cycle by working to reestablish relationships in the family.

I suggest that adolescent problem behavior be viewed along a continuum from mild to moderate to severe.

- When the problem behavior is *mild*, the adolescent tests limits but generally has maintained positive relationships with the family. At this level, I recommend that therapy focus not on strategies to eliminate the problem behavior but rather on helping the family members adapt to the developmental transitions they are facing. Build on existing family strengths to encourage conflict resolution and to expand dialogue among the family members.

- When the problem behavior is *moderate*, there is a more persistent pattern of defiance. The adolescent might be abusing drugs or alcohol, might be sexually promiscuous, or might be chronically truant. Despite frequent arguments with parents, the adolescent has never been violent at home. At this level, the key principle is to redirect the parents' efforts away from trying to control the youth. Discourage control-based methods of influence and emphasize the parents' emotional investment in the youngster. Explore with the adolescent and the family how it came to be that the parents' feelings and wishes became unimportant to the adolescent and how the bond between them could be repaired or strengthened.

- *Severe* problem behavior presents a threat of harm to self or others. The adolescent is engaging in dangerous, destructive, or violent behavior. At this level of severity, the main principle is to find a balance between supporting the parents and supporting the adolescent. Restore authority to the parents without alienating the kid. Help the parents to regain some control over their own lives, and then shift the emphasis to helping the parents provide age-appropriate nurturance to the youngster. The recommended procedure involves separate parallel meetings with the parents and adolescent. In the sessions with the parents, the therapist works to help them regain a sense of control over their own lives and home, and establish clear and realistic expectations and consequences for the adolescent's behavior. In the sessions with the adolescent, the therapist strives to uncover the "softer" feelings of hurt or sadness beneath the anger and defiance. Finally, the family is reunited in sessions during which the adolescent talks with the parents about ways in which they have contributed to his or her feelings of hurt, sadness, or abandonment. After listening nondefensively, the parents make a commitment to take concrete and specific steps to repair the relationship with the child.

9

Psychosis

Throughout this book, I have emphasized that interpersonal isolation, overt and covert, contributes to and results from the development of symptoms in adolescence. Every syndrome we have considered—eating disorders, depression, and aggressive and defiant behavior—has been related to a cycle of interactions that has at its core the experience of isolation for both the symptomatic adolescent and for the other family members. The symptomatic adolescent's isolation results from being misunderstood, controlled, or marginalized in the family. The isolation of the other family members comes from the constriction in their lives that has resulted from the consequences of the symptom or their efforts to change or control the behavior of each other. We now consider psychosis, admittedly a rare symptom among adolescents but one with far-reaching consequences.

Psychosis is almost synonymous with profound isolation. Individuals experiencing psychotic symptoms have retreated into a private world populated by terrifying voices and frightening images. They are wracked with uncertainty about what is real—the world around them or the world inside of them. Delusional beliefs about other people contribute to the feeling that they are completely alone in a dangerous world. Their speech is unintelligible and their loose associations make it impossible for them to communicate about their experiences with others. Their bizarre behavior frightens other people and drives them away.

THEORETICAL PERSPECTIVES

Family Dynamics

In post-Freudian psychoanalytic theory, psychosis was thought to result from severe disturbances in the relationship between the infant and his or her "schizophrenogenic" mother (Fromm-Reichmann, 1948). The pioneers of family therapy sought to break from this tradition by emphasizing more complex interactions that involved both parents and the child. For example, Theodore Lidz and his colleagues identified the patterns of *marital schism* and *marital skew* in families with schizophrenic children (Lidz, Cornelison, Fleck, & Terry, 1957). Martial schism involved mutual undermining by the parents and competition for the child's loyalty. In marital skew, one spouse was weaker and dependent on the other spouse, who appeared stronger but who actually bullied the weaker spouse into submission. Murray Bowen (1978) described families with schizophrenic children as an *undifferentiated ego mass*, characterized by intense emotional reactivity and triangulation. Lyman Wynne and his colleagues (Wynne, Ryckoff, Day, & Hirsch, 1958) emphasized the dynamic of *pseudomutuality* in psychotic families, whereby all family members were invested in maintaining rigid interactional patterns at the expense of developing an individual identity.

Other early family models of psychosis emphasized the disturbed patterns of communication in these families. Gregory Bateson, Don Jackson, Jay Haley, and John Weakland (1956) proposed the well-known *double-bind theory*, according to which the presence of irreconcilable contradictory messages ultimately led to a retreat from reality on the part of the psychotic individual. Margaret Singer and Lyman Wynne asserted that a disordered style of communication, known as *communication deviance*, was the defining characteristic of families with young adult schizophrenics (Singer, Wynne, & Toohey, 1978).

Mara Selvini-Palazzoli (1986) described a step-by-step process by which psychosis evolves in families, termed the *family game*. According to this model, the child becomes embroiled in a long-standing battle between the parents, each of whom uses the child's symptoms as a way of gaining advantage over the other parent. Selvini-Palazzoli advocated use of the *invariant prescription*, by which parents are given the instruction to go out alone without telling the children where they are going, meanwhile recording scrupulous observations on any events in the family that seem to be related to this prescription.

Biological Factors

In reaction to perceived efforts on the part of the professional community to blame parents (especially mothers) for psychotic symptoms, the pendulum has swung in the other direction so that many families now militantly rebel against the idea that parents play a role in the development of psychotic symptoms among their offspring. The growing body of literature linking psychosis to genetic and other biological causes has reinforced this position. There has been a movement to medicalize psychosis and treat it as an illness that can be managed, but not cured.

Although biological factors play an important role in psychosis, those who view psychosis as a strictly biological disorder run the risk of ignoring important interpersonal interactional patterns that can contribute to the emergence or exacerbation of symptoms. On the other hand, ignoring or minimizing biological factors or treatments can prolong suffering and can be harmful. There is speculation that the symptoms of psychosis can interact with the biology of the nervous system in a cyclical manner, such that the symptoms alter the biology of the brain, which then produces more symptoms (Harrop, Trower, & Mitchell, 1996). Thus, failure to treat the symptoms could increase the biological vulnerability for future psychotic episodes.

A middle ground between a strictly biological and strictly psychological model for psychosis is one that integrates the effects of biology and environment. According to this model, termed the *diathesis–stress model*, genetic factors determine the degree to which a person is predisposed or vulnerable to developing psychosis (Gottesman, 1991). Whether psychotic symptoms actually emerge depends on the amount of environmental stress that the individual experiences. Symptoms appear once the combination of genetic vulnerability and stress exceeds a theoretical threshold. Those with minimal biological vulnerability require a substantial amount of environmental stress before showing psychotic symptoms, while those with a higher vulnerability require less stress. In other words, individuals with a high genetic predisposition to psychosis are more likely to show psychotic symptoms under relatively lower degrees of stress.

Integrated Approaches

One of the consequences of the diathesis–stress model has been a de-emphasis on single modes of treatment and a greater emphasis on integrating biological and psychosocial treatments. There has been a shift from identifying the family patterns that presumably cause psychosis to identifying factors that influence the course and prognosis of the disorder. For example, relapse rates in schizophrenia have been linked to a family pattern known as *high expressed emotion* (Hooley, 2007; Leff & Vaughn, 1981). These families are emotionally overinvolved with one another, overtly critical of the patient, and express hostility in a rejecting manner. There is evidence that high levels of expressed emotion are associated with relapse in bipolar disorder as well (Hooley, 2007; Miklowitz, 2007; Miklowitz et al., 2006).

One example of an integrated approach to treating psychosis is the *psychoeducational* model, originally developed by Carol Anderson

(1983) and Michael Goldstein and his colleagues (Kopeikin, Marshall, & Goldstein, 1983). According to this model, family members are helped to identify and change the interactional patterns that are presumed to exacerbate the psychotic symptoms, even though these patterns are not necessarily seen as etiological. Family members are encouraged to view the psychosis as an illness in order to promote feelings of sympathy and helpfulness toward the patient rather than anger or resentment. They are coached to interact with one another in ways that minimize levels of conflict and negative affect in the family. The psychoeducational model has proven to be a valuable adjunct to medications for preventing relapse of schizophrenia and bipolar disorder (McFarlane et al., 2003; Miklowitz, 2008; Miklowitz et al., 2006).

PSYCHOSIS AND ISOLATION

I also advocate an integrated approach to treating psychosis that includes both medication to relieve the psychotic symptoms and family therapy to help the family members change the way they interact with one another. As I have argued in previous chapters, members of families where there are severe symptoms are often profoundly isolated from one another. As the family members become increasingly focused on the symptoms, they neglect other aspects of their relationships with one another, thus breeding more isolation and more symptomatic behavior in a mutually reinforcing process known as the symptomatic cycle. Psychosis represents the most extreme form of this isolation, where the presence of delusions, hallucinations, and bizarre behavior constitutes a private world to which others have no access. Thus, the treatment of psychosis must include not only amelioration of the psychotic symptoms but also work with the family members to reduce their isolation from one another and from their community. The following case illustrates these principles.

Melissa, age 15, lived with her mother, Barbara, an overwhelmed single parent. Melissa's father had left the family when she was an infant, and his whereabouts had been unknown for years. Barbara had a strained relationship with her own mother, Nina, who did not have a high opinion of her daughter's parenting capabilities. When Barbara and Nina were together, they often fought bitterly. When Melissa was doing well and not experiencing psychotic symptoms, she was a typical teenager, who tested her mother's patience and bickered with her. After a few weeks of these skirmishes, Barbara would begin to feel overwhelmed. In response, she would distance herself from Melissa, hide out in her own room, and when they were together she would act coldly toward her. Melissa would then begin to act strangely and talk about hearing voices. Terrified by these symptoms, Barbara would call Nina, who would move in for a few days until things settled down. When Melissa improved, Nina would move back home, but the cycle would start again a few weeks later.

In this family, the symptomatic cycle took the following form:

- *Step 1*. As long as Barbara feels capable, she parents Melissa alone, with Nina on the periphery.

- *Step 2*. Gradually, Barbara becomes overwhelmed by the responsibility of parenting Melissa alone, and responds by distancing herself from the girl.

- *Step 3*. Cut off from a relationship with her mother, Melissa's symptoms intensify.

- *Step 4*. Barbara calls Nina for help.

- *Step 5*. Nina moves in, giving Barbara a respite. Barbara, now feeling less overwhelmed, reconnects with Melissa, who improves.

- *Step 6*. After Melissa appears to be doing better, Nina returns to her own home, leaving Barbara and Melissa alone again, thus leading back to Step 1 in the cycle.

In this case, the emergence of Melissa's psychotic symptoms appeared to be linked to her experience of disconnection from her mother, who would distance herself from Melissa when she felt overwhelmed with the responsibilities of parenting. Grandmother's presence allowed Melissa and Barbara to reconnect, and Melissa's symptoms waned in response. One of the treatment goals was to promote a stronger connection between Barbara and Nina, so that Nina would be engaged on a more consistent basis and not only when Melissa became symptomatic. This required helping Barbara and Nina address their own unresolved conflicts, develop mutual respect, and learn to collaborate.

Professionals could easily become inducted into a symptomatic cycle such as this one. For example, a therapist might interpret Nina's involvement as intrusive and undermining of Barbara's parental authority. To support Barbara's role as parent and to shore up the family's boundaries, the therapist might keep Nina at a distance and block her efforts to get involved with Barbara and Melissa. However, this intervention would be a mistake, since the distance between Nina and Barbara would serve only to increase Barbara's isolation and make it more likely that she would disengage from Melissa when she felt overwhelmed.

One way to assess the role of family dynamics is to observe how the adolescent's psychotic symptoms wax or wane in reaction to family events.

For example, Melissa's psychotic symptoms were linked to the strength of her connection with Barbara. When Barbara withdrew, Melissa would become symptomatic. When Nina's presence alleviated Barbara's stress, Barbara would reconnect with Melissa, who subsequently improved. The following case illustrates how a boy's experience of abandonment by his father led to an exacerbation of his psychotic symptoms.

Gabe Flynn, a 16-year-old boy with a diagnosis of bipolar disorder, was belligerent and disrespectful to the other family members. The boy's father had always remained peripheral, aligned in a covert coalition with the boy against his mother, who had taken most of the responsibility for parenting, and did so in a rather heavy-handed manner. Initially, family sessions focused on helping Mr. Flynn become more involved in co-parenting. Mr. Flynn, however, took the opposite extreme—in order to avoid the breakup of his marriage when his wife gave him an ultimatum that he either take a stronger position with Gabe or face losing her, Mr. Flynn flipped over to supporting his wife, which left the boy feeling abandoned and encouraged an exacerbation of his symptoms. The boy's hostility toward his mother increased, and as Mr. Flynn persisted in supporting his wife, Gabe began directing hostility toward his father. Gabe became more disorganized in his behavior and speech, and claimed to be hearing voices. Nevertheless, Mr. and Mrs. Flynn continued to view Gabe's behavior as "bad" rather than "crazy" and kept punishing him. Eventually, the boy became so symptomatic that he needed to be hospitalized.

In Gabe's case, two factors were related to the exacerbation of his psychotic symptoms. First, he experienced abandonment by his father when his father joined his mother in disciplining him. Second, his behavior was misunderstood by his parents as willfully defiant, which also contributed to Gabe's feeling disconnected and disregarded by his parents. While the coalition between Gabe and his father was ineffective from a structural point of view, the intensity of their relationship helped to calm Gabe and kept his bizarre symptoms in check. Father's inability to maintain a relationship simultaneously with his wife and son led him to abandon Gabe completely when he decided to support his wife to prevent her from leaving him.

The solution required shifting the parents' attention away from setting limits to developing ways to manage conflict without escalating it. I encouraged Mr. and Mrs. Flynn to see Gabe as temporarily under the influence of "bipolar disorder," which would pass with appropriate treatment and management. The parental coalition was solidified not by exhorting them to remain firm against the boy, but by prompting them to talk with each other about ways that they could be more helpful to Gabe and more supportive of each other when Gabe's behavior got out of control. Toward this end, I suggested ways to deescalate family conflicts by using techniques such as distraction, focusing on points of agreement, and avoiding unproductive arguing. I also encouraged both the father and mother to foster a relationship with Gabe. Initially, Gabe was opposed to a relationship with his mother, but she persisted, and eventually they were able to spend some time together without fighting. Father was coached on how to support and encourage Gabe without appearing to side with him against his wife.

In both of these cases, the adolescent's functioning deteriorated when he or she felt isolated and disconnected from family members. This is not to imply that the experienced abandonment *caused* the psychosis. Rather, the family's response to milder symptoms contributed not to alleviating or containing these symptoms but rather to intensifying them. Therapy should focus on these interactional patterns, not with the goal of discovering "why" the psychosis occurred, but rather with the goal of promoting better family functioning as a way to reduce stress on the adolescent. It is important to help the family members discover ways to facilitate the adolescent's progress and prevent the symptoms from intensifying.

Melissa's case illustrates how the girl's symptoms were kept in check by helping her mother and grandmother to work effectively together as a team. In Gabe's case, I needed to support the parental subsystem while also promoting stronger connections between Gabe and each of his parents. The focus remains on helping the adolescent function as well as possible despite the psychotic symptoms. Changes in the family relationships are encouraged for the purpose of helping the adolescent to function better. It is important to help the family members navigate between the poles of underestimating and overestimating the psychotic youngster's competence. If family members underestimate the youth's competence, they might encourage too much dependency. If family members overestimate the youth's competence, they might fail to provide the support he or she needs when faced with a developmental demand that appears minor but that might be a substantial stressor for an adolescent vulnerable to psychosis. In other cases, as we saw in Gabe's family, the family members might misattribute the adolescent's behavior to willful defiance and therefore respond in a way that exacerbates the problem.

REDUCING ISOLATION IN PSYCHOTIC SYSTEMS

Listening to the Adolescent's Voice

Psychotic adolescents might be paranoid or so self-involved that they cannot enter into a relationship in the usual sense of the term. The challenge is to remain engaged in spite of the absence of the usual kinds of emotional reciprocity one experiences in a relationship. Relationships with psychotic individuals will have a different "feel," so therapists should not base their assessment of the quality of the relationship on their subjective experience of it. The adolescent's involvement in the therapeutic process is a better indicator of the quality of the relationship with the therapist. Some questions to consider include: Does the adolescent come to sessions? Does the adolescent seem interested in what the therapist says? Does the adolescent follow the therapist's suggestions? How does the adolescent's relationship with the therapist compare to other relationships in the adolescent's life?

As part of building a relationship with the adolescent, it is necessary to exert more effort than usual to listen to the adolescent and try to decipher what he or she is trying to say. It is a mistake to assume that disorganized ways of communicating disqualify the adolescent from having a voice. In fact, it should be assumed that the adolescent has something very important to say. It is the therapist's job to understand the adolescent and to help the family to understand the youth. It is important to take what the adolescent is saying seriously, even if it seems to be unintelligible or tangential at first. It is then possible to help the adolescent to express him- or herself in a way that is more readily comprehensible.

Sometimes the emergence of symptoms is an indirect request for help. For example, a boy who had experienced three psychotic episodes would become disorganized toward the end of sessions when it was time for him to take the subway home. The boy expressed his fear of taking the train alone by becoming disorganized and bizarre in his speech. When the meaning of this message became clear to me, I wanted to communicate to the boy that I understood. I acknowledged his fear and offered to walk with him to the subway station and wait with him until his train arrived. Over the next few sessions, I worked to expand the boy's sphere of independence, first by walking him to the station and not waiting for the train, then eventually by walking him halfway to the station, until eventually he was traveling to sessions on his own. Over the course of these sessions, the boy was able to communicate his fear intelligibly and appropriately and no longer relied on symptoms as a way of expressing his need for help.

It is important to wait for moments of lucidity and then amplify these moments by paying attention to them and helping the family members to pay attention to them. Sometimes, the message that the adolescent wants to communicate is not one that the family is ready to hear. Let's return to the case of Melissa for an example.

Melissa had been doing well for several months and was discovering her voice. At a family session, Melissa confronted Nina on the way she treated Barbara and asked her to try to act "nicer." Nina, who usually viewed herself as the victim of Barbara's irrational anger, uncharacteristically lashed out at Melissa and accused her of disrespect and ingratitude. She said that she was "through" with Melissa and Barbara and would stop seeing them.

I realized that I needed to support both Melissa and Nina, and do so in a way that did not alienate Barbara. Melissa was expressing her concerns in an age-appropriate way, rather than in disorganized speech or erratic behavior. On the other hand, Nina had a point: Neither Melissa nor Barbara really acknowledged how much she had done and continued to do for them. She felt used and understandably hurt when Melissa implied that she had to do more by assuming responsibility for her conflicts with Barbara.

I intervened by first acknowledging how hard it was for Melissa to speak up, because she loved her grandmother and did not want to hurt her. I praised her for her courage in taking the risk to express herself. I then turned to Nina and acknowledged how hurt she must feel. As I expressed my appreciation for her efforts and apologized for not having done so sooner, I turned the focus to our relationship. Did Nina believe that I viewed her as a capable, caring, generous woman? Did she believe that I had helped her family? She answered both questions in the affirmative, and I asked a third: Was she angry at me for any reason? She initially said that she was not angry with me, but as I pushed a bit she eventually admitted that she felt that I did not always appreciate how much stress she was under and how difficult it was for her to work with Barbara. I apologized again, and asked if she would be willing to give me another chance to help her feel more appreciated in the family. I reminded Nina that leaving Barbara and Melissa meant leaving me, and I wanted another chance. She reluctantly agreed, and even said that she would try to keep her anger at Barbara in check.

I then turned to Barbara and asked her if she could think of any way that she and I could show Nina how much we appreciated all that she had done. Barbara noted that Nina would be turning 65 next month, and she suggested that she give a party as a way of thanking her. I commended her on this idea and offered to help her organize it. I had also been working to help reduce this family's isolation from their community. Nina had a few friends, but she saw them rarely. I suggested that Barbara include Nina's friends on the guest list and think of other ways to bring Nina's friends into their lives.

Building Relationships with Family Members

If a family has a psychotic member, the other family members might be sensitive about being blamed for the psychotic person's problems. This concern is understandable, given some of the early models that attributed psychosis to parental behavior. To engage the family members in treatment, it is important to avoid implying that they are to blame for the adolescent's condition. Rather, it is necessary to communicate empathy for the stress the symptoms have placed on the family. The therapist must look beyond any apparent dysfunction in the family to the ways in which the family members have demonstrated concern and loyalty for one another and for the psychotic youngster.

It is important to show interest in each member of the family as an individual, and not reduce him or her to a role as a family member of a psychotic adolescent. Whenever a person's complexity is reduced and one facet is emphasized over all others, the person is likely to feel misunderstood, alienated, and marginalized. In psychotic families, the symptoms are so powerful that they command the family's attention. In response, family members' needs are likely to be neglected, while they give top priority to helping the psychotic youngster. Family members might feel that they have no right to pursue other interests as long as the youngster is psychotic. They might be ashamed of the adolescent's behavior, so they withdraw from social contact and isolate themselves from the community.

Therapists must communicate respect and interest in each family member, get to know him or her as an individual, and show that they care about his or her unique needs. The family members should be encouraged to work together to help *each other*, rather than concentrate exclusively on the psychotic member. Thus, sessions should focus on relationships among all family members, not just on the relationships of the family members with the psychotic adolescent. Other family relationships might be neglected as the family members strive to help the symptomatic adolescent. Therapy should work against this tendency and put emphasis on each family member's needs and concerns, whether or not they appear to be directly related to the psychotic symptoms.

Sometimes, family members who are overwhelmed by the stress within the family might look outside the family for support. This move can be a positive one if it alleviates stress or helps the family member feel valued and respected by another individual. However, it is also possible that relationships outside the family could be detrimental, both to the family member who is involved as well as to the relationships within the family. This problem was exemplified in Melissa's family.

As Barbara began to feel more confident and comfortable in her parenting role, she began to venture out and expand her social network. She began to date a man whom Nina did not like, because he used drugs and threatened Barbara with physical violence. At one session a crisis erupted when Nina announced that she would not be returning to sessions and would break off further contact with Barbara because she refused to end the relationship with her boyfriend. I realized that we were on a tightrope. On the one hand, it was a positive step for Barbara, who had never had many friends, to pursue relationships with other adults. On the other hand, it was difficult to disagree with Nina's opposition to Barbara's boyfriend's behavior. I addressed this impasse by asking Barbara to talk openly about her loneliness while Melissa and Nina listened. Then, I asked Barbara to listen to Nina's concerns without defending her boyfriend, and instead see if they could find a common ground. By the end of the conversation, Barbara had told her mother how much she needed her, and Nina had acknowledged Barbara's desire for male companionship, even though both women agreed that her current boyfriend was not a good influence on Melissa.

Supporting the Family's Competence

As Haley (1997) and Madanes (1981) have pointed out, family members who are dealing with severe symptoms often attempt to abdicate their parental role by declaring themselves incompetent to deal with the problem. They might try to shift responsibility to the professionals, who are viewed as more knowledgeable and competent. If the professionals accept this responsibility, the family's dependency is reinforced and their belief in their inability to handle their own problems is strengthened. The pitfall of assuming that the problem is too complex for the family to handle must be avoided. Instead, it is important to consider what additional resources or skills the family might need in order to handle the problem more effectively. This perspective keeps the family in an appropriately central role and affirms their competence, while also recognizing that families will need the help of extended family, friends, and professionals.

For example, when Barbara began to worry that Melissa was becoming symptomatic and might need to be hospitalized, she would call me for help. If I were to take over or encourage Barbara to take Melissa to the hospital, then the goal of promoting better collaboration between Barbara and Nina could be thwarted. Instead, I proposed the following plan: Barbara should immediately contact Nina, and they should discuss together what should be done. If they thought that hospitalization might be necessary, before going to the hospital, Barbara and Melissa should go to Nina's house and the family should simulate an "Emergency Room" there, contacting me by phone to receive advice and support. If after 24 hours of being in this "Emergency Room" at Nina's home the family still wanted Melissa to be hospitalized, then we would meet for a crisis session and decide on the next steps. Barbara reluctantly agreed to this plan, but after a few hours at Nina's house, Melissa seemed better and hospitalization was averted.

The purpose of this intervention was to encourage the family members to rely on their own resources and not turn responsibility over to the professionals. As we saw above, reconnecting with Nina would often alleviate Barbara's anxiety over Melissa's symptoms. Encouraging Barbara to take Melissa to Nina's house, rather than to the hospital, brought Barbara and Nina together, helped to reduce Barbara's anxiety, and enabled both women to avert the crisis by working together. On the other hand, if I were to agree that Melissa should be hospitalized at the first sign of symptoms, the family's competence would be undermined. Moreover, hospitalizing Melissa could contribute to increased isolation from her family, when what she actually needed to feel more secure was stronger connections with them.

Fostering Collaboration among Helpers

In treating psychosis, it is likely that other professionals will be involved with the family. The problem of coordination then comes to the fore. In some cases, the therapist might be in the role of case manager and head of the treatment team. Ideally, all members of the team will share a common view of the treatment goals, decisions will be made collaboratively, and periodic meetings with the family and the team will be arranged. As team leader, the therapist must attend not only to his or her relationship with the family, but also to the relationships among the members of the team. Conflicts among team members can undermine effective treatment and must be resolved.

In some cases the family therapist is not head of the treatment team and might feel left out when major decisions are being made. In these cases, the therapist must find a way to work with the other professionals for the benefit of the patient and the family. Cultivating relationships based on mutual respect rather than competition is essential. Therapists might conceptualize their role as that of consultant to the team in matters pertaining to family dynamics and effective team coordination. As with any consultant, the other team members are free to accept or reject the therapist's suggestions and the therapist should not take this personally.

Therapists who have a conflict with another team member must be careful not to triangulate the family by attempting to win the family over to their side. It is also important to watch out for attempts by the family members to triangulate the therapist into conflicts between the family and another team member. Rather than assuming the role of mediator in these conflicts, it is more beneficial to help the family to deal directly and effectively with the member of the team with whom the family is in conflict.

For example, Barbara began to complain to me about the psychiatrist who was monitoring Melissa's medications. Barbara felt that the psychiatrist was not respectful of her, ignored her input, and acted as if Nina were the person in charge of taking care of Melissa. Nina disagreed with Barbara's assessment. She found the psychiatrist competent, if a bit businesslike, and thought that Barbara was often disrespectful of the psychiatrist. I could understand why Barbara and Nina had these feelings. In my dealings with the psychiatrist, I sometimes felt that she was a bit brusque and spoke about Barbara in a condescending way. However, I also knew that Barbara could take an immature, disrespectful tone toward authority figures.

Before jumping to the conclusion that the psychiatrist was undermining my treatment plan, I wondered if I had explained clearly enough my rationale for my treatment goals. I decided that I would contact the psychiatrist, not to report Barbara's complaints, but rather to invite her to share her impressions of the family and then to share mine. I also wanted to encourage Barbara to express her concerns directly to the psychiatrist and not mediated through me, but it was important that she do so in a mature and respectful manner. I asked Nina if she would be willing to help Barbara talk with the psychiatrist about her feelings. Nina agreed, and Barbara and I spent the next several minutes discussing how she might bring up her issues in a way that did not simply reinforce the psychiatrist's opinion of her as impulsive and irrational. My conversation with the psychiatrist went well, and at the next session Barbara and Nina reported that they had spoken with the psychiatrist, felt that she had listened, and believed that she took Barbara seriously. The psychiatrist apologized for giving Barbara the impression that she did not value her opinion, and resolved to be more sensitive to this issue in the future.

SUMMARY

Patience and persistence are the keys to working with psychotic adolescents and their families. Many of the same principles discussed in previous chapters can be applied to working with these families. Here is a summary of the major points covered in this chapter:

- Therapy should focus on improving the adolescent's functioning, and not simply removing or alleviating psychotic symptoms.
- Do not imply that family dynamics caused the psychosis. Focus on altering family patterns with the goal of helping the psychotic youngster to function better and avoid relapse.
- Listen carefully to the psychotic adolescent's voice, and show

particular attention at those times when the adolescent communicates lucidly.

• Develop relationships with each member of the family. Treat each member as a unique individual, not just as a family member of a psychotic patient.

• Improve the family's capacity to cope with the psychotic symptoms by strengthening relationships with each other and with members of their community.

• Encourage and support the family members' ability to handle crises on their own rather than immediately turning to professionals.

• Avoid triangulation on the treatment team. Help the family members resolve conflicts with other team members on their own rather than relying on the therapist to mediate the conflicts.

10

Underachievement and Other School-Related Problems

It was only the fourth week of the school year and Dave, age 13, had been suspended for the third time because he had been fighting on school grounds and "mouthing off" disrespectfully to teachers. It was Dave's father, Carl, who contacted me and requested help. The school was considering a referral to a special school program for disruptive students, and Carl believed that "it would kill Dave if he had to go to that program."

Both parents, Dave, and Dave's quiet, studious, younger brother attended the first session. Carl, a sincere, gentle man, opened the session by recounting a long list of school problems starting in the third grade. Dave interjected at several points to clarify details of time, place, or sequence. Dave's mother, Bernice, remained silent, but her expression betrayed her frustration.

After listening to Carl for a while, I invited Bernice to comment. She burst out, "I've had it! This kid doesn't respect anyone—least of all me. He's headed to reform school, and there's nothing I can do about it."

Carl jumped in. "Well, honey, that's why we're here. We're here to find out what we are doing that's making Dave act this way." Bernice sighed and looked away, defeated.

It seemed likely that this scene had played out before: The father, the reasonable, supportive parent, wanting to help his son so much that he was willing to accept the blame for the boy's actions, and the mother, the tired, frustrated parent who was reluctantly cast in the role of reminding Carl how out of control Dave was.

I learned that the dynamics were even more complicated when

I contacted the school. The school counselor confided in me that she believed that Bernice was "the problem." She thought "something was up" with the mother, and that Dave was acting out at school because he was displacing onto teachers and other students his aggression against his mother. At school conferences, just as in our family session, Bernice remained silent and allowed the father to do the talking. When she did speak, she expressed herself in a way that seemed critical of the school. The school counselor believed that the father was the more reasonable parent, since he was able to be calm at the school conferences and agreed with the school that Dave's fighting was a reflection of "underlying issues."

Many families come to therapy with a school problem as the presenting complaint. Usually, the concern is the child's "underachievement" (i.e., the youngster's academic performance is falling short of his or her capabilities). Behavioral problems, such as truancy or noncompliance with school rules, might or might not accompany underachievement.

Harry Aponte (1976a) was one of the first family therapists to recognize that effective family therapy must also include work with the larger system or *ecosystem* of which the family is a subsystem. For school-related problems, Aponte advocated working with the family and school together rather than with the family alone. Evan Imber-Black (1991) also extended traditional family therapy concepts to the larger system or *macrosystem*. She made two observations that are particularly relevant to the relationship between the family and the school:

1. Neither system (i.e., family or school) need be inherently dysfunctional in order for problems to arise in their interaction. This point extends to larger systems the principle that relationships within the family might be dysfunctional even in the absence of individual psychopathology.
2. Patterns of relationship between the family and larger systems might replicate existing patterns within the family. This is known as *isomorphism*. For example, in a case reported by Power and Bartholomew (1985), detouring of conflict between the parents through the symptomatic child was isomorphic to the pattern of detouring conflict between the parents and the school through the child.

I believe that academic underachievement is usually the result of multiple factors that interact with one another. Rather than attempting to isolate a single "cause" of the school problem, I recommend that the relative importance of all of the following common contributors to academic difficulties be considered in order to arrive at the appropriate intervention strategy.

FACTORS CONTRIBUTING
TO ADOLESCENT UNDERACHIEVEMENT

Learning Disability

Learning disability might be present when a student fails to master academic skills despite adequate intellectual ability (Chalfant, 1989; Lipka & Siegel, 2006). In many cases, learning disability will be identified during the early grades, although in some cases it will not be detected until adolescence. Adolescents with an undiagnosed learning disability often compensate for their deficits during the early school years but falter when work demands increase. Because they had been successful at school in the past, these adolescents are frequently not considered learning disabled but rather are viewed as inadequately motivated. Students who appear to be unmotivated might have given up because they feel overwhelmed and view themselves as incompetent.

Learning disability can accompany any of the other problems discussed in this chapter. Since learning disability in adolescence can have substantial importance for academic planning, the therapist should consider consulting with a qualified psychologist to determine if a complete psychoeducational evaluation is indicated.

Attention-Deficit/Hyperactivity Disorder

Attention-deficit/hyperactivity disorder (ADHD) is a syndrome of presumed but unknown neurological etiology that affects the capacity to direct and sustain attention to tasks (Barkley, 2006). In some cases, learning disability might also be present. In many cases, the child will also exhibit problematic behavior associated with the impulsivity and hyperactivity that are part of this syndrome (Wender, 1995). Follow-up studies of children and adolescents with ADHD have shown that they are at higher risk for antisocial behavior and other forms of marginal adjustment in adulthood (Barkley, Fischer, Smallish, & Fletcher, 2006; Gittelman, Mannuzza, Shenker, & Bonagura, 1985; Mannuzza & Gittelman, 1984; Mannuzza, Klein, Bonagura, & Malloy, 1991; Young, 2000).

Three subtypes of ADHD are identified in the DSM-IV-TR (American Psychiatric Association, 2000): the predominantly inattentive type, the predominantly impulsive type, and the combined type. Although most adolescents with ADHD will exhibit signs of impulsivity and hyperactivity, it is important to note that an adolescent might have an attentional problem even though signs of hyperactivity are absent. This *inattentive* subtype of ADHD might be mistaken for depression and can be differentiated from it by the absence of other symptoms characteristic of a depressive syndrome and the presence of attentional deficits on psychological testing.

In many cases, treatment with stimulant medication such as methylphenidate can improve the student's attention span, although it is important to evaluate the potential for abuse of the medication. Cognitive-behavioral methods to train youngsters to modulate their impulsivity have also been effective (Kendall, 1991), as well as psychoeducational interventions (Barkley, Guevremont, Anastopoulos, & Fletcher, 1992).

The procedure for diagnosing ADHD includes taking a careful history, gathering behavioral ratings of the student by parents and teachers, and psychological testing to rule out a coexisting learning disability (Barkley, 2006). Even with comprehensive testing, ADHD can be difficult to detect, particularly when it occurs comorbidly with other disorders, or when it is embedded in a context of other social or interpersonal problems. When the diagnosis is uncertain, a trial on medication might be undertaken, although some experts caution against this practice, pointing out that stimulants can improve performance even when true ADHD is not present.

Motivational Factors

Although motivation and academic performance typically decline when kids enter high school (Elmen, 1991), students who are more oriented toward intrinsic goals and more confident in their abilities are more likely to demonstrate persistence and eventual success on academic tasks (Ames & Archer, 1988; Ginsburg & Bronstein, 1993). Providing tangible rewards (e.g., money for grades achieved) tends to reduce intrinsic motivation, while a cognitively stimulating home environment tends to increase intrinsic motivation (Deci, Koestner, & Ryan, 1999; Gottfried, Fleming, & Gottfried, 1998).

Academically successful students tend to attribute their success to internal factors ("I studied hard"), while underachieving students are more likely to attribute their success to external factors ("The test was easy"; Carr, Borkowski, & Maxwell, 1991). Some students believe that their achievement is not under their control and so feel helpless in response to failure (Dweck & Licht, 1980). Underachieving students might not benefit from feedback regarding their academic performance because they don't see a connection between success and their own efforts or study strategies. Teacher perceptions and expectations of a student's academic abilities can also influence how well the student performs in school. This *self-fulfilling prophecy* appears to exert a stronger influence on performance for low-achieving than high-achieving students (Madon, Jussim, & Eccles, 1997).

Motivational factors are particularly relevant for students from certain cultural minority groups. For African American adolescents, school achievement is negatively affected by the belief that discriminatory practices limit their employment opportunities (Taylor, Casten, Flickinger, Roberts, & Fulmore, 1994). African American students can also be affected by *stereotype threat* (Steele, 1997), whereby exposure to negative stereotypes about the academic abilities of African Americans can depress their performance on cognitive tests (Kellow & Jones, 2008). Girls, too, are vulnerable to stereotype threat. For example, girls who are exposed to the stereotype that girls are not as good as boys on math tests perform more poorly on these tests than girls who are not exposed to this message (Spencer, Steele, & Quinn, 1999).

Many students have never learned how to study, lack basic academic skills, and spend insufficient time on their studies. In particular, those adolescents who are above average in intelligence might have been able to succeed in elementary school without exerting much effort. When they get to middle school, where more independent work is required, their grades plummet. The shock of encountering failure for the first time can begin a downward spiral of underachievement beginning in middle school and continuing into high school.

It is important to differentiate low motivation in school from low motivation in general. Students who are not academically oriented might nevertheless be highly motivated in another area, such as sports or the arts. Students who appear unmotivated in general are more likely to experience other individual and interpersonal problems in addition to academic difficulties. The possibility of depression should be considered if the low-achieving adolescent is exhibiting a pattern of low motivation in many areas of life. Depression can contribute to low motivation, which in turn contributes to poor performance, which in turn reinforces and intensifies the depression. Reactions of the family members and the school staff can contribute to this pattern as well.

The School Environment

Jacquelynne Eccles and her colleagues (1993) have pointed out that the typical middle school is often unsuited to the needs of the developing adolescent. Compared to elementary school teachers, middle school teachers are less likely to trust their students and more likely to emphasize control and discipline in the classroom. They are also likely to be perceived by their students as less friendly, less supportive, and less caring than elementary school teachers. A poor fit between the adolescent's needs and the school environment can be a major factor contributing to academic underachievement.

Conflicts within the faculty or between the faculty and the administration can also undermine a school's effectiveness in meeting students' needs (Fisher, 1986). Teachers who feel overworked or unappreciated might displace some of their frustration onto students, who, in turn, might personalize the teacher's attitude and respond in ways that only serve to intensify the teacher's frustration.

One obviously bright girl told me that she deliberately failed a course because she "hated" the teacher and refused to do any work "for her." For this girl and many other adolescents, achievement is strongly influenced by the quality of their relationships with teachers. Erratic performance at school, with a wide range of grades and no consistency in patterns of high and low grades, suggests that the personal relationship with a teacher could be an important factor in an adolescent's academic performance.

Peer Relationships

Students who associate with high achievers are likely to value high achievement, while students whose friends are underachievers are likely to underachieve as well (Epstein, 1983). Undermining of academic competence by peers is particularly intense for African American students, whose peers might accuse them of "acting white" when they get high grades (Fordham & Ogbu, 1986).

Students who are strongly oriented toward peers tend to perform more poorly in school, but the strength of an adolescent's peer orientation depends on the quality of his or her relationship with parents (Fuligni & Eccles, 1993). Adolescents who are most strongly oriented toward peers are those who come from authoritarian homes in which they are afforded few opportunities for decision making. Studies have shown that authoritative parenting (warm but firm) is associated with school success (Steinberg, Lamborn, Dornbusch, & Darling, 1992), while strict and punitive parenting is associated with diminished school achievement (DeBaryshe, Patterson, & Capaldi, 1993).

Another feature of the adolescent peer context is the socialization pressures experienced by girls and boys at school. Mary Pipher (1994) has called attention to the prevalence of sexual harassment of girls by boys in middle school, a practice that can poison the entire school experience for some girls. Boys are also subject to gender-specific socialization pressures at school, such as intimidation and violence among the male peer group (Denborough, 1996). Boys who deviate from culturally pre-scribed standards of masculinity face ostracism or victimization by other boys, male coaches, and male teachers (McLean, 1996; Pollack, 1998). The myth that boys must be independent can lead to the emotional aban-donment of boys by parents, especially mothers, thus intensifying boys' alienation from the family and amplifying the dynamics of the male peer culture (Silverstein & Rashbaum, 1994).

Problems within the Family

In the early days of family therapy, any symptom, school-related or otherwise, was considered to be a sign of internal family dysfunction. As family therapy matured into a more ecosystemic view, the lens was broadened to include other factors. School-related problems were no lon-ger necessarily considered symptomatic of internal family dysfunction, but could be maintained by problematic interactions between the family and school.

The error of assuming that academic problems reflect internal fam-ily dysfunction is a particular risk when a family is referred to treatment by the school. Jorge Colapinto (1988) warned of this "common pitfall in compulsory school referrals" and cautioned therapists against assum-ing that the school problem was caused by problems within the family. Colapinto advised therapists to concentrate on fostering better teamwork between the family and school rather than focusing on internal family dynamics that were presumed to be encouraging or maintaining the stu-dent's problem at school.

While a narrow focus on family dynamics can distract the therapist from seeing the complex interrelationships among the child, family, and school that could be contributing to the problem, an ecosystemic view avoids either/or formulations and considers the possibility that the stu-dent's problems at school could be symptomatic of problematic interac-tions within the family. In making a careful assessment of the academic problem, the therapist should observe the family interactions and con-sider ways that these internal family dynamics might be contributing to or maintaining the problem. The manner in which some families handle noncompliance with homework is an example of this pattern.

Homework Problems

Some families get into battles around a child's failure to complete home-work assignments. The parents see the problem as the child's "laziness" or willful noncompliance, while the child insists that the parents' overinvolvement is the cause of the problem. A power struggle can ensue: The parents demand that the child complete homework and impose consequences for noncompliance; the child refuses to comply or begins to act out in other ways.

If a family does not readily respond to simple and commonsense advice on how to handle homework more effectively, then it is possible that the child's refusal to comply with homework is a symptom of a wider family problem. The case of 14-year-old Michelle illustrates this point. Michelle had just received three failing grades on her report card, and teachers commented that the reason for the grades was her failure to turn in homework. Taking the problem at face value at first, I recommended a few standard strategies: Arrange a specific time and place for homework, help the child get organized and then back off, check to be sure the work has been done after the homework time is over, and regularly communicate with teachers regarding assignments and their completion. These strategies did not work. Michelle became angrier at her parents, and the parents became more frustrated with Michelle.

As I observed the family interactional patterns around the problem I noticed that the parents were ignoring Michelle's anger at them. Instead, they kept insisting that they were in charge and she had to follow their rules. Their position only served to make Michelle angrier. When talking with her parents about this issue, Michelle would often say, "You don't really care about me." At one point, I interrupted the interaction among the family members and asked Michelle to talk more about her feeling that her parents didn't care about her. She said that her parents didn't understand how unhappy she was and cared only about her grades. She hated school and most of her teachers and believed that she didn't have any friends whom she could trust.

It was also clear that Michelle's mother was overwhelmed. She had a medical illness that caused chronic fatigue. She worked outside the home, and had no energy left for Michelle when she came home from school. Michelle's father's job required frequent trips away from home. He felt guilty about leaving his wife and children, but felt he had no other career options at this time. To compensate for his guilt, when he was home he zealously tried to support the mother, but did so by taking an authoritarian position with Michelle.

In a private session, Michelle's mother revealed that her own mother had physically and emotionally abused her. She was hurt at Michelle's accusations that she didn't care about her, because she had tried so hard to be more loving and attentive than her own mother was. She realized, though, that she had been dismissive of Michelle and overly critical of her because she didn't have the energy to give Michelle the attention she needed.

I orchestrated a conversation between Michelle and her mother during which Michelle told her mother how she was feeling and her mother was able to listen nondefensively. Mother was willing to take this step because I had expressed that I understood how overwhelmed she felt and I did not blame her for Michelle's problems. I then helped Michelle's mother tell Michelle that she did care about her, but that her own background made it very difficult for her to be as sympathetic to Michelle as she knew she should be. Michelle's mother was able to acknowledge that she had made mistakes and validated Michelle's anger at her. Father was able to do the same: He acknowledged that he came down hard on Michelle because of his desire to protect the mother, and that his doing so was not helpful to Michelle but rather made her feel even more misunderstood.

As happens in many cases when parents can drop their guard and show their humanity and frailty, Michelle rose to the occasion. She listened sympathetically to her parents, acknowledged that she was rude to them, and apologized. Often, youngsters have little understanding of a parent's own struggles because the parents have been unwilling to share these struggles with them, either to protect the child or to avoid appearing weak. However, when parents share the reasons behind the behaviors that have frustrated the child, the child will often respond in a sympathetic and mature manner that demonstrates their caring for the parent. They are willing to accept their parent's weaknesses, as long as the parent has the courage and honesty to admit them. In turn, they are willing to acknowledge their own shortcomings. While these favorable events don't happen in all cases, they happen far more often than we might expect. It happened in Michelle's family, and the unproductive arguments over homework ended. Michelle, her parents, and I were able to collaborate more effectively on solutions that would work for them.

Problems Involving the Adolescent, the Family, and the School

At times, a dysfunctional relationship among the adolescent, the family, and the school contributes to the academic problem. Here are some examples:

1. The parents undermine the school by giving the student overt or covert messages that the school personnel are not competent. For example, a parent criticizes a teacher in the presence of the student or repeatedly complains to the school administration about the teacher.

2. Parents become overinvolved in micromanaging the student's academic work. One parent whose son had a long history of underachieve-

ment despite above-average intellectual abilities would "help" her son with his homework by agreeing to do half of it for him if he would agree to do the other half. She would plead with the school to give her son extensions on assignments that he had left to the last minute. Routinely, on the eve of the renegotiated due date, she would sit with her son at the word processor, liberally "editing" what he dictated to her to help the paper "flow better." Not only did this practice undermine the school's expectation that the boy accept responsibility for his own assignments, but it also gave the message to the boy that he was incapable of doing his work without his mother's help.

3. A problematic interaction between the family and school could be maintained by the school's perspective that the parents are responsible for the student's problem because they are creating obstacles to implementing what the school believes is the best solution. The more the school personnel insist on their point of view, the more the parents resist. Therapists can get inducted into this pattern, particularly if they are referred a case by the school or directly hired as a consultant by the school. At the end of this chapter, I offer suggestions for identifying and avoiding the traps of triangulation in situations such as these.

4. Sometimes the parents and school are locked in intense conflict over what is best for the student. Rather than working collaboratively to help the student succeed, the parents and school battle with one another over whose approach is right. In these cases, the student's failure and the family–school conflict elicit one another. To the extent that the parents and school are distracted by their conflict with one another, they are less available to support the student. Consequently, the student is more likely to fail, which elicits more intense conflict between the parents and school. The cycle might end with the student changing schools, only to repeat itself in the next school the student attends.

5. The school might undermine the parents' authority in more subtle ways by failing to maintain communication with the home or discounting the parents' perspective, values, or priorities. Through well-intentioned offers of support, school counselors could lend credence to a student's complaints about the parents without getting the parents' perspective. For example, a teacher would routinely allow a female student to visit her on weekends, go on trips with her, and join her for meals. The well-intentioned teacher felt genuine compassion for the child, who lived in an economically impoverished household where her needs and those of her seven siblings were often neglected. The teacher, believing that the student's academic success depended on her being safe and appropriately nourished, attempted to compensate for the apparent neglect in her family. Unfortunately, the more the girl confided in the teacher about the

conditions at home, the more disrespectful the child became to her own parents, to the point that whenever they tried to discipline her, she threatened to run to the teacher's house and report them for abusing her.

6. Sometimes, the parents and school have a benevolent attitude toward the student and view themselves as allies. However, in attempting to present a unified front, the parents and school might fail to involve the student. School conferences might involve the parents and exclude the adolescent. While this practice communicates to students that the adults in their lives are working together on their behalf, excluding them can also give the message that the adults will assume responsibility and they need not. It is small wonder that many students in this position fail to apply themselves to their schoolwork. Having been given the message that their opinions regarding their education are not important, they comply by abdicating responsibility for their own academic success. The adolescent's failure in school elicits only more concern from the parents and school, who redouble their efforts to close ranks to "help" the student.

In all of these examples, a problematic relationship among the family, school, and student contributes to maintaining the academic difficulties. In the next section, I discuss strategies for intervention in these cases and highlight how common pitfalls can be avoided.

STRATEGIES FOR INTERVENTION

The first step in developing an appropriate intervention strategy is to *consider whether a learning disability or ADHD is contributing to the underachievement*. Either of these conditions can have a significant impact on academic performance, so it is prudent to consider these conditions whenever underachievement is the presenting problem. In some cases, learning disability or ADHD might already have been identified, in which case it is important to determine whether the school is providing the appropriate remedial education. In other cases, learning disability or ADHD has not been diagnosed before, and it will be necessary to refer the student for a comprehensive psychoeducational evaluation. The presence of learning disability or ADHD does not mean that systemic dynamics do not also contribute to the adolescent's underachievement. However, neglecting to consider the possibility of learning disability or ADHD can create unnecessary frustration and vitiate other interventions.

The second step is to *assess the family* and consider whether the student's problems at school might be symptomatic of other problems within the family, or whether the family's strategy for solving the aca-

demic problem is actually making it worse. If the student's academic difficulties can be attributed to internal family dynamics (as in the case of
Michelle, discussed earlier), then intervention efforts should be directed
at altering these dynamics by working with the family as a whole.

The third step is to *assess the relationship patterns among the adolescent, the family, and the school* in order to identify the level of involvement the therapist should assume with each system. I shall describe three
strategies that represent different degrees of involvement by the therapist
in the family–school macrosystem. Each of these strategies has advantages and pitfalls. In *coaching*, the therapist refrains from direct contact
with the school and directs all interventions through the adolescent or
parents. In *mediation*, the therapist has contact with both the family and
the school but does not attempt to intervene directly in the relationship
between the two systems. In *direct intervention*, the therapist convenes
the family and school personnel together in order to intervene directly to
change the problematic relationship patterns between the two systems.
These strategies are depicted in Figure 10.1.

In general, it is wise to select the least intrusive method of intervention that is appropriate to the problem at hand; that is, first evaluate
whether the problem can be resolved from the position of coaching and
consider moving to a more intensive level of involvement only if coaching
has not been effective.

Coaching

Coaching the Adolescent

The therapist can coach the student in ways of handling problems at
school more effectively. If the parents are involved, they remain in a supportive role but allow the adolescent to take the lead in solving the problem. The following case illustrates this approach.

Beth, a 17-year-old senior, was struggling in her math class. She was
typically a mediocre student in math, but had never before been in danger
of failing. To make matters worse, she had been poorly motivated at the
beginning of the school year, hadn't turned in several assignments, and
had lost favor with the teacher. Beth had tried on her own to approach
the teacher, but she felt the teacher was unresponsive to her. Now, Beth
was convinced that she would fail the course because the teacher didn't
like her. Beth's parents were prepared to intercede for her, but I believed
that it would be more appropriate if Beth handled the problem on her
own.

I listened sympathetically as Beth explained in detail her frustration
with the class and her anger at the teacher. At first, the two feelings were

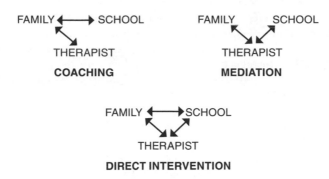

FIGURE 10.1. Three models of intervention for school-related problems.

merged in her experience, but, as we talked, she began to differentiate them. Beth was a bright, intuitive girl, and it did not take her long to recognize that her feelings toward the teacher were fueling her frustration with the subject matter. We then explored several options. She decided that she would write the teacher a note in which she would apologize for not working at the beginning of the year and ask if she could meet with him after class to try to convince him that she was now serious about passing the course. I wondered aloud how Beth might feel if the teacher did not respond to her note. Beth replied that she would feel hurt, but that she would try to put her feelings aside and approach the teacher in person a few days later to ask what he thought about her note. As a last resort, if the teacher still seemed unwilling to help, then Beth would ask her school counselor to intercede.

Coaching the adolescent is most appropriate when the school problem is relatively circumscribed and does not appear to be related to dysfunctional interactions within the family or between the family and school. It is likely to be most suitable for older adolescents who are able to take some distance from the conflict and not personalize the teacher's behavior. This approach is essential for adolescents with a learning disability or ADHD who are preparing to enter college, and who will need to advocate for themselves in order to receive the appropriate academic supports.

Coaching the Parents

If the adolescent is not motivated to handle the problem independently, or if the problem requires parental involvement, coaching the parents might be the appropriate strategy. This approach has been described by Mary Eno (1985):

Parents can be coached to work with schools, that is, to learn how to get the kind of information they need, how to evaluate that information, and how to negotiate with school staff members for specific changes. This therapeutic approach is in line with the guidelines of minimal intervention—the parents are nudged to do as much of the work as possible themselves. (p. 166)

I used the strategy of coaching to help the family of Todd, a 13-year-old boy who was failing three courses. Todd had assured his parents that he was doing well, despite the fact that they never observed him doing any homework. When they approached Todd to talk about the failure notice, Todd protested that the teachers were being "unfair." He insisted that he was doing his work, and that he did not deserve the failure notice. He also assured his parents that his grades had improved, and that his most recent test grades in all three courses were A's. Todd's parents were not convinced. They phoned the teachers and heard a different story. Not only was Todd getting failing grades on tests and quizzes, but he was not participating in class and not turning in assignments.

I first considered the possibility of a previously undiagnosed learning disability or ADHD. However, Todd did not fulfill the criteria for ADHD, and his previous academic performance was exemplary. The challenge was to help the parents and school close ranks so that Todd would not be able to split them.

I encouraged Todd's parents to make contact with the school counselor, who could be a resource to them and a liaison to the faculty. I suggested that the parents discuss with the counselor the possibility of instituting a procedure whereby Todd would write down his assignments in a special notebook at the end of class and check them with the teacher for accuracy. Todd would then show his assignment book to his parents every night. They would expect him to complete all of his homework and they would sign the assignment book after the work was completed.

The counselor agreed to the plan and the teachers welcomed the parents' involvement. Todd balked at being treated "like a little kid," but his parents reminded him that they would consider discontinuing the plan as soon as he demonstrated that he was capable of monitoring his school performance on his own. They confiscated his cell phone and told him that he would not be permitted to watch television or talk on the telephone until his assignments for the night were completed satisfactorily. If Todd "forgot" to bring his assignment book home, then he would not be allowed to watch television, use the computer, or talk on the telephone at all that night, and he would still need to spend 2 hours in his room studying or reading. Over the next few weeks, the parents and school worked out the "glitches" in the plan, and by the end of the marking period, Todd was passing all of his courses.

Pitfalls of Coaching

When therapists do not have direct contact with the school, they must rely on the family's potentially biased report as an accurate account of the interactions taking place between the family and school. This pitfall can be minimized by requesting the parents to bring in report cards, notes, or other written evaluations by teachers.

While it might seem that relying on the family's account of the interactions with the school will put the family in a favorable light and cast the school in the role of culprit, it is also possible that the school might be contributing to the problem in ways not apparent to the family. For example, there might be a conflict between the student's teachers about how best to handle the student. The school might be failing to intervene in harassment of the adolescent by peers or by a teacher. If one of these situations is suspected, then more direct involvement with the school (e.g., mediation or direct intervention) might be appropriate.

A second pitfall of coaching occurs when parents and the school avoid conflict with each other by blaming the therapist for not being able to solve the problem. If the therapist believes that this might be occurring, the therapist can request a single meeting with the family and school to clear up the "miscommunication." In this case, the therapist must be prepared to move to a more intensive level of involvement if it appears difficult to return to the less involved position of coaching.

Mediation

Mediation represents a step up in the level of involvement between a therapist and the school. In coaching, the therapist avoids direct contact with the school. In mediation, the therapist engages directly with the school in the role of liaison or go-between.

Mediation is similar to the approach advocated by Don-David Lusterman (1985) for "situations in which negative contact between the school and the family has increased pressure on the parents to produce change in the child's school behavior, but has in fact produced more negative behavior, and exacerbated existing problems in the home" (p. 24). Lusterman proposed a five-step process:

1. The therapist advocates complete disengagement between the family and the school.
2. The therapist contracts with the family and school that, for a

specified period of time, the school will not contact the family if the student has difficulties in school, but rather will contact the therapist, who will then work with the school to develop appropriate school-based interventions for the problem.

3. The therapist works with the family on problems not related to school.

4. When the home situation has improved, the therapist gradually reintroduces contact between the parents and school, adopting the position of coach for the family.

5. The therapist withdraws when it is clear that the family and school are working together more productively.

The case of 15-year-old Mike represents an example of mediation. Mike's parents were getting almost daily phone calls from the school complaining about Mike's disruptive behavior and poor academic performance. When Mike's parents tried to talk with him about the school's concerns, within a few minutes they'd be shouting at one another. The argument would escalate, and Mike would storm out of the house, only to return hours later after his exhausted parents had gone to bed.

It appeared that the parents and the school had developed a dysfunctional cycle of interactions: The parents' efforts to solve the school problem were increasing the tension at home and making it less likely that Mike would change his behavior at school. Mike himself agreed that he was very upset about the tension in the house, and he wished that he and his parents could get along better. He claimed that he was often so upset by the arguments of the night before that he had a "bad attitude" in class the next day and displaced his frustration onto the teachers.

I decided that I might be able to disrupt this pattern by inserting myself between the parents and the school. Adopting Lusterman's (1985) strategy, I negotiated a contract with the parents and the school that stipulated that they would have no contact with each other for 6 weeks. Instead, the school would contact me if Mike misbehaved, and I would provide consultation to the school on ways to handle the problem without contacting the parents. The family signed releases that permitted me the freedom to speak with the school about Mike.

Meanwhile, I encouraged the parents to "back off" and allow Mike to decide how he would manage his school responsibilities. I worked with Mike and his parents to draft a contract specifying that Mike would be expected to bring home passing grades in all of his subjects and not be suspended from school for any reason. For 6 weeks, any discussion about school would be "off limits." If Mike needed advice on how to handle a problem at school, he was to contact me. I would work with the family on other issues, such as balancing supervision and autonomy for Mike in other areas of his life, helping the parents work more collaboratively as a team, and encouraging the parents to resume some of the outside activities that they had been neglecting because they had been so consumed by Mike's school problems.

Privately, I challenged Mike to prove to his parents that he didn't need them to monitor his schoolwork. At the beginning of each session, I spent a few minutes alone with Mike, checking in with him about his progress and coaching him on ways he could handle problems at school. The remainder of the session was focused on other family issues. Twice a week, I contacted Mike's school counselor for a report on Mike's behavior and to offer suggestions on how the school might respond when Mike was uncooperative. I met with Mike's teachers and helped them to develop a consistent strategy for working with him.

Gradually, the relationships between Mike and his parents improved. At the end of the 6-week period, Mike had brought up his grades, even though he was still failing one subject. I decided to use this as an opportunity to reinvolve the parents with the school. I suggested that the parents contact Mike's teacher to find out why he was failing. After gathering this information, we would discuss how Mike's parents could help him if he was interested in passing the course. I emphasized that passing the course was Mike's responsibility, and that his parents would take neither the credit if he passed nor the blame if he failed. They would not, however, sign permission for him to take a part-time job after school unless he passed all of his subjects.

When to Use Mediation

In many cases, poor boundaries between the family and school can underlie family–school conflict. Mediation is an appropriate strategy to consider when the parents are either too involved with the school or not involved enough. As Lusterman (1985) points out and Mike's case illustrates, by serving as mediator the therapist can reduce the tension and associated reactivity between the parents and school. It is possible to draw a clearer distinction between "home" problems and "school" problems, restoring the former to center stage in the family sessions and moving the adolescent to a more central role in dealing with the latter.

Mediation has an advantage over coaching in that the mediating therapist has direct contact with both family and school and is thus able to see the problem from both perspectives rather than relying exclusively on the family's account. From the position of mediator, the therapist can positively reframe the actions of the family and school to each other, thus countering biased perceptions that can contribute to heightened conflict. It is possible to selectively underscore points of agreement between the family and school to foster collaboration between them, while ensuring that the student is not scapegoated.

Pitfalls of Mediation

A pitfall of mediation is the possibility that either family or school could cede all authority to the therapist. Either or both systems could refuse to engage in the process of negotiation and instead appeal to the therapist's "expertise," while abdicating responsibility for the consequences of the decisions.

To avoid this pitfall, therapists should clearly negotiate their role with both the family and the school at the outset of the mediation process. Therapists should adopt the position of advocate for the student and use this position as leverage to effect a change in the family's relationship with the school. For example, if the parents are protecting the student from appropriate consequences at school, the therapist can support the school's position by blocking messages from the school to the family and instead arrange to be the go-between for all communication.

Direct Intervention

Of the models discussed in this chapter, direct intervention requires the greatest degree of involvement by a therapist in the family's relationship with the school. In coaching, the therapist works only with the family. In mediation, the therapist works simultaneously with the family and the school. In direct intervention, the therapist works conjointly with the family and school together.

Harry Aponte's (1976a) "ecostructural" approach is an example of direct intervention in a conflict between a family and school. Aponte held the initial family session at the school and included in this session the student, parents, and relevant school personnel. The goal was to foster greater collaboration between the family and the school, facilitate conflict resolution, and encourage the development of specific plans to assist the student. Mary Eno (1985), while generally supporting a principle of minimal intervention in order to respect the boundaries between family and school, nevertheless endorsed direct intercession at the "interface" of the family and school in those cases when coaching was ineffective. Power and Bartholomew (1985) presented a case in which a series of direct interventions with the family and the school promoted a restructuring of a dysfunctional family–school relationship. Charles Fishman (1993) described a very intensive model of intervention called the "enhanced home–school partnership." According to this model, "parents become intimately involved in the child's education" (p. 183). This involvement could include maintaining daily communication with the school or even accompanying the child to school to help the teachers elicit greater compliance from the child.

Advantages of Direct Intervention

Direct intervention has a number of advantages. First, since all the "key players" are together in one place, communication of information is more efficient, and it is easier to negotiate a shared definition of the problem that is acceptable to all. Second, rather than relying on reports of interactions between the family and school, the therapist can observe these interactions directly. Third, the therapist has more leverage to alter these interactional patterns. As long as both systems have agreed to utilize the therapist as a resource, the therapist can address dysfunctional interactions not only between the systems, but also within each system.

Pitfalls of Direct Intervention

Therapists who choose this strategy must be skilled at tracking both content and process in large groups. It is not unusual for a family–school meeting to have a dozen participants, each with a different agenda. Therapists must be comfortable enough with their role in these meetings to allow all issues to be aired while preventing the meeting from degenerating into chaos. It can help if both the parents and the school agree at the outset that the therapist will be in charge of the meeting.

One disadvantage of direct intervention is that the parents might feel intimidated in a large meeting attended by many professionals. Parents might express their intimidation in different ways. Some become overly submissive, others passively resistant, and still others attack counterphobically. It is important to avoid drawing conclusions about family dynamics from the way family members behave at these meetings, because this behavior might not be typical of the way they usually act, but rather a reaction to the unique context of the family–school meeting. It is possible to help parents feel less intimidated by encouraging the parents to speak first, actively soliciting their input, recounting ways in which they have tried to be helpful to the student in the past, and focusing on positive steps they could take to be helpful in the future.

Another pitfall is that school personnel might feel intimidated and react defensively if they think that the therapist is aligned with the family against them. This reaction is understandable if the therapist has been working with the family for some time and only recently has initiated contact with the school. Therapists can avoid this pitfall by making an effort to join with the school at the outset of the meeting. To prevent family members from feeling betrayed or abandoned if the therapist seems to be more aligned with the school's point of view than they had anticipated, therapists should explain their intentions to the family in advance.

In order for direct intervention to be effective, the following principles should also be kept in mind:

- The therapist should make sure that both the family and school are open to the therapist's involvement.
- The purpose of the meeting should be framed as serving the needs of the student.
- The therapist should acknowledge the important contributions that the parents and school are each making to the student's welfare.
- The therapist should state explicitly that the goal of the meeting is to help the family and school work more effectively as a team for the student's sake.

Case Example: "You Know He Tries to Split Us Apart."

In the case of Dave, introduced at the beginning of this chapter, I concluded that lack of collaboration between the parents and the school was blocking them from finding an effective solution to Dave's fighting. I suggested a meeting at school with the following goals: (1) to help the school counselor see Bernice in a more positive light, (2) to help the parents and school personnel take a more consistent position toward Dave's fighting, and (3) to break the apparent coalition between Carl and the school counselor by strengthening the parental team.

Prior to the school conference, I met with the parents to bring out Bernice's voice in a way that was more likely to be heard by Carl. I told the parents that I had telephoned the school and had learned that the school was concerned that Dave's fighting and temper outbursts could pose a danger to other students. Because of this concern, they were considering a referral to a special program for disruptive students. Carl expressed his strong opposition to the school's idea of referring Dave to this program.

I then invited Bernice to express her ideas. She stated that she agreed with Carl that Dave should remain in the regular classroom, but she also understood that he was disruptive in class and could pose a danger to the other students because of his temper. I noted that Bernice was more appreciative of the school's dilemma than was Carl, even though she had been cast in the role of the "more difficult" parent by the school. I encouraged Bernice to elaborate on her understanding of the school's dilemma and asked if I could invite her to express these ideas at the start of the school conference. I hoped that by articulating her appreciation of the school's position, Bernice would elicit a more positive view from the school counselor.

Bernice stated that she believed that Dave needed "more consistency." Often, there were no consequences at home for his disruptive behavior at school. Carl began to disagree, but I interrupted him and reminded him that our goal was to keep Dave from placement. Maybe school personnel would be more willing to give Dave another chance if they were convinced that the parents would support them by enforcing consequences at home when Dave misbehaved at school.

As is often the case, the frustrated parent softens toward the more lenient parent when he or she feels that the therapist understands his or her plight. Bernice turned to her husband and said in a calm voice, "You know he tries to split us apart. He takes advantage of any disagreement between us." Carl, now able to hear his wife, agreed and said that he would work with her and the school to enforce consequences at home.

The meeting at school was attended by the parents, the principal, and the school counselor. We agreed that the adults would meet first, and then Dave would be asked to join the meeting later. As the parents and I had planned, I began by inviting Bernice to present her understanding of the school's dilemma, while Carl took a back seat. Bernice then asked school personnel if there was anything the school would like them to do to support their expectations of Dave. The principal replied that he appreciated the parents' involvement and would find it helpful if the parents could hold Dave accountable at home for his behavior at school. Before the parents could reply, the school counselor interjected, "Yes, but we shouldn't lose sight of the fact that Dave is a very troubled boy who needs more than just discipline. He needs help."

The school counselor's statement implied that the triangle in the home was isomorphic to a triangle at the school. Bernice and the principal were in the role of enforcers, while Carl and the counselor were in the role of protectors. Each faction could try to enlist me against the other or triangulate me into the conflict. The latter is what happened: Carl turned to me and said, "Well, what do *you* think? Should we be harder on Dave, or do we need to be more permissive because he has problems that we don't fully understand?"

Fortunately, I was prepared for this question and was ready with a response: "I don't think the issue is whether to be tougher or more permissive with Dave. I think the issue is to make sure that all of the adults who care about him are working together as a team to help him do the best he can."

I picked up on Bernice's nodding and asked the parents if they could find out from the principal what he had in mind when he asked them to reinforce at home the school's expectations of Dave. In response to their question, the principal said that it would be helpful if the parents could tell Dave that they believed that his fighting at school was a serious problem and that they supported the school's rules against it. The parents agreed and also promised to contact the school every Friday to obtain reports about Dave's behavior, so that they could reinforce the school's expectations at home. I suggested that Carl should take the responsibility for contacting the principal to receive these reports. In making this recommendation, I hoped that this arrangement would engage Carl, a member of the "protective" faction, with the principal, a member of the "discipline" faction.

I had to find a way to link the two factions together. If I appeared to be siding with one position to the exclusion of the other, the excluded faction could redouble its efforts to be heard and thus perpetuate the polarization. To do so, I would have to acknowledge the other faction's position: that Dave resorted to fighting because he had no other way of expressing anger or resolving conflicts. Could the team work together to help Dave find other alternatives to fighting?

The principal suggested that the school counselor could meet with Dave to help him explore ways of handling conflicts with teachers and other students without losing his temper or resorting to fighting. I supported this suggestion, and the school counselor agreed to it. I then pointed out that until Dave learned new ways of handling conflicts, he would probably continue to use old methods. One method he used to avoid being held accountable for his own actions was to take advantage of any apparent disagreement between the authority figures and enlist one in a coalition against the other. This could happen, for example, if Dave complained to the counselor about a problem he was having at home with his parents.

All agreed that it would be helpful if the counselor discouraged Dave from complaining to her about his parents and instead focused on Dave's relationships with teachers and other students. She would instruct Dave to bring family problems to me, and I would help him and his parents resolve their conflicts. To reinforce this message, the counselor would tell Dave that she would notify Bernice if he continued to complain to her about problems between him and his parents.

The factions appeared to be dissolving. The parents and school personnel seemed to be working more effectively as a team. One more step was necessary. I suggested that Dave be invited to join the meeting so that he could hear what had been decided. I asked if the principal could start by telling Dave what the school expected of him. Then, Carl would reinforce the principal's message by informing Dave that he would be in frequent contact with the principal, and that there would be consequences at home for disruptive behavior at school. Next, Bernice would verbalize agreement with Carl's message. She would then tell Dave that she believed that he needed to find different ways of expressing his anger rather than holding in feelings or exploding in rage. Finally, the counselor would express agreement with Bernice, offer to help Dave explore other ways of dealing with conflicts at school, and tell him that she would not discuss problems Dave was having at home with his parents. The team also agreed to meet again in one month to review the plan and to make any necessary adjustments.

This case demonstrates how a carefully planned meeting involving the parents and school personnel promoted better teamwork and encouraged new patterns of interaction among the family, the school, and the adolescent. Sometimes, the parents and school are simply disengaged from one another, and the therapist need only facilitate greater engagement between them. At other times, the relationship between the parents and school is so fraught with conflict that each system triangulates another party to help them deal with the other system. Therapists can sometimes get caught in these patterns of triangulation.

IDENTIFYING AND AVOIDING TRIANGULATION

Triangulation is a hazard whenever a therapist becomes involved in working with multiple systems. In work with families and schools, some common patterns of triangulation include the following:

1. *One system (family or school) invites the therapist into a coalition against the other.* For example, the parents complain to the therapist about the school and vice versa. Or, the school could disclose information to the therapist that the school does not want the therapist to share with the parents.

2. *The therapist encourages a coalition with one system against the other.* For example, the therapist adopts the role of the family's protector against the school. Or, the therapist joins with the school in blaming the parents for the student's school problems.

3. *Both systems join forces against the therapist.* For example, the family and school avoid conflict with each other by scapegoating the therapist, or the parents and school repeatedly discount the therapist's input while complaining that therapy isn't helping.

4. *Conflicts in each system's relationship with the therapist are replicated isomorphically in the therapist's relationship with the other system.* For example, the therapist's difficulty developing a relationship with an authoritarian father could be replicated in the therapist's difficulty devel-

oping a relationship with an authoritarian principal. A mother's tendency to confide in the therapist rather than in her husband could be replicated in a teacher confiding in the therapist rather than in the principal. In other cases, the relationship between the therapist and one system might be complementary to his or her relationship with the other system. For example, the therapist might adopt a submissive role with the school and a dominant role with the family. Or, the therapist might avoid conflicts with the family by scapegoating the school.

Here are some suggestions for avoiding the pitfalls of triangulation:

• Be clear about one's role and act at all times in ways consistent with this role.

• Remain connected and concerned about the (possibly conflicting) agendas of the involved parties, without feeling the need to find an ideal solution that is acceptable to all. One of the most common ways that therapists become triangulated is by being recruited into assuming full responsibility for solving the problem. Therapists who accept this role will often feel frustrated or inadequate if they are unable to resolve an impasse between conflicting parties who are not motivated to negotiate a solution themselves.

• Avoid becoming invested in any particular outcome or solution, but instead intervene to facilitate a more productive collaborative *process* between the family and school. Strive to get the family and the school to talk directly with one another and negotiate a solution that is acceptable to both of them, rather than providing them with the solution.

When a School Requests a Consultation

While parents often take the initiative in seeking help for a child's school problem, sometimes it is the school that enlists the therapist's help with a problem. This arrangement poses its own potential pitfalls.

It is essential in these situations for therapists to be clear about their role and what is being asked of them. If the therapist is hired by the school, then the therapist is working for the school, not the family (or, for that matter, the student). Nevertheless, it is important to make sure that the parents have authorized the therapist's involvement. Meeting with minors without parental informed consent could violate ethical and legal guidelines.

Ideally, therapists should negotiate a role whereby they provide suggestions to the school regarding ways to handle problematic situations involving students. The school is free to accept or reject these suggestions, but the school (not the consultant) retains the responsibility for solving the problem that precipitated the consultation.

Therapists who are hired as consultants by schools should be wary of getting pulled into coalitions between competing factions. Therapists might be hired with the understanding that they will provide recommendations to the school regarding ways to help a particular student. Therapists might then find out that their recommendations have become fodder in political or philosophical battles among school personnel. Members of each conflicting faction might attempt to engage the therapist in a coalition against the other. For example, a counselor who believes that a particular teacher is insensitive to the emotional needs of students might attempt to gain ascendancy in the conflict by using the therapist's suggestions as support for his or her position.

To deal with challenging situations such as these, it is important to pay attention to the relationship patterns and history of conflicts within the school. When hired as a consultant by a school, before meeting with a student or family, the therapist should first meet with the school personnel who are involved with the student. The purpose of the meeting is not simply to gather information about the student, but also to assess the nature of the relationships among the members of the student's team. While therapists are usually not in a position to address any systemic problems discovered in this process, they can take care to frame their recommendations in a way that avoids being perceived as entering into a coalition with one party or faction against another.

SUMMARY

Here's a summary of the main points to keep in mind when working with school-related academic or behavioral problems:

- School-related problems can be the outcome of many interacting factors. Long-standing academic difficulties might be the result of a learning disability or ADHD. If either of these conditions is suspected, the student should be referred for a comprehensive psychoeducational evaluation.

- Academic difficulties can also be a "proxy" for other problems, including depression or anxiety. If internal family dynamics are contributing to the academic problems, or if the academic problems are an adolescent's way of communicating distress to the parents, then the appropriate focus of intervention is to work with the family as a whole.

- Sometimes a problematic relationship between the parents and school is contributing to the adolescent's problems at school. I described three different levels of involvement for the therapist: coaching, mediation, and direct intervention.

• In *coaching*, the therapist refrains from direct contact with the school and directs all interventions through the adolescent or family.

• In *mediation*, the therapist has contact with both the family and the school but does not attempt to intervene directly in the relationship between the two systems.

• In *direct intervention*, the therapist convenes the family and school personnel together in order to intervene directly to change the problematic relationship patterns involving the two systems.

• Each of these methods has advantages and pitfalls. In selecting among these methods, it is best to choose the one that will have the maximum impact while being least intrusive on the family.

• Whenever working with multiple systems, it is necessary to be alert to and avoid the possibility of triangulation.

11

Leaving Home

The high school senior who misses the deadline for filing college applications....

The college freshman who "flunks out" after his first semester....

The recent high school graduate who has no plans to attend college and no job....

The college student who withdraws midway through her second semester because she "can't take the pressure."

Cases like these are often viewed as problems of "leaving home." According to the theory of the family life cycle (Carter & McGoldrick, 2005), families face a significant transition at the end of adolescence when the children move out of the parental home. While this step usually occurs following high school graduation when the young person either leaves for college or begins working full time, there is considerable variability in the manner in which families negotiate this transition.

Leaving home is not a single event, but rather a process that can span several years. Adolescents go through a process of gradual individuation and increasing independence throughout the teenage years, and college students continue to maintain ties to the parental home by returning during weekends or vacations. What is most important is whether the adolescent and family have been able to negotiate a successful transition that permits the young adult more independence while remaining connected to one another.

Sometimes a young person has difficulty leaving home because the parents have difficulty letting go. At other times, problems associated with leaving home can be traced to a process that has been too abrupt rather than too prolonged. The culturally prescribed timetable that dictates high school graduation as the dividing line between dependence on and independence from parents is simply not applicable to some adolescents and families. These adolescents, particularly boys, fall prey to our societal equation of maturity and independence, as Silverstein and Rashbaum (1994) point out:

> With all the focus on facilitating a departure, too little consideration is given to the possibility that getting sick, or getting into serious trouble, might be a young man's only means of being able to come home again, and perhaps a sign that he needs to *be* home. Unfortunately, the mental health field has managed to convince us that there is something wrong with any boy who is not ready to "leave the nest" on schedule. But human development is vastly more complex and variable than that of the birds who inspired this metaphor. (p. 160, emphasis in original)

The family's ethnic background and local community norms must also be taken into account. In certain cultures (e.g., Southern European), families value physical proximity and prefer children to remain at home until marriage (McGoldrick, Giordano, & Garcia-Preto, 2005). In these families, transition from adolescence to young adulthood is generally less abrupt and is usually not accompanied by a physical separation from the parents. These families might find it difficult to accept a child's departure from home, and conflicts could arise when the young person tries to leave and the family discourages it.

It is a mistake to assume that all problems that arise during late adolescence mean that the family is having difficulty with the adolescent leaving the family home. The family might come to therapy because of a problem that appears to have arisen *de novo* during the later years of adolescence, but upon further discussion with the family it becomes apparent that the roots of the problem extend back many years. Perhaps there has been a history of academic difficulties, failure to meet responsibilities, or parental overprotectiveness that had been just mild enough for everyone to ignore until the time came for the adolescent to make a decision about what to do after high school graduation.

Keeping these points in mind, I believe that there are certain signs that suggest that problems of late adolescence are tied to the family's difficulty in making the developmental transition to the "launching" phase of the life cycle:

1. The family's primary concern is the adolescent's leaving home and there is no evidence of other significant issues in the family.

2. The parents are treating the young adult in the same way they

would treat a much younger adolescent. Sometimes parents work too hard to protect their child from failure and thus deprive the young person of the opportunity to learn how to handle problems independently. For example, if the adolescent's grades are dropping during senior year, the parents go into overdrive to monitor the youngster's homework, use concrete rewards or punishments for grades, or convene meetings with teachers that don't include the student.

3. Neither the parents nor the adolescent seem in a particular hurry for the young person to leave, and so the adolescent seems stuck in his or her own development. For example, an 18-year-old boy of average intelligence and adequate social skills graduated from high school without any plans for seeking employment. Three months later he's still watching soap operas in his pajamas, and no one in the family seems concerned.

4. The young person makes several "false starts" or failed attempts to leave home. For example, the young person might have dropped out of several colleges or repeatedly moved in and out of the parental home.

5. An eldest or youngest child in the family develops symptoms that appear to have come on suddenly during the last year of high school, shortly after graduation, or upon leaving for college. These symptoms might have arisen because the young person is having difficulty separating from the parents, the parents are reluctant to let the child go, or the parents are pushing the young person to assume more independence than he or she is ready to assume.

PERSPECTIVES ON LEAVING HOME

The family therapy literature has proposed a number of theories to explain difficulties associated with the process of leaving home. Jay Haley (1997) asserted that a young adult might be unable to leave home because the child's presence is necessary to regulate the level of tension between the parents. Haley recommended that therapists push parents to require the adolescent to function more independently and set a deadline for the child to leave home. The therapeutic work should focus on helping the parents remain united and firm in their expectations. According to Haley, the therapist should relentlessly pursue this agenda, even when the family raises other seemingly important concerns (e.g., marital conflict), and view attempts to divert attention to these issues as yet another effort to delay the adolescent's departure.

Cloe Madanes (1981) pointed out that parents' efforts to help the young person reinforce the young person's helplessness, which elicits more helpfulness from the parents in an endless cycle. Similar to Haley, Madanes advised the therapist to challenge the parents to state explicitly what they expect of the young person and then to hold him or her accountable.

Eron and Lund (1993) suggested that a network of reciprocally confirming beliefs, expectations, and actions can transform a mild developmental difficulty with initial separation into a "narrative of failure." Well-intentioned offers of support from the parents can undermine an adolescent's self-confidence as the young person interprets the parents' expressions of concern as evidence that they view him or her as not competent to manage independently. Eron and Lund gave an example: A college freshman calls home frequently to express worry about failing academically and socially. The child's anxiety evokes the parents' anxiety, who respond with expressions of worry and concern about the child. The young person interprets the parents' anxiety as confirmation of the validity of his worries and evidence that they agree that he's not competent to manage the situation on his own. As a result, the young person's anxiety increases and his confidence in himself decreases. Eventually, his concerned parents suggest that he return home, thus contributing to a "narrative of failure."

Taking a different view, Carl Whitaker (1975) argued that the young person's failure to separate from the family is the result of a rupture in family relationships that prevented the parents from providing the adolescent with the appropriate context for successful individuation. Whitaker advised the therapist to reengage the young person with the family and then help all family members to work through the issues that precipitated the adolescent's premature departure.

Ivan Boszormenyi-Nagy and Muriel Spark (1973) suggested that adolescents will not be able to leave home if they have been saddled with disproportionate responsibility for the welfare of the parents. Sometimes, the child's self-sacrifice on behalf of the parents can result in extreme symptoms, such as delinquency, psychosis, or suicide, which become the ostensible reason why the adolescent can't leave. These authors recommended that the therapist help the parents acknowledge the child's efforts on their behalf and help the child to find more appropriate and less self-defeating ways of demonstrating care for them.

According to Helm Stierlin (1973; Stierlin, Levi, & Savard, 1971), the young person could be tied to the parents through covert, unconscious processes such as projective identification. For example, parents who have not integrated their own terrifying impulses (such as aggression) might project these impulses onto the child, and then induce the child to act in accordance with these projections. In order for this defense to function, the child must be present, so the parents unconsciously thwart the child's efforts to leave home. Successful treatment requires the parents to recognize and reown their split-off impulses, thus freeing the child from the bonds of projective identification. According to Stierlin (1973), some families (*centripetal*) delay the adolescent's separation and block moves toward autonomy and independence, either by fostering the young person's dependency on the family or by inducing extreme guilt at any hint of separation. Other families (*centrifugal*) push the adolescent into premature autonomy and separation, which often results in failure because the young person has not been sufficiently prepared for independence.

ASSESSMENT

Each of these theories has something to offer for understanding problems of leaving home. The approach I propose integrates elements from the above perspectives. The first step in helping these families is to assess both the adolescent's readiness for more independence as well as the family's readiness to allow it.

Assessing the Young Person

Difficulties with leaving home do not necessarily imply dysfunctional family dynamics. Other obstacles might be preventing the young person from adjusting to life away from the parents. In assessing a young adult who is having difficulty at college, it is important to consider whether an undiagnosed learning problem might be interfering with adjustment to college. For example, a college sophomore was in danger of failing out of college. After talking with him and his family, I found no apparent difficulties associated with the developmental transition. Both parents seemed to be handling the boy's leave taking well, and there did not appear to be marital conflicts. However, it did turn out that the boy had a previously undiagnosed attention-deficit disorder that made it difficult for him to concentrate on lectures. In addition, because he had managed to "get by" with little studying in high school, he had no idea of how to prepare for tests. The boy agreed to take medications, attended a class on study skills, managed to pass the semester, and did well the following semester.

Some adolescents feel pushed out of the family home before they are ready to leave. These young people are not on the same timetable as their peers, yet might be embarrassed to discuss their reservations about leaving home for fear of not meeting real or imagined parental expectations. For example, a high school senior was procrastinating on filling out his college applications, while still professing a desire to attend a college in another state. He and his parents were locked in conflict around his "lack of responsibility." When I raised the possibility that the boy might not be sure whether he wanted to go to college right away, he at first rebuffed this idea, but as I pursued it he hesitantly admitted that he was "confused" about what he wanted to do and wished he could have more time to think it over. Eventually, the boy decided to attend a 2-year college close to home.

In other cases, the parents have not prepared the adolescent for the separation because they have been overly protective of the child. For example, a boy with a history of severe learning disabilities began to experience panic attacks 1 month before he was scheduled to leave for college. It turned out that the boy had never written a paper on his own because his mother had written all of his papers for him during high school. He was now understandably anxious that he could not handle the writing demands of the college he was planning to attend.

In another family, a very high-achieving but shy young man who had done well through high school became depressed soon after leaving for college 4 hours from home. The young man attributed his depression to missing his family and feeling lonely. The parents, well-meaning but a bit naive, had not pushed this shy boy to expand his social network during high school, interpreting his preference for being alone as evidence of his studiousness. In this case, the goal was to block the parents from rescuing the boy. Instead, I urged them to encourage him to persist, reiterate their confidence in his ability to adjust to living away from home, and arrange for him to receive counseling at college. By the second semester, the boy reported feeling better, had made a few friends, and was looking forward to returning for his second year.

In the case of the boy who was procrastinating on his college applications, it was clear to me that he really had not thought through the decision to attend college, and instead was being carried along by encouragement from teachers and parents. Thus, I believed that it was important to slow down the process to allow the boy a "moratorium" on the college decision rather than pushing for premature "foreclosure" based on the wishes of his family. In the case of the shy boy who became depressed when separated from his family, it was clear that this boy really wanted to attend college, had done well academically through high school, and simply wished that he could feel better so that he could make the most of his college experience. He needed some help in developing social skills. Following the advice of Eron and Lund (1993), I also believed that the parents needed to communicate to the boy their confidence that he could succeed if he persisted.

Assessing the Family

The Parents Need the Adolescent

Sometimes parents who have been overly focused on parenting have not developed a support network for themselves. They fail to encourage the young person's independence because they fear being left alone. In these cases, it is important to help the parents develop relationships and activities outside of the home.

Take the case of a young man who dropped out of college after his first year, took and promptly quit a series of jobs, and was now sitting at home while his widowed mother supported them both. I suspected that the mother was willing to condone the boy's behavior because she was worried about how she would manage if he left home. I told the mother and the boy that I believed that the boy seemed to be taking advantage of the mother's generosity, and that she should keep a record of how much she was spending on his support so that he could repay her when he eventually got a job. Meanwhile, I encouraged the mother to develop her own social network, to accept offers to go out on dates, and to spend some evenings away from home, using the rationale that she needed to prepare for the boy's inevitable departure from home as soon as he "got on his feet again." As the mother's connections outside the family expanded, she began to expect more from the boy, and eventually gave him the choice either to find a job within 30 days or to move out of the house. Once the mother had taken a stand to support the boy's growing up, I shifted my support to the boy. I coached him on job-seeking skills, and encouraged him to take aptitude and interest tests in order to define clearer career goals.

The Family Is Distracted by Other Stressors

In some cases, the family is distracted by other stressors or another family member who is symptomatic. For example, the parents could be experiencing failing health. An older child might be going through marital problems and depending more on the parents who, distracted by their older child's problems, withdraw too much from the adolescent at a time when he or she still needs their support. Or, the parents could be preoccupied with their own aging parents whose increasing dependency on them might coincide with the adolescent's graduation from high school.

The Child Feels Responsible for the Parents

In some cases, the young person might delay leaving home out of a sense of responsibility. For example, a family presented with three problems: a daughter who had become intensely "homesick" and was unable to complete her college work, a mother with a history of depression who would periodically retire to her room for weeks at a time, and marital conflict that was managed primarily through mutual avoidance. The family came to therapy asking for help with the daughter's problem.

When I met with the girl alone, it was obvious that she was not so much homesick as worried about her mother. I encouraged her to share her concern about her mother with her parents at the next family session. After she had done so, I turned to the parents and asked, "Can you convince your daughter that you can get along without her?" Toward the end of a tearful discussion, during which I repeated my question four times, the mother agreed to treatment for her own chronic depression and both parents agreed to marital therapy. The parents thanked the girl for her concern, assured her that they would take better care of themselves, and gave her permission to leave.

INTERVENTION

Regardless of the reasons for the adolescent's or parents' difficulty with the transition, it is important to keep the family on the track toward increasing independence for the young person. This is not to say that the adolescent must be pushed in a particular direction, nor even that the young person must be forced into a physical separation from the family. Rather, *the therapist should encourage the parents to help the young person take the next developmental step for which he or she is ready*. Keep the momentum toward maturity going, either by unblocking a stuck process or discouraging the parents from prematurely rescuing the adolescent.

Framing the Problem

It is important to frame the problem as one involving the transition toward greater independence and avoid a frame that would imply that the problem is one more typical of an earlier life stage. For example, take the case of Tyrone, discussed in Chapter 8, as an example of mild problem behavior. Tyrone's mother was primarily concerned with what she called Tyrone's "lack of responsibility" because he repeatedly came home late from dates with his girlfriend. I reframed the problem as one reflecting the difficulty Tyrone was having "saying good-bye" to his girlfriend, and then talked with him and his mother about the series of "good-byes" he was about to face as he prepared to leave for college. If I had accepted that Tyrone's "lack of responsibility" was the problem, I might have precipitated a power struggle between him and his mother, which would enact a dynamic more characteristic of a younger adolescent and distract Tyrone from the important process of mourning the losses associated with leaving home.

Expanding Support Networks

Both the young adult and the parents often need support from sources other than each other. Building upon the young person's peer networks can help, as well as engaging the support of other adults outside of the immediate family. As discussed above, some parents have led constricted lives and have relied excessively on the young adult for companionship. Encouraging these parents to develop connections beyond the immediate family or strengthening the parental bond can help to ease the transition.

Dealing with Mourning and Loss

Every leave taking involves mourning. It is important to deal head-on with the issues of mourning and loss that accompany a young adult's leaving home. This point is an important one that is often overlooked by families as the adolescent excitedly prepares to go away to college. In their haste to support the adolescent's maturity, parents might fail to acknowledge the losses they and the adolescent are facing.

For example, a young man and his divorced father were locked in conflict regarding the expensive phone bill the boy had incurred talking nightly to his girlfriend who was attending a month-long college orientation program 6 hours away. The boy also had not found a summer job and was, in father's view, "pining away" for his girlfriend. During one of their typically unproductive arguments, the father cried, "I thought we had a great relationship, but I don't think so anymore. You obviously care more about her than you care about my feelings."

I interjected at this point to offer a different explanation: The boy cared a great deal about his father, and the fact that his relationship with his girlfriend seemed to be coming between them was evidence that the emotions connected with saying good-bye to her were so overpowering that it led him to act in a way that hurt his father. It was not that he didn't care enough about his father, but rather that his mourning over the loss of his girlfriend was so intense that it impeded his judgment.

The boy agreed that, no matter how hard he tried, he could think of little else than how much he missed his girlfriend. I asked him and his father to talk about how his dad might help him through this difficult experience. This discussion led us to consider the other losses this boy was about to face, including the loss of daily contact with his father, to whom he was strongly attached.

After several tearful conversations, the boy decided that he needed to end his relationship with his girlfriend because it was draining too much energy from the task of getting ready for college. We spent the final weeks of the summer helping him and his father plan a "ritual of leave taking" that would include an opportunity for them to reminisce about the past, affirm their relationship in the present, and talk about how their relationship would change as the boy grew older.

Meanwhile, I talked with the boy about his relationship with his girlfriend, and learned that he felt very insecure about her affection for him. His mother had left him and his father when the boy was 11. Although he continued to see his mother regularly, they were not close. He and his mother had never talked about the divorce. I suggested that the intensity of the boy's longing for his girlfriend might be related to unresolved feelings of abandonment by his mother. He agreed that he had never felt sure about his mother's feelings for him, and that he frequently wondered "how a mother could just up and leave her kid like that."

I proposed that the "unfinished business" between him and his mother could be an obstacle to his leaving home successfully, since he might be tempted to keep "hanging on" in hopes of finally getting the affection from her that he had never received as a child. I suggested that we arrange a few sessions for him to talk with his mother about his feelings, not with the goal of necessarily receiving any particular response from her, but rather to help him acknowledge the loss and move on.

SUMMARY

As I have emphasized in this chapter, when an adolescent and family appear to be stuck in the developmental process known as "leaving home" it is important to assess the context carefully before assuming that the therapeutic task is to force the separation to occur. Sometimes (but not always) the adolescent's leaving home threatens a family's rigid organization, and it is necessary to facilitate the reorganization of the family in order to allow the young person to leave. Other times, less malignant dynamics are at work, and it is these cases that I have tried to highlight in this chapter.

In closing and by way of summary, I suggest the following four steps for treating problems of leaving home:

• Assess the adolescent's developmental readiness to leave home, and then support whatever steps seem appropriate given the young person's level of maturity.

• Try to get the parents to take a supportive and encouraging stance with the adolescent by which they clearly communicate their confidence that the young person will ultimately succeed at being more independent.

• If the parents express resistance to this approach, it is likely that they are having difficulty "letting go" of the adolescent. It is essential that these issues be acknowledged and addressed, but only if the previous step has failed. Don't imply that the parents are holding back the young adult before giving the parents a fair chance to support the transition.

• Continue to maintain a positive and optimistic position about the young person's potential for success and the family's ability to make the transition. Decrease the mutual dependence of the adolescent and the parents by enlisting support for both of them from outside the immediate family. Deal directly with issues of mourning and loss that accompany the change in family structure.

12

Families with
Multiple Problems

Before the session had even begun, Rosa appeared exhausted from trying to control her six children in the waiting room. Now, sitting in my office, she could hardly complete a sentence without having to reprimand one of the children. A single mother, she was referred by the Department of Child Protection after the school reported suspicious bruises on the legs of Inez, Rosa's 11-year-old daughter. During the preliminary investigation, Rosa admitted that she often slapped her children, but she denied abusing them. The child protection worker, however, assessed Rosa as a "high-risk parent" and informed her that she would be under observation and have to attend therapy.

Rosa's six children ranged in age from 2 to 13. Rosa's oldest child, Ramon, now 13, had seen a counselor for a few sessions after it was discovered that he had been sexually abused by one of Rosa's former boyfriends. Ramon continued to have nightmares and flagrantly disobeyed his mother. He was failing all of his classes and was frequently truant from school. Inez was a good student but very quiet and withdrawn. The third child, Carlos, had been suspended three times since school started 2 months earlier, and was being considered for transfer to a special class. Next in line was Enrique, who was in the first grade and had already been identified by the school as possibly having "learning problems." The school psychologist had placed him on a waiting list for a psychological evaluation. Still at home were Carmen, age 4, and Rosita, age 2. Rosa admitted that she often had difficulty controlling the youngest children, and reported a recent incident when she found Carmen playing with matches.

Only Ramon and Inez had the same father, who was now incarcerated for dealing drugs. The other four children all had different fathers. Two of these men were incarcerated; one for murder. Rosa was unsure of the whereabouts of the third, and the fourth had been expelled from her home when she discovered that he had abused Ramon. Rosa had admitted to the child protection worker that these men had beat her up, sometimes in the presence of the children. Her present boyfriend lived with his mother around the corner, but often spent nights at Rosa's tiny apartment, sleeping with her in the same room as three of the younger children. The three older children shared a sofa bed in the living room.

Rosa had lived on public assistance since she came to the mainland from Puerto Rico when she was 17. At that time, she already had one child and was pregnant with her second. She had two sisters who lived in the area; one was addicted to crack, and the other was married and worked part time. Rosa's father left her mother when Rosa was 9. She reported that her father was often drunk and would beat their mother and "touch" the girls, including Rosa. After her father left, Rosa's mother decided to come to the mainland, because she felt there was more opportunity for employment. Rosa's mother had a stroke 2 years ago and lived in a squalid nursing home too far from Rosa's house to permit regular visits.

Rosa had never worked outside the home. She still struggled with English, but pointed out that she could read English and often helped her children with their homework. She never finished high school, but hoped one day to earn her general equivalency diploma and then study cosmetology. She spent her day taking care of the two youngest children, who had not yet started school. Most days, Rosa's boyfriend, who was also unemployed, kept her company. She evaded my question about whether her boyfriend was hitting her, and she became defensive when I asked whether he was using or selling drugs. She indignantly denied that she would allow drugs in her home, where her children could be exposed to them.

The day after our first session, the child protection worker called me and asked for my "impressions" of the family. The worker told me that she felt that "something was going on" in this family, and she hoped I could find out what it was. She would need a written report from me within 60 days, "with recommendations" (she emphasized). Two days later, I received a call from Ramon's school. Rosa had told them that I was working with Ramon. They were calling to ask my advice because they had run out of strategies for dealing with Ramon's behavior. They asked whether I could come to a meeting at the school to discuss what they should do next.

The following week, Rosa called an hour before the scheduled appointment to say that she could not come to the session because Rosita was sick. We rescheduled for the following week at the same time. Rosa arrived 40 minutes late for the rescheduled appointment. We had barely started when my next family arrived for their appointment. Rosa said that she understood and made another appointment for the following week.

Rosa did not appear for the appointment and did not call in advance. Since she had no phone, I was unable to reach her. The day after the appointment, the child protection worker called me to ask how the family was progressing and to remind me that my written report would be due in a few weeks. When I told the worker that it had been difficult to schedule a meeting time with the family, the worker said that she would visit the family at home and remind them that if they did not come to therapy, then there was a good chance that the children could be placed in a foster home.

Increasingly, therapists are called upon to work with families, like Rosa's, who have multiple problems. These families are overwhelmed by too many demands and too few resources. Many of these families live in economic poverty and are supported by public assistance. Often they have come into contact with a variety of helping professionals such as counselors, social workers, child advocates, and foster parents. Many of these families are immigrants or members of cultural and linguistic minorities.

There is little doubt that poverty is associated with a variety of negative outcomes for children and adolescents (Bradley & Corwyn, 2002; McLoyd, 1998; Seccombe, 2000; Wadsworth, Raviv, Compas, & Connor-Smith, 2005). In addition to the direct effects on a youngster's sense of security, mastery, and well-being (Conger, Conger, Matthews, & Elder, 1999), growing up in an economically impoverished environment affects child development indirectly through the impact of economic deprivation on parents. Parents who are overburdened tend to experience themselves as less competent as parents and engage in more coercive or neglectful parenting strategies, which in turn contribute to poorer parent–child relationships (Conger, Ge, Elder, Lorenz, & Simons, 1994; Goosby, 2007; Gutman, McLoyd, & Tokoyawa, 2005; McLoyd, Jayaratne, Ceballo, &

Borquez, 1994; Mistry, Vanderwater, Huston, & McLoyd, 2002; Myers & Taylor, 1998). On the other hand, positive and supportive family relationships serve as protective factors and buffer against the negative effects of living in economically deprived conditions (Eamon & Mulder, 2005; Farrell & White, 1998; Li, Nussbaum, & Richards, 2007; Richards, Miller, O'Donnell, Wasserman, & Colder, 2004). Family factors might even be more strongly associated with child and adolescent outcomes than are neighborhood factors (Leventhal & Brooks-Gunn, 2000). Thus, efforts to promote stronger family ties and more positive family interactions will have a favorable impact on youth who live in high-stress, low-income urban environments.

Over 40 years ago, Salvador Minuchin and his colleagues broke new ground in working with low-income families with the publication of *Families of the Slums* (Minuchin, Montalvo, Guerney, Rosman, & Schumer, 1967). In this work, based upon their experiences at the Wiltwyck School for Boys, a correctional facility in New York, the authors described their attempts to develop a model of therapy that was more suited to urban low-income families than techniques based on reflection and insight. The result of their efforts was the action-oriented model of treatment that became known as structural family therapy.

Harry Aponte (1976b) later expanded on this work by articulating the particular issues posed by therapy with low-income families:

> There is another problem that comes with poverty, and certainly not the exclusive possession of the poor, which is related to social organization. Social organization is an aspect of social ecology. It can be weakened at every socioeconomic level, but it is particularly vulnerable to dysfunction under the social conditions linked to poverty and other forms of powerlessness. Some call the cluster of organizational problems that poor families often have *disorganization*; I prefer to call it *underorganization*, to suggest not so much an improper kind of organization, as a deficiency in the degree of constancy, differentiation, and flexibility of the structural organization of the family system. This kind of internal underorganization is accompanied by a lack of organizational continuity of the family with the structure of its societal context, that is, its ecology. (1976b, p. 433, emphasis in original)

In the three decades since Aponte's article was published, families who live in economic poverty have become even more disenfranchised. Low-income families are subject to disorganizing forces from both inside and outside. The rising rates of drug addiction, sexual abuse, adolescent pregnancy, and child neglect have taxed the already underorganized resources in these families. Furthermore, the environment in which these families live is hardly conducive to effective family functioning. Surrounded by violence, despair, homelessness, and drug addiction, these families understandably experience the world as a threatening place. The involvement of well-intentioned social agencies threatens the family's integrity, undermines their autonomy, and encourages dependency.

On the other hand, characteristics of successful and functional families who live in low-income urban environments have been identified. According to Burton and Jarrett (2000), these factors include:

- The involvement of supportive members of the extended family.
- Family role flexibility, characterized by interdependence and teamwork.
- Structured family routines, including household maintenance and regular mealtimes.
- Protection strategies that minimize contact between family members and dangerous elements in the neighborhood.
- Rejection of "street values."
- Commitment to family relations and humanistic values such as self-respect, dignity, and concern for others.
- A strong family identity and belief in one's family as "distinct."
- Parents' commitment to their parenting roles.
- Clear generational role boundaries.
- Efforts by parents to locate resources for their children and advocate on their children's behalf.
- Consistent monitoring of children's activities.

These characteristics of successful and functional families provide aspirational goals for working with overburdened, low-income families. This list also provides a template for family assessment and can alert therapists to potential strengths that already exist in the family.

Many useful resources exist for therapists who work with overwhelmed, low-income families (e.g., Aponte, 1994; Madsen, 2007; Minuchin, Colapinto, & Minuchin, 2007; Walsh, 2006). In this chapter, I highlight some of the most important considerations to keep in mind when working with these families.

PRINCIPLES FOR WORKING WITH OVERWHELMED, LOW-INCOME FAMILIES

Since a strong family buffers youth from many of the disruptive effects of economic poverty, the most important principle for working with low-income families is to strengthen the family. This is accomplished by helping to shore up the overburdened executive subsystem, which in many instances is a single parent. Thus, the focus of work with these families is on joining with the parent and providing the parent with the support he or she needs to create a supportive family context for the children.

Joining with Parents

In working with overwhelmed, low-income families, therapists should assume that any apparent dysfunction in the family is related to the family's economic and social circumstances. What might appear to be ineffective parenting might be surrender of an overwhelmed single parent to the social networks that appear to exert more influence over the children than he or she does. Pushing a parent in these circumstances to "take charge" of the children can alienate the parent, who will feel blamed for his or her children's behavior. Instead, it is important to join with the parent, pay attention to his or her own unique needs as an individual, and strengthen the parent's connection with other adults before pushing for a more hierarchical and/or nurturing relationship with his or her children (cf. Becker & Liddle, 2001). This principle is illustrated when I return to discussing Rosa's family. In working with this family, I did not focus on modifying the behavior of the "problem child" Ramon. Instead, I directed my efforts toward supporting Rosa. Before addressing parenting issues directly, I attended to her needs as an individual, thereby communicating to her my belief in her as a person with strengths and resources.

Accentuating Strengths and Competence

Throughout this book, I have emphasized the idea that therapists should amplify existing family strengths as a way of solving problems. This principle is particularly important with members of overwhelmed, low-income families, who are often unaware of their strengths or discount their significance. Many families have been recruited into negative societal narratives about them. These narratives describe low-income families as unsophisticated, uneducated, powerless, irresponsible, and in need of supervision from others. Therapists, too, can be unwitting participants in these narratives, and might bring to therapy certain assumptions about work with low-income families. As a result, a therapist and family can participate in a problem-saturated narrative (White & Epston, 1990) that depicts low-income families as helplessly entangled in a web of problems from which there is little hope of escape.

Therapists must be astutely attentive to signs of competence. For example, a parent might set limits firmly but kindly, acknowledge a child's voice, or show pleasure at a child's accomplishments. By calling attention to their strengths, therapists can help families construct new narratives about themselves, in which they have more emotional resources and more control over their own lives than the dominant societal narratives assert. One way to demonstrate belief in the family's intangible resources is to attend to particular ways in which a family's cultural origin might enrich a family's experience.

Cultural Sensitivity and Multicultural Competence

Since many overwhelmed, low-income families are members of minority cultures, cultural sensitivity and competence are essential in working with these families. Therapists must be familiar with the values and mores of the family's culture, as well as the impact of discrimination on the family members' individual lives, relationships with each other, and relationships with representatives of the dominant culture. Attention to acculturation is essential in work with immigrant families. In particular, generational differences in acculturation must be considered in deciding how to intervene in cases of parent–child conflict. Even within the spousal subsystem, differences in acculturation might be relevant (cf. Inclan, 2001).

Attention to the family's culture also means attention to differences between the therapist's cultural experiences and those of the family. Therapists who are members of the dominant culture must be prepared to address this difference openly and directly, as failure to acknowledge these differences could imply to the family that their experiences as cultural minorities are being minimized. Therapists must acknowledge their membership in a dominant and sometimes hostile culture along with the perceived and real power differential between them and the family. These issues are all relevant to the family's ability to trust the therapist and the therapeutic process. Therapists must also be honest with themselves regarding their own prejudices and values and how these could influence their relationship with the family.

On the other hand, it is also important to feel free to challenge family interactional patterns that appear to be contributing to or helping to maintain the problem for which the family is seeking help. A way to do so while being respectful of the family's culture is to explore with the family alternative ways of relating to one another that might be consistent with the family's cultural values. A collaborative approach such as this, rather than a prescriptive one, communicates respect for the cultural differences between the therapist and family while at the same time opening up the possibility for change.

Although therapists must honestly acknowledge the limits of their familiarity with a family's culture, therapists cannot rely on families to teach them about their cultural experiences and values. It is incumbent on therapists to obtain adequate training and supervised experience with clients who are members of cultures that are commonly encountered in their geographical area. A number of excellent resources have been published that address the role of culture and ethnicity in family life and treatment (e.g., Bean, Perry, & Bedell, 2001; Boyd-Franklin, 2003; Falicov, 1998; McGoldrick et al., 2005).

The Importance of Understanding Power Dynamics

Some of the cherished concepts of systems theory need to be modified in order to be applicable to families who live in poverty. Feminist family therapists (e.g., Goldner, 1985, 1988; Lucpnitz, 1988) have pointed out that the concepts of circularity and complementarity, integral to systems theory, assume that all members of the system have equal power. It is only by modifying a systems view with one informed by an awareness of hidden power differentials that therapists can avoid reinforcing the inequality among members of the system.

When working with low-income families, it is essential to keep in mind the pervasive powerlessness experienced by these families by virtue of racial and economic discrimination in our society. Failing to acknowledge the importance of these issues in the lives of these families risks perpetuating the social order by implying that these issues are not relevant. It is necessary to recognize that the family members are almost always "one down" relative to the social agencies that have become involved in their lives. There might also be power differentials within the family based on who controls the family's finances. Interactions that appear dysfunctional to a therapist can appear adaptive when these issues are taken into account.

For example, a therapist might notice that a mother fails to take a stand against the intrusive remarks and actions of her own mother. The therapist identifies this interaction as evidence of a dysfunctional hierarchy in the family and decides to work on increasing the mother's authority in the system. It is only when the mother's mother refuses to return to therapy sessions that the therapist realizes the error. The mother lives rent-free in the grandmother's home, and the grandmother also contributes financial support to the mother and the grandchildren. Were the mother to leave the grandmother's home, she would sacrifice her own and her children's standard of living and jeopardize their safety by having to move to a dangerous neighborhood.

While the mother might be open to the possibility of renegotiating her relationship with her mother, it is the grandmother who determines how much this relationship will actually change. Had the therapist been aware of the mother's economic dependence on the grandmother, he or she might have taken a different approach. For example, rather than joining with the mother in a coalition against the grandmother, the therapist might have joined with the grandmother to help her to see that her intrusive efforts to help her daughter contribute to her daughter's dependency on her. By recognizing the power differential in the family, it is no longer rendered invisible, and its implications can be fully explored. If the therapist had acknowledged the grandmother's tangible contributions to the welfare of her daughter and grandchildren, he or she might have had more leverage to induce the grandmother to wield her power more benevolently.

Powerlessness, subjugation, and violence are not simply "environmental stressors" in the lives of low-income families. They are inescapable elements of the context in which these families live. A therapist who aspires to be systemic recognizes that each family's context is unique, constituted not only by the immediate interactions in the room but also by the family's own history, as well as the history and politics of the society in which the family lives. Families are shaped not only by interactions among the family members, but also by value systems and political forces that keep them marginalized. As a relatively more powerful member of society simply by virtue of being well educated, if not male and/or Caucasian, the therapist is in a unique position either to support or subvert these societal discourses that strip power from individual family members and from the family collectively.

Goal Setting: Empowering the Parents

Therapy must help to empower families who have been disempowered by the system. These families do not see themselves as having much influence over what happens to them. They view the source of their problems as residing in others and the resolution of these problems as beyond their control. The notion that they can and should take responsibility for their own change seems to ring true to them in principle, but is difficult to implement in practice because they feel so powerless to accomplish anything that has much impact on their lives.

It is important to stimulate in family members the experience that they can influence something that matters to them, that they can affect something significant in their lives. In setting goals, it is essential to follow the family's lead. It is a good idea to start by identifying a simple, concrete goal that is attainable quickly, in order to build hope and confidence in the efficacy of therapy (Boyd-Franklin, 2003).

It is essential to involve families in the process of making decisions all along the way. Whenever decisions are to be made, therapists should consult the family members and encourage them to participate collaboratively in the decision-making process. It is important to avoid acting unilaterally, but rather work under the direction of family members on their behalf. In this way, it is possible to join with the family by taking a temporary leadership position that is based on shared power rather than hierarchy.

We should work *through* and *with* the parent(s) and family members, not *for* them. The more active therapists are in solving problems for families, the less opportunity families have for learning to make better use of the resources at their disposal, however limited these resources seem to be. Rather than asking, "What can I as the therapist do to solve this problem?" it is preferable to ask, "What is preventing this family from solving the problem? How can I help family members confront these obstacles and utilize their resources more creatively?" These questions orient therapists to helping families take the next attainable step in the process of achieving more independence.

Coordinating the Helpers

One of the important tasks for therapists who work with low-income families is coordinating the efforts of the multiple helpers who are involved with the family. In their well-intentioned efforts to help, social agencies often exacerbate the structural problems in low-income families (Colapinto, 1995). Most social service agencies have missions that target individuals (e.g., abused children, battered wives) and see their job as working to help these individuals rather than supporting the entire family. Low-income families who experience problems with their children are often subject to scrutiny by child protection agencies mandated by law to remove children from the home if there is evidence of abuse or neglect. Welfare laws encourage the peripheral status of fathers and husbands by cutting benefits if an able-bodied adult male resides in the household. The ascendance of "home-based" services (e.g., Markowitz, 1992; Seelig, Goldman-Hall, & Jerrell, 1992; Tavantzis, Tavantzis, Brown, & Rohrbaugh, 1985), intended to make therapy more available to isolated families, can also inadvertently contribute to the deterioration of the boundary between the family and the social service team.

Therapists who work with low-income families must be prepared to confront the issues posed by the participation of the family in multiple extrafamilial systems. Therapists must broaden their lens beyond the family to the larger system that includes the family plus all of the systems that have become attached to the family over time. Often a problem that seems to be localized within the family can be linked to a problem between the family and the larger system. It is a logical extension of the systems metaphor that the relationship between the family and social service agencies can be dysfunctional without the dysfunction being localized either within the family or within the agency (Imber-Black, 1991).

For example, a mother requested help with a defiant and oppositional adolescent girl. The mother, a single parent, had been reported to the Department of Child Protection for having slapped the girl during an argument some months ago. The mother complained that the child defied her rules, lied to her, and threatened to report her to the child protection worker whenever the mother tried to discipline her.

While the possibility of physical abuse must be investigated, it would be an error to ignore the potential impact of the larger system in contributing to the weak hierarchy in the family that led the mother to feel powerless. In exploring the role of the child protection worker, I realized that the worker had unwittingly invited the adolescent into a coalition with her against the mother. The worker, eager to establish a trusting relationship with the girl, had gone so far as to take her out to lunch and listen attentively as she recounted the "injustices" perpetrated on her by her mother. Concerned that the adolescent might be in danger of abuse, the worker gave the girl her card and invited her to call at any time. Feeling empowered by her alignment with the worker, the girl was actually more apt to be defiant toward her mother, which only increased the risk that her mother could lose control and physically abuse her. Meanwhile, the worker, a single, childless woman 20 years the mother's junior, reported to me that she was frustrated because the mother seemed "resistant" to her suggestions about how to treat the girl. The worker, dedicated and well-intentioned, seemed oblivious to her contribution to the symptomatic cycle.

In order to work effectively in situations such as these, the therapist must have strong relationships with both the family and the representatives of the social agencies. The goal is to help them to collaborate toward accomplishing common goals in an atmosphere of teamwork and mutual respect. It is not helpful for the therapist to adopt a position as the family's advocate *against* the representatives of the social agencies. Rather, it is important to acknowledge the family's distrust of the system and help the representatives of the agencies understand that apparent lack of cooperation on the part of the family members can be a product of mistrust born from powerlessness and experienced disrespect.

In the example above, the therapist must acknowledge both the worker's anxiety about the child's safety as well as the mother's fear of losing the child or being upstaged by a younger, more educated, and more affluent woman who is a member of the majority culture. It is not just the mother who must come to trust the worker; the worker must also trust the mother's competence and concern for the child. The worker must help to empower the mother by involving her in decision making; the mother must understand that the worker is simply trying to do the job she has been hired to do. Mutual trust can be stimulated by facilitating opportunities for the worker and the mother to interact in positive ways that involve them as equal participants working toward common goals.

Helping families achieve more independence from the external agents who have become involved with their lives goes hand in hand with enhancing their abilities to function more effectively. Both goals must be addressed simultaneously. As families develop a greater repertoire of problem-solving capacities, they can function more and more independently of monitoring by external agencies. Similarly, to stimulate families to use their resources more creatively, it is important to discourage them from relying too much on external agencies for the solutions to their problems and instead mobilize resources in their extended family and community when they need assistance.

Mobilizing Resources in the Community

One of the factors that promotes effective functioning in families living in low-income neighborhoods is the presence of social support from extended family or social networks (Taylor & Roberts, 1995; Taylor, Seaton, & Dominguez, 2008). In addition to providing the children with opportunities to have more adults in their lives, the presence of a supportive kin network indirectly benefits children by promoting the mother's well-being. Support from her siblings appears to be especially important in promoting mental health of low-income mothers (Bassuk, Mickelson, Bissell, & Perloff, 2002).

On the other hand, intense or frequent conflict with members of the kin network can have a detrimental effect on single mothers (Bassuk et al., 2002; Taylor et al., 2008). Mothers who are burdened with the responsibility of providing emotional or concrete assistance to extended kin are further depleted and have fewer resources available for their children (Lindblad-Goldberg & Dukes, 1985). Thus, it is important to assess the extended family network carefully and selectively include members of the network who can provide support rather than increase stress on the mother.

Beyond the kin network, there are other potential sources of support within the community including friends, churches, and schools (Jarrett, 1995). After decades of office-based practice, many family therapists are taking to the streets. Therapists who work with low-income families have become increasingly aware of the importance of building stronger social communities in the areas in which these families live (e.g., Rojano, 2004). This movement addresses the disruptive effects of the neighborhood environment at its roots by working with families in "catalytic community partnerships" that are "driven less by therapist-defined problems and professional expertise, and more by community-defined problems and families' own expertise" (Doherty & Beaton, 2000, p. 149).

CASE EXAMPLE: TWO TOKENS

After some research, I learned that Rosa could obtain a transportation grant that could help pay carfare to the nursing home where her mother was staying. I wrote Rosa a short note telling her that I had found out that some money could be available to her for transportation, and that I would tell her more about it when next we met. I also wrote that the child protection worker had been pressing me for information, and I wanted to discuss with Rosa what information (if any) I would release.

When a week had passed and I had not heard from Rosa, I phoned the child protection worker and asked whether she could bring the family to the next therapy session. The worker protested that she was too busy to transport the family, and that it was up to the family to find transportation to the sessions. I then asked whether I could accompany the worker to her next home visit. The worker gave me the time of the next scheduled visit and told me that if I wanted to be present, I could meet her at the family's home. I wrote another note to Rosa, stating that I would like to visit her at home. If she objected, she should call me before the visit to tell me not to come. I then contacted the child protection worker to ask her for a specific list of the information she needed from me, as well as detailed criteria that her agency would use to decide whether Rosa was complying with the department's mandates.

I did not hear from Rosa, so I arranged to be free for 2 hours on the date of the scheduled home visit. I planned to arrive at Rosa's apartment 30 minutes before the child protection worker was scheduled to arrive. I had received from the worker the list of questions I was being asked to answer and the criteria by which Rosa's fitness as a parent would be judged. I intended to discuss these items with Rosa during the 30 minutes prior to the worker's arrival.

Rosa greeted me like an old friend. Neither she nor I brought up the topic of the missed therapy appointments. She did, however, apologize for not responding to my "nice letter" and explained that she was very busy with the children and her mother. She ushered me into the small but clean living room and offered me a cup of tea. Sipping tea together, I told Rosa how she could apply for the transportation grant. She was grateful and told me that she would try to come to therapy again. I asked her whether she knew the purpose of the meeting with the child protection worker. Not surprisingly, she didn't really understand why we were meeting. I explained that I was being asked to provide evidence that Rosa was complying with treatment and making changes in the way she disciplined her children. I asked Rosa whether she would help me decide what I should tell the worker. At first, Rosa protested, claiming, "I can't do that—I don't know anything."

I persisted, insisting that Rosa knew far more than I about what was best for her and for her family. Rosa then timidly suggested that perhaps I could help her convince the worker that she really was a good mother, and that she did not abuse her children. I saw this as an opportunity to share with Rosa the criteria I had received from the worker. At first defensive, Rosa eventually accepted the criteria, which included cooperating with the investigation, working to develop new parenting skills, and keeping the children safe.

I said that I thought I could help if Rosa would be willing to negotiate a contract to work with me toward meeting these criteria. I would tell the worker that I believed Rosa was actually making progress toward these goals even though she had been unable to attend therapy sessions regularly. With Rosa's help, I listed Rosa's strengths as a parent and cited several specific examples that demonstrated that she loved and took care of her children.

I asked Rosa whether she could attend therapy every week. Rosa became a bit defensive, arguing that she did not have the time or money to come to therapy every week. As a compromise, I proposed that Rosa could attend therapy sessions at my office every other week. Once a month, I would make a home visit and hold therapy at Rosa's apartment. In addition, Rosa would telephone me weekly at a specific time, and I would also telephone Rosa at a specific time at her sister's house.

The latter would require Rosa to ask her sister for help, something she was initially reluctant to do, until I convinced her that a stronger relationship with her sister could help her case with the child protection worker.

When the worker arrived a few minutes later, I noted with interest how coolly Rosa greeted her. She was nevertheless polite and offered the worker a cup of tea, which she declined. The worker immediately got down to business. She told Rosa that she knew that Rosa was not attending therapy, and that there was a strong possibility that her children would be taken from her. I asked the worker whether Rosa could share with her what she and I had just been discussing. The worker looked surprised, but she agreed. Rosa then gave the worker a sketch of the plan we had devised, as I prompted her with reminders. The worker seemed satisfied but skeptical. All agreed that another home visit would be scheduled in 3 months to evaluate Rosa's progress.

After the worker left, I congratulated Rosa on remaining calm even though I could see that she was not fond of the worker. I then brought up the phone calls I had received from Ramon's school. I told her that they were asking me for advice on how best to help Ramon in the classroom. Would Rosa like me to be involved in this way? She agreed that Ramon needed help and expressed her frustration with him. I asked what she thought could help Ramon to do better in school. She came up with a few ideas, which I conspicuously wrote down. I then asked whether Ramon could come to the next session, so that I could ask him whether he had any additional ideas. Rosa agreed and we parted cordially. The next therapy session was scheduled for the following week. Immediately after returning to my office, I dashed off a short note reminding Rosa of the appointment and included two subway tokens for transportation. I mailed the note on the way home.

Rosa showed up on time for the family session, accompanied by Ramon and a modestly dressed, stately woman who appeared slightly older than she. Rosa introduced the visitor as her sister Julia and explained that Julia had offered to drive them to my office. Rosa offered to return the tokens, but I said she should keep them in her purse in case Julia was not available to drive them to our next appointment. Rosa asked whether Julia could join the session, and I enthusiastically agreed. We discussed how we could help Ramon at school and came up with a few more ideas that I added to the list. At the end of the session, I asked Rosa whether she would allow me to ask Julia for her telephone number, so that I had someone to call if I needed to reach Rosa between the sessions. Rosa agreed.

Over the next several weeks, my relationship with Rosa continued to improve. Although she occasionally missed therapy sessions, she remained about 80% faithful to the contract we had negotiated. One day, Rosa came to a session with a black eye, and it immediately occurred to me that she might have missed previous therapy sessions because she was afraid that I would suspect that she was being beat up by her boyfriend.

When I first asked about her black eye, Rosa was evasive. I then asked her directly whether her boyfriend was hitting her. Rosa burst into tears and admitted that her boyfriend was violent and she was afraid of him. She couldn't move in with Julia, because he knew where Julia lived, and Rosa didn't think she or the children would be safe there. I suggested that we contact the child protection worker, tell her about Rosa's dilemma, and see whether the worker could arrange for Rosa to go to a shelter for battered women.

A few weeks later, Rosa's mother's condition worsened. I suggested that one of our scheduled therapy sessions be held at the nursing home, an idea Rosa wholeheartedly supported. Julia was willing to drive us all to the nursing home. At the bedside of the frail, dying woman, I helped Rosa to grieve and say good-bye to her mother.

Although the family continued to have crises, although the children continued to have trouble at school, and although Rosa continued to miss about one out of every four therapy sessions, she nevertheless provided the Department of Child Protection with satisfactory evidence of her fitness as a parent, and they closed her case. By then, however, Rosa had come to see me as a resource and agreed to continue in therapy even though it was no longer mandated.

SUMMARY

In this chapter, I have discussed the challenges and potentials of working with overwhelmed low-income families with multiple problems. The following are important principles to keep in mind to avoid therapist burnout and to empower the family to make the most of therapy:

- Concentrate on family strengths.

- Provide emotional and physical support to the parent by acknowledging his or her struggles and helping to access resources to shore up his or her role as the person in charge of the family.

- Build hope and confidence in therapy by working first on a concrete, readily attainable goal that benefits the parent.

- Attend to cultural issues and the power dynamics within the larger system.

• Work *with* and *through* the family members rather than *for* them. Empower the family members to achieve their own goals and insist that the family members take active roles in making decisions that affect them.

• Help family members and representatives of helping agencies work collaboratively in an atmosphere of mutual respect.

• Help to mobilize potential resources in the extended family and community.

• Contribute time to addressing communitywide needs and help to build systems that address neighborhood needs.

Epilogue: The ARCH

"I don't want to be here. I'm here only because my parents made me come. They said that I wasn't part of the family anymore and if I wanted to get back in, I had to come here."

I asked the scruffy 16-year-old what he meant by not being "part of the family anymore."

He just shrugged and said, "I don't know. It's just what they said. They'll feed me and give me a place to live but that's all."

I was surprised to hear this bland recital of what sounded like a major rejection by the family. I wondered how the situation at home had deteriorated to this point. The boy's mother sounded nice enough on the telephone a few days earlier when she called to ask me to see Steve.

"I know you work with families," she said, "but Steve said he wouldn't go with us. If he has to see someone, he wants to go alone. Will you do it?"

Sometimes you have to size up a clinical situation quickly, on the basis of very little information. The mother sounded sincere, and I thought perhaps I could convince Steve to allow the rest of the family to come in after I had a chance to connect with him. However, I needed more information before deciding how to proceed. I asked Mrs. O'Brien to tell me more about the problem.

She related a not-unfamiliar story. Steve was a junior in a Catholic high school and was doing marginal work. He had just failed two subjects at midyear and didn't seem to care. What concerned her most, however, was that Steve had been in trouble with the police three times since the beginning of the school year: once for writing graffiti on a wall, once for stealing a cigarette lighter from a store, and once for pelting cars with eggs on Halloween. He was doing community service for the first charge and was awaiting hearings on the other two.

Mrs. O'Brien also suspected that Steve was smoking marijuana, although she didn't think that he was using any other drugs. She said that Steve's father had "read him the riot act" the night before, told him that he'd be sent to public school if he didn't improve his grades, and grounded him for a month. They had tried family therapy before, but after a few visits Steve refused to attend. He was "open" to the idea of seeing a counselor now, but insisted that his parents not be part of the meetings.

I knew there were risks involved in agreeing to see Steve alone, but I decided to go ahead anyway. I realized that I could be inducted into a coalition with Steve against his parents, or that Steve could disclose information to me that he didn't want them to know but that I thought they needed to know. I might fall into the trap of trying to replace his parents and he'd let me by having a better relationship with me than with them. Maybe we'd develop a bond that his parents could precipitously sever if his behavior did not improve, thus exposing him to the trauma of losing a relationship that had grown to be important to him.

On the other hand, Steve had expressed a clear preference to be seen alone. His parents were willing to agree that our sessions would be confidential, and that they would defer to my judgment regarding when they should be apprised of anything Steve had disclosed to me. They also recognized that it would take time for me to build a relationship with Steve, so they shouldn't necessarily expect to see any major changes right away. If they wanted therapy to end, for any reason, they would allow me at least one additional session to meet with Steve alone so that we could terminate comfortably.

Steve arrived promptly for his session late one January afternoon, a sturdy boy with wild hair that just grazed his shoulders, dressed in a torn T-shirt and shorts beneath his winter coat, and lime green high-top sneakers. He reluctantly shook the hand I offered him, sat down, and, without waiting to be asked, made his announcement about not wanting to be in therapy and needing to come in order to "get back in the family."

I told Steve that I appreciated knowing where I stood, and that I sympathized with the bind he was in. I asked him if there was anything he wanted to talk about, and was not really surprised when he smirked and replied in the negative, glaring at me as if daring me to offend him. I got the same response when I asked him whether he wanted to ask me any questions about myself.

Feeling a little anxious now, I related to Steve what his mother had told me on the phone and asked him whether he had any comment. Another smirk and grunt. I asked him why he didn't want his parents to come to therapy.

"We tried it once," he said with a frisson of contempt in his voice, "but it didn't do any good. My parents won't change."

I got another grunt when I asked him how he wanted his parents to change. I then asked him whether he had ever talked with a therapist or counselor alone.

"Once," he said, "they made me go see this other guy. He asked me why I was there, and I said I didn't know. He asked me if I wanted to work on anything, and I said 'no,' so he told me I could leave. I was there about 10 minutes. I don't think he liked me very much."

I had no way of knowing whether Steve realized that he had given me good advice on how not to do therapy with him. I couldn't repeat my colleague's mistake, even if Steve was baiting me to dismiss him from my office in frustration. It was up to me to find a way to have a relationship with him.

I asked him about school. "What's it like there?" I asked, with genuine curiosity. I hadn't worked with any kids who had attended his school, and I had some fond and not-so-fond memories of my own high school, an all-male Catholic prep school, similar to the one Steve was attending.

Perhaps sensing my real curiosity, Steve seemed to let his guard down a bit. He said he liked the school, but he hated taking Latin, and he thought some of the teachers were "jerks." I asked him whether there were any classes he liked. He told me that he liked art and added that he had been taking art classes on weekends since he was in elementary school. His smirk in response to my question about participation in school sports told me not to go there, but he added on his own that he was on the chess team and often went out of town to play tournaments with the team. Jumping at what seemed to be an opening, I suggested that maybe we could play a game of chess at our next session.

"No thanks," Steve sneered.

I asked him how he liked going to an all-boys school, and he said that he didn't mind because he had no trouble meeting girls outside of school. But he didn't have a girlfriend right now, and he didn't care to.

"There's plenty of time for that," he said. "Right now I just like hanging out with my friends."

I asked him what he liked doing with his friends.

"Just hanging out," he said, "playing a little ball, listening to music, you know."

Risking our fragile conversation, I asked whether he ever smoked any "weed" with his friends. I was surprised when he answered, without a beat. "Yeah, sometimes," he said, "but not as much as my parents think."

The conversation continued in this way for the next 30 minutes, and by the end of our session, I had learned quite a bit about Steve. In addition to what I have already related, I also learned that he got straight A's in math, that he liked math and found it challenging, that he had been working 20 hours per week at a gas station since he was in the ninth grade, and had even begun saving money in an IRA. He grunted when, at the end of our session, I said I'd see him next week at the same time, but I really didn't doubt that he'd be back.

Not only did Steve come back the following week, but he came on time every week for the next 3 months. His grades had improved, and while he wasn't exactly delightful to live with, he occasionally had dinner with the family, did his chores more or less regularly, and followed the house rules most of the time. It was his father who suggested that maybe Steve didn't need to come anymore. He was doing much better and he was involved in a lot of activities during the last month of school. Steve, of course, "didn't mind" stopping, since (he reminded me) he didn't want to come in the first place. But we had had some interesting conversations over those 3 months.

Reflecting on our time together, I remembered that the first breakthrough came when I decided that I'd open up a bit more than I usually do about my own life and my own experiences as a teenager attending a Catholic high school not unlike his own. Steve actually started asking me questions; an event that I chose to interpret as his beginning to have an interest in me. I told Steve that I enjoyed talking with him.

He parried back, "Yeah, sure, you're getting paid for it."

"You're right. I am getting paid," I admitted. "But I'm not paid to like you. And I do. And I don't like everyone I work with."

Steve didn't answer, but for the first time he was speechless, not just silent.

At our sixth session, I asked Steve how he was feeling about our meetings.

"Just like I thought," he replied. "A waste of time and money. I'm not going to change, and you can't make me change."

A bit surprised, I asked Steve if he thought that I was trying to change him. He answered, "That's what you're supposed to be doing, ain't it?"

I even surprised myself at the spontaneity of my reply: "Maybe. But I'm not doing it with you. I'm just trying to get to know you. So far, I like what I see and even if I could (and I can't), I wouldn't want to change you."

A few sessions later, Steve sardonically remarked that "you adults" were interested only in "showing us kids that we gotta do whatever you say."

I asked him to elaborate, and he told me that the weekend before, he and his friends were "hanging out" in a parking lot, just tossing a football around, and they were chased away by the police.

"We weren't using drugs or anything, I swear," Steve said with indignation. "The cop thought we were going to cause trouble just because we were a bunch of teenagers."

Steve went on to tell me about other such experiences, and I began to remember some long-forgotten feelings from my own youth, when I felt that I didn't have any rights and that I was a "second-class citizen" in an adult world.

It occurred to me that Steve was a member of a minority group, and, like many minorities, he was subject to prejudice based on stereotypes. I thought about this idea a lot after the session, and when we met the following week, I thanked Steve for teaching me this valuable lesson. I apologized to him "on behalf of all adults" for the times we were disrespectful and unreasonable in our dealings with teenagers. Steve glared at me suspiciously.

"I really mean it," I added. "And I just needed to say that to you whether you believe me or not."

He fidgeted in his chair, and I thought I might have seen a glisten of moisture in his eyes.

Our sessions had a spontaneous quality. I never knew what would be the topic of the day. One week, we debated politics; I took the role of asking questions that forced Steve to articulate his position. Another week, Steve gleefully told me about his mock campaign for the class presidency. Toward the end, he finally showed me some of his artwork. I asked questions (again, genuinely curious) and told him what I liked about his work.

So what did we accomplish? I was glad that Steve wasn't a managed care case, because I don't know how I would have provided adequate justification for the "medical necessity" of his treatment or the treatment goals I was pursuing. All I knew was that we were developing a relationship, I genuinely liked this boy, and he seemed to be calming down. He was beginning to differentiate himself from his peers and take fewer affronts at his parents' expectations of him.

He never mentioned it, but I assume he "got back in" the family. When his dad (whom Steve always spoke of with a mixture of contempt and fear) asked me whether Steve could stop coming to therapy, I sensed a very different tone in Mr. O'Brien's voice, one that told me that he was less frantic and more confident that Steve would be OK.

I'll remember Steve as one of my best teachers. He taught me to be more spontaneous in my sessions, to draw on parts of myself that I don't usually draw on in therapy. At various times, I was peer (when I told him stories of my own adolescence), adult (when I apologized for the way adults treated kids, when I told him what it feels like to be an adult, what our fears and insecurities are), student (when I thanked him for helping me to see the prejudice kids experience just for being kids), advocate (when I offered to speak with his parents on his behalf), and, yes, even therapist (when I helped him articulate his feelings of humiliation at having to show his homework to his father every night, which led to his confronting his father verbally rather than in passive–aggressive refusal to comply with his father's directive).

Because I was forced to modify my typical therapeutic stance in order to offer this boy a lifeline that he was willing to grasp, because I had to admit that I couldn't force Steve to change, I was left only to be myself, to respond to him not out of any theoretical or technical principles, but out of my genuine liking and care for him. What he had for those 15 sessions was my undivided attention, my honesty, my willingness to be vulnerable, and my unconditional acceptance of him—all ultimately based on my conviction that I had something to offer him if he would just stick it out long enough.

Steve taught me that, after all is said and done, after all the pages are read and written, theory and principles can take us only so far. The rest comes from the heart of therapy, the relationship, one firmly supported by the ARCH—Acceptance, Respect, Curiosity, and Honesty.

References

Adam, K. S., Sheldon-Keller, A. E., & West, M. (1996). Attachment organization and history of suicidal behavior in clinical adolescents. *Journal of Consulting and Clinical Psychology, 64*(2), 264–272.

Adams, G. R., & Berzonsky, M. D. (Eds.). (2003). *Blackwell handbook of adolescence.* Malden, MA: Blackwell.

Adams, G. R., Gullotta, T., & Montemayor, R. (Eds.). (1992). *Adolescent identity formation.* Newbury Park, CA: Sage.

Ainsworth, M. D. (1989). Attachments beyond infancy. *American Psychologist, 44*(4), 709–716.

Alberts, A., Elkind, D., & Ginsberg, S. (2007). The personal fable and risk-taking in early adolescence. *Journal of Youth and Adolescence, 36*(1), 71–76.

Allen, J. P., Insabella, G., Porter, M. R., Smith, F. D., Land, D., & Phillips, N. (2006). A social-interactional model of the development of depressive symptoms in adolescence. *Journal of Consulting and Clinical Psychology, 74*(1), 55–65.

Allen, J. P., & Land, D. (1999). Attachment in adolescence. In J. Cassidy & P. Shaver (Eds.), *Handbook of attachment: Theory, research, and clinical applications.* New York: Guilford Press.

Allen, J. P., Marsh, P., McFarland, C., McElhaney, K. B., Land, D. J., Jodl, K. M., et al. (2002). Attachment and autonomy as predictors of the development of social skills and delinquency during midadolescence. *Journal of Consulting and Clinical Psychology, 70*(1), 56–66.

Allen, J. P., McElhaney, K. B., Kuperminc, G. P., & Jodl, K. M. (2004). Stability and change in attachment security across adolescence. *Child Development, 75*(6), 1792–1805.

Allen, J. P., Moore, C., Kuperminc, G., & Bell, K. (1998). Attachment and adolescent psychosocial functioning. *Child Development, 69*(5), 1406–1419.

Allgood-Merten, B., Lewinsohn, P. M., & Hops, H. (1990). Sex differences and adolescent depression. *Journal of Abnormal Psychology, 99,* 55–63.

Amato, P. R., & Fowler, F. (2002). Parenting practices, child adjustment, and family diversity. *Journal of Marriage and Family, 64,* 703–716.

American Psychiatric Association. (1999). Position statement on psychiatric treatment and sexual orientation. *American Journal of Psychiatry, 156,* 1131.

American Psychiatric Association. (2000). *Diagnostic and statistical manual of mental disorders* (4th ed., text rev.). Arlington, VA: Author.

American Psychological Association. (1998). Resolution on appropriate therapeutic responses to sexual orientation in proceedings of the American Psychological Association, Incorporated, for the legislative year 1997. *American Psychologist, 53,* 882–939.

Ames, C., & Archer, J. (1988). Achievement goals in the classroom: Students' learning strategies and motivational processes. *Journal of Educational Psychology, 80,* 260–270.

Anderson, C. M. (1983). A psychoeducational program for families of patients with schizophrenia. In W. R. McFarlane (Ed.), *Family therapy in schizophrenia.* New York: Guilford Press.

Aponte, H. (1976a). The family–school interview: An eco-structural approach. *Family Process, 15,* 303–311.

Aponte, H. (1976b). Underorganization in the poor family. In P. Guerin (Ed.), *Family therapy: Theory and practice.* New York: Gardner.

Aponte, H. (1994). *Bread and spirit: Therapy with the new poor.* New York: Norton.

Arbona, C., & Power, T. G. (2003). Parental attachment, self-esteem, and antisocial behaviors among African American, European American, and Mexican American adolescents. *Journal of Counseling Psychology, 50*(1), 40–51.

Archer, S. L. (1989). Gender differences in identity development: Issues of process, domain, and timing. *Journal of Adolescence, 12,* 117–138.

Archibald, A. B., Graber, J. A., & Brooks-Gunn, J. (2003). Pubertal processes and physiological growth in adolescence. In G. R. Adams & M. D. Berzonsky (Eds.), *Blackwell handbook of adolescence.* Malden, MA: Blackwell.

Arnett, J. J. (1999). Adolescent storm and stress, reconsidered. *American Psychologist, 54*(5), 317–326.

Ary, D. V., Duncan, T. E., Duncan, S. C., & Hops, H. (1999). Adolescent problem behavior: The influence of parents and peers. *Behaviour Research and Therapy, 37*(3), 217–230.

Aseltine, R. H. (1995). A reconsideration of parental and peer influences on adolescent deviance. *Journal of Health and Social Behavior, 36*(2), 103–121.

Asseltine, R. H., Jr., Gore, S., & Colton, M. E. (1994). Depression and the social developmental context of adolescence. *Journal of Personality and Social Psychology, 67*, 252–263.

Attie, I., & Brooks-Gunn, J. (1989). The development of eating problems in adolescent girls: A longitudinal study. *Developmental Psychology, 25*, 70–79.

Barkley, R. A. (2006). Attention-deficit hyperactivity disorder. In D. A. Wolfe, & E. J. Mash (Eds.), *Behavioral and emotional disorders in adolescents*. New York: Guilford Press.

Barkley, R. A., Fischer, M., Smallish, L., & Fletcher, K. (2006). Young adult outcome of hyperactive children: Adaptive functioning in major life activities. *Journal of the American Academy of Child and Adolescent Psychiatry, 45*(2), 192–202.

Barkley, R. A., Guevremont, D. C., Anastopoulos, A. D., & Fletcher, K. E. (1992). A comparison of three family therapy programs for treating family conflicts in adolescents with attention-deficit/hyperactivity disorder. *Journal of Consulting and Clinical Psychology, 60*, 450–462.

Barrett, P. M., Dadds, M. R., & Rapee, R. M. (1996). Family treatment of childhood anxiety: A controlled trial. *Journal of Consulting and Clinical Psychology, 64*(2), 333–342.

Barrett, P. M., Fox, T., & Farrell, L. J. (2005). Parent–child interactions with anxious children and with their siblings: An observational study. *Behaviour Change, 22*(4), 220–235.

Bartholomew, K., & Horowitz, L. M. (1991). Attachment styles among adults: A test of a four-category model. *Journal of Personality and Social Psychology, 61*(2), 226–244.

Basow, S. A., & Rubin, L. R. (1999). Gender influences on adolescent development. In N. G. Johnson, M. C. Roberts, & J. Worell (Eds.), *Beyond appearance: A new look at adolescent girls*. Washington, DC: American Psychological Association.

Bassuk, E. L., Mickelson, K. D., Bissell, H. D., & Perloff, J. N. (2002). Role of kin and nonkin support in the mental health of low-income women. *American Journal of Orthopsychiatry, 72*(1), 39–49.

Bateson, G., Jackson, D. D., Haley, J., & Weakland, J. H. (1956). Toward a theory of schizophrenia. *Behavioral Science, 1*, 251–264.

Baumrind, D. (1978). Parental disciplinary patterns and social competence in children. *Youth and Society, 9*, 239–276.

Bean, R. A., Perry, B. J., & Bedell, T. M. (2001). Developing culturally competent marriage and family therapists: Guidelines for working with Hispanic families. *Journal of Marital and Family Therapy, 27*(1), 43–54.

Becker, D., & Liddle, H. A. (2001). Family therapy with unmarried African American mothers and their adolescents. *Family Process, 40*(4), 413–427.

Bem, S. (1975). Sex-role adaptability: One consequence of psychological androgyny. *Journal of Personality and Social Psychology, 31,* 634–643.

Bergman, S. J. (1995). Men's psychological development: A relational perspective. In R. F. Levant & W. S. Pollack (Eds.), *A new psychology of men.* New York: Basic Books.

Berman, A. L., & Jobes, D. A. (1991). *Adolescent suicide: Assessment and intervention.* Washington, DC: American Psychological Association Press.

Berndt, T. (1979). Developmental changes in conformity to peers and parents. *Developmental Psychology, 15,* 608–616.

Bingham, C. R., & Crockett, L. J. (1996). Longitudinal adjustment patterns of boys and girls experiencing early, middle, and late sexual intercourse. *Developmental Psychology, 32,* 647–658.

Blair, C., Freeman, C., & Cull, A. (1995). The families of anorexia nervosa and cystic fibrosis patients. *Psychological Medicine, 25,* 985–993.

Blos, P. (1962). *On adolescence: A psychoanalytic interpretation.* New York: Free Press.

Blos, P. (1967). The second individuation process of adolescence. *Psychoanalytic Study of the Child, 22,* 162–186.

Boergers, J., Spirito, A., & Donaldson, D. (1998). Reasons for adolescent suicide attempts: Association with psychological functioning. *Journal of the American Academy of Child and Adolescent Psychiatry, 37*(12), 1287–1293.

Bogels, S. M., & Siqueland, L. (2006). Family cognitive behavior therapy for children and adolescents with clinical anxiety disorders. *Journal of the American Academy of Child and Adolescent Psychiatry, 45*(2), 134–141.

Bogels, S. M., van Oosten, A., Muris, P., & Smulders, D. (2001). Familial correlates of social anxiety in children and adolescents. *Behaviour Research and Therapy, 39,* 273–287.

Booth, A., Johnson, D. R., Granger, D. A., Crouter, A. C., & McHale, S. (2003). Testosterone and child and adolescent adjustment: The moderating role of parent–child relationships. *Developmental Psychology, 39*(1), 85–98.

Boszormenyi-Nagy, I., & Spark, M. (1973). *Invisible loyalties.* New York: Harper & Row.

Bouchey, H. A., & Furman, W. (2003). Dating and romantic experiences in adolescence. In G. R. Adams & M. D. Berzonsky (Eds.), *Blackwell handbook of adolescence.* Malden, MA: Blackwell.

Bowen, M. (1978). *Family therapy in clinical practice.* Northvale, NJ: Aronson.

Bowlby, J. (1988). *A secure base: Clinical applications of attachment theory.* London: Routledge.

Boyd-Franklin, N. (2003). *Black families in therapy: Understanding the African American experience* (2nd ed.). New York: Guilford Press.

Bradley, R. H., & Corwyn, R. F. (2002). Socioeconomic status and child development. *Annual Review of Psychology, 53,* 371–399.

Brendler, J., Silver, M., Haber, M., & Sargent, J. (1991). *Madness, chaos, and violence: Therapy with families at the brink.* New York: Basic Books.

Brent, D. (2007). Antidepressants and suicidal behavior: Cause or cure? *American Journal of Psychiatry, 164*(7), 898–991.

Brent, D. A., Kolko, D. J., Allan, M. J., & Brown, R. V. (1990). Suicidality in affectively disordered adolescent inpatients. *Journal of the American Academy of Child and Adolescent Psychiatry, 29,* 586–593.

Brent, D. A., Moritz, G., Liotus, L., Schweers, J., Balach, L., Roth, C., et al. (1998). Familial risk factors for adolescent suicide: A case-control study. In R. J. Kosky, H. S. Eshkevari, R. D. Goldney, & R. Hassan (Eds.), *Suicide prevention: The global context.* New York: Plenum Press.

Brooks-Gunn, J., Graber, J. A., & Paikoff, R. L. (1994). Studying links between hormones and negative affect: Models and measures. *Journal of Research on Adolescence, 4*(4), 469–486.

Brooks-Gunn, J., & Reiter, E. (1990). The role of pubertal processes. In S. Feldman & G. Elliott (Eds.), *At the threshold: The developing adolescent.* Cambridge, MA: Harvard University Press.

Brown, B. B. (1990). Peer groups and peer cultures. In S. Feldman & G. Elliott (Eds.), *At the threshold: The developing adolescent.* Cambridge, MA: Harvard University Press.

Brown, B. B., Mounts, N., Lamborn, S. D., & Steinberg, L. (1993). Parenting practices and peer group affiliation in adolescence. *Child Development, 64,* 467–482.

Brown, L. M., & Gilligan, C. (1992). *Meeting at the crossroads.* New York: Ballantine.

Browning, S., Collins, J. S., & Nelson, B. (2005). Creating families: A teaching technique for clinical training through role-playing. *Marriage and Family Review, 38,* 1–19.

Bruch, H. (1982). Anorexia nervosa: Therapy and theory. *American Journal of Psychiatry, 139,* 1531–1538.

Bruch, H. (1988). *Conversations with anorexics.* New York: Basic Books.

Buchanan, C., Eccles, J., & Becker, J. (1992). Are adolescents the victims of raging hormones?: Evidence for activational effects of hormones at adolescence. *Psychological Bulletin, 111,* 62–107.

Buhrmester, D., & Furman, W. (1987). The development of companionship and intimacy. *Child Development, 58,* 1101–1113.

Buist, K. L., Dekovic, M., Meeus, W., & van Aken, M. A. G. (2004). The reciprocal relationship between early adolescent attachment and internalizing and externalizing problem behaviour. *Journal of Adolescence, 27,* 251–266.

Burton, L. M., & Jarrett, R. L. (2000). In the mix, yet on the margins: The place of families in urban neighborhood and child development research. *Journal of Marriage and the Family, 62,* 1114–1135.

Byng-Hall, J. (1995). Creating a secure family base: Some implications of attachment theory for family therapy. *Family Process, 34*(1), 45–58.

Carl, D., & Jurkovic, G. J. (1983). Agency triangles: Problems in agency-family relationships. *Family Process, 22,* 441–451.

Carpenter, S. (2001). Sleep deprivation may be undermining teen health. *Monitor on Psychology, 32,* 42–45.

Carr, M., Borkowski, J. G., & Maxwell, S. E. (1991). Motivational components of underachievement. *Developmental Psychology, 27,* 108–118.

Carris, M. J., Sheeber, L., & Howe, S. (1998). Family rigidity, adolescent problem-solving deficits, and suicidal ideation: A mediational model. *Journal of Adolescence, 21*(4), 459–472.

Carter, B. (1988). Fathers and daughters. In M. Walters, B. Carter, P. Papp, & O. Silverstein (Eds.), *The invisible web: Gender patterns in family relationships.* New York: Guilford Press.

Carter, E. A., & McGoldrick, M. (Eds.). (2005). *The expanded family life cycle: Individual, family, and social perspectives* (3rd ed.). Boston: Allyn & Bacon.

Cartwright-Hatton, S., Roberts, C., Chitsabesan, P., Fothergill, C., & Harrington, R. (2004). Systematic review of the efficacy of cognitive behaviour therapies for childhood and adolescent anxiety disorders. *British Journal of Clinical Psychology, 43*(4), 421–436.

Casey, B. J., Getz, S., & Galvan, A. (2008). The adolescent brain. *Developmental Review, 28,* 62–77.

Caspi, A., & Moffitt, T. E. (1991). Individual differences are accentuated during periods of social change: The sample case of girls at puberty. *Journal of Personality and Social Psychology, 61,* 157–168.

Chalfant, J. C. (1989). Learning disabilities: Policy issues and promising approaches. *American Psychologist, 44,* 392–398.

Chao, R. (1994). Beyond parental control and authoritarian parenting style: Understanding Chinese parenting through the cultural notion of training. *Child Development, 65,* 1111–1119.

Colapinto, J. (1988). Avoiding a common pitfall in compulsory school referrals. *Journal of Marital and Family Therapy, 14,* 89–96.

Colapinto, J. (1995). Dilution of family process in social services: Implications for treatment of neglectful families. *Family Process, 34,* 59–74.

Colby, A., Kohlberg, L., Gibbs, J., & Lieberman, M. (1983). A longitudinal study of moral judgment. *Monographs of the Society for Research in Child Development, 48* (Serial No. 200).

Cole, D. A., & McPherson, A. E. (1993). Relation of family subsystems to adolescent depression: Implementing a new family assessment strategy. *Journal of Family Psychology, 7,* 119–133.

Cole-Detke, H., & Kobak, R. (1996). Attachment processes in eating disorder and depression. *Journal of Consulting and Clinical Psychology, 64,* 282–290.

Collins, W. A. (2003). More than myth: The developmental significance of romantic relationships during adolescence. *Journal of Research on Adolescence, 13*(1), 1–24.

Compas, B. E., Ey, S., & Grant, K. E. (1993). Taxonomy, assessment, and diagnosis of depression during adolescence. *Psychological Bulletin, 114,* 323–344.

Conger, R. D., Conger, K., Matthews, L. S., & Elder, G. H. J. (1999). Pathways of economic influence on adolescent adjustment. *American Journal of Community Psychology, 27*(4), 519–541.

Conger, R. D., Ge, X., Elder, G. H., Lorenz, F. O., & Simons, R. L. (1994). Economic stress, coercive family process, and developmental problems of adolescents. *Child Development, 65,* 541–561.

Cook, W. L. (2000). Understanding attachment security in family context. *Journal of Personality and Social Psychology, 78*(2), 285–294.

Cook, W. L. (2001). Interpersonal influence in family systems: A social relations model analysis. *Child Development, 72*(4), 1179–1197.

Coyne, J. C. (1976). Depression and the response of others. *Journal of Abnormal Psychology, 85,* 186–193.

Coyne, J. C. (1999). Thinking interactionally about depression: A radical restatement. In T. Joiner & J. C. Coyne (Eds.), *The interactional nature of depression: Advances in interpersonal approaches.* Washington, DC: American Psychological Association.

Cramer, P. (1979). Defense mechanisms in adolescence. *Developmental Psychology, 15,* 476–477.

Crick, N. R., Casas, J. F., & Nelson, D. A. (2002). Toward a more comprehensive understanding of peer maltreatment: Studies of relational victimization. *Current Directions in Psychological Science, 11*(3), 98–101.

Crisp, A. H. (1983). Some aspects of the psychopathology of anorexia nervosa. In P. L. Darby, P. E. Garfinkel, D. M. Garner, & D. V. Coscina (Eds.), *Anorexia nervosa: Recent developments in research.* New York: Liss.

Crockett, L. J., Raffaelli, M., & Moilanen, K. L. (2003). Adolescent sexuality: Behavior and meaning. In G. R. Adams & M. D. Berzonsky (Eds.), *Blackwell handbook of adolescence.* Malden, MA: Blackwell.

Cross, W. E. J. (1991). *Shades of Black: Diversity in African American identity.* Philadelphia: Temple University Press.

Culbertson, F. M. (1997). Depression and gender: An international review. *American Psychologist, 52,* 25–31.

Dadds, M. R., Marrett, P. M., & Rapee, R. M. (1996). Family process and child anxiety and aggression: An observational analysis. *Journal of Abnormal Child Psychology, 24*(6), 715–734.

Darby-Mullins, P., & Murdock, T. B. (2007). The influence of family environment on self-acceptance and emotional adjustment among gay, lesbian, and bisexual adolescents. *Journal of GLBT Family Studies, 3*(1), 75–91.

Darling, N., & Steinberg, L. (1993). Parenting style as context: An integrative model. *Psychological Bulletin, 113*, 487–496.

D'Augelli, A. R., Hershberger, S., & Pilkington, N. (1998). Lesbian, gay, and bisexual youth and their families: Disclosure of sexual orientation and its consequences. *American Journal of Orthopsychiatry, 68*, 361–371.

DeBaryshe, B. D., Patterson, G. R., & Capaldi, D. M. (1993). A performance model for academic achievement in early adolescent boys. *Developmental Psychology, 29*, 795–804.

Deci, E. L., Koestner, R., & Ryan, R. M. (1999). A meta-analytic review of experiments examining the effects of extrinsic rewards on intrinsic motivation. *Psychological Bulletin, 125*(6), 627–668.

Denborough, D. (1996). Step by step: Developing respectful and effective ways of working with young men to reduce violence. In C. McLean, M. Carey, & C. White (Eds.), *Men's ways of being*. Boulder, CO: Westview.

DeWilde, E. J., Kienhorst, I. C., Diekstra, R. F., & Wolters, W. H. (1993). The specificity of psychological characteristics of adolescent suicide attempters. *Journal of the American Academy of Child and Adolescent Psychiatry, 32*(1), 51–59.

Diamond, G., & Josephson, A. (2005). Family-based treatment research: A 10–year update. *Journal of the American Academy of Child and Adolescent Psychiatry, 44*(9), 872–887.

Diamond, G. S., Reis, B. F., Diamond, G., Siqueland, L., & Isaacs, L. (2002). Attachment-based family therapy for depressed adolescents: A treatment development study. *Journal of the American Academy of Child and Adolescent Psychiatry, 41*(10), 1190–1196.

Diamond, G. S., Serrano, A., Dickey, M., & Sonis, W. (1996). Empirical support for family therapy. *Journal of the American Academy of Child and Adolescent Psychiatry, 35*, 6–16.

Diamond, G. S., & Stern, R. S. (2003). Attachment-based family therapy for depressed adolescents: Repairing attachment failures. In S. M. Johnson & V. E. Whiffen (Eds.), *Attachment processes in couple and family therapy*. New York: Guilford Press.

Diamond, L. M. (1998). Development of sexual orientation among adolescent and young adult women. *Developmental Psychology, 34*, 1085–1095.

Diamond, L. M. (2000). Sexual identity, attractions, and behavior among young sexual-minority women over a two-year period. *Developmental Psychology, 36*, 241–250.

Diamond, L. M., & Savin-Williams, R. C. (2003). The intimate relationships of sexual minority youth. In G. R. Adams & M. D. Berzonsky (Eds.), *Blackwell handbook of adolescence*. Malden, MA: Blackwell.

Dishion, T. J., Capaldi, D., Spracklen, K. M., & Li, F. (1995). Peer ecology of male adolescent drug use. *Development and Psychopathology*, 7(4), 803–824.

Dishion, T. J., & Loeber, R. (1985). Adolescent marijuana and alcohol use: The role of parents and peers revisited. *American Journal of Drug and Alcohol Abuse*, 11(1–2), 11–25.

Dishion, T., Patterson, G., Stoolmiller, M., & Skinner, M. (1991). Family, school, and behavioral antecedents to early adolescent involvement with antisocial peers. *Developmental Psychology*, 27, 172–180.

Doherty, W. J., & Beaton, J. M. (2000). Family therapists, community, and civic renewal. *Family Process*, 39(2), 149–161.

Dorius, C. J., Bahr, S. J., Hoffman, J. P., & Harmon, E. L. (2004). Parenting practices as moderators of the relationship between peers and adolescent marijuana use. *Journal of Marriage and Family*, 66, 163–178.

Dubow, E. F., Kausch, D. F., Blum, M. D., Reed, J., & Bush, E. (1989). Correlates of suicidal ideation and attempts in a community sample of junior high and high school students. *Journal of Clinical Child Psychology*, 18, 158–166.

Dunphy, D. (1963). The social structure of urban adolescent peer groups. *Sociometry*, 26, 230–246.

Dweck, C., & Licht, B. (1980). Learned helplessness and intellectual achievement. In J. Garber & M. Seligman (Eds.), *Human helplessness*. New York: Academic Press.

Eamon, M. K., & Mulder, C. (2005). Predicting antisocial behavior among Latino young adolescents: An ecological systems analysis. *American Journal of Orthopsychiatry*, 75(1), 117–127.

Eccles, J. S., Midgley, C., Wigfield, A., Buchanan, C. M., Reuman, D., Flanagan, C., et al. (1993). Development during adolescence: The impact of stage–environment fit on young adolescents' experiences in schools and families. *American Psychologist*, 48, 90–101.

Eisler, I., Dare, C., Hodes, M., Russell, G., Dodge, E., & le Grange, D. (2000). Family therapy for adolescent anorexia nervosa: The results of a controlled comparison of two family interventions. *Journal of Child Psychology and Psychiatry and Allied Disciplines*, 41(6), 727–736.

Eisler, J., Dare, C., Russell, G. F., Szmulker, G., le Grange, D., & Dodge, E. (1997). Family and individual therapy in anorexia nervosa: A five-year follow-up. *Archives of General Psychiatry*, 54(1), 1025–1030.

Elkind, D. (1967). Egocentricism in adolescence. *Child Development*, 38, 1025–1034.

Elliott, D. S., & Ageton, S. S. (1980). Reconciling race and class differences in self-reported and official estimates of delinquency. *American Sociological Review*, 45, 95–110.

Ellis, L. (1996). Theories of homosexuality. In R. C. Savin-Williams & K.

M. Cohen (Eds.), *The lives of lesbians, gays, and bisexuals: Children to adults*. Fort Worth, TX: Harcourt.

Elmen, J. (1991). Achievement orientation in early adolescence: Developmental patterns and social correlates. *Journal of Early Adolescence, 11*, 125–151.

Emslie, G., Wagner, K. D., Kutcher, S., Krulewicz, S., Fong, R., Carpenter, D. J., et al. (2006). Paroxetine treatment in children and adolescents with Major Depressive Disorder: A randomized, multicenter, double-blind, placebo-controlled trial. *Journal of the American Academy of Child and Adolescent Psychiatry, 45*(6), 709–719.

Eno, M. M. (1985). Children with school problems: A family therapy perspective. In R. L. Ziffer (Ed.), *Adjunctive techniques in family therapy*. New York: Grune & Stratton.

Epstein, J. (1983). The influence of friends on achievement and affective outcomes. In J. Epstein & N. Karweit (Eds.), *Friends in school*. New York: Academic Press.

Erikson, E. (1950). *Childhood and society*. New York: Norton.

Erikson, E. (1959). Identity and the life cycle. *Psychological Issues, 1*, 1–171.

Erikson, E. (1968). *Identity: Youth and crisis*. New York: Norton.

Eron, J. B., & Lund, T. W. (1993). How problems evolve and dissolve: Integrating narrative and strategic concepts. *Family Process, 32*, 291–309.

Evans, C., & Street, E. (1995). Possible differences in family patterns in anorexia nervosa and bulimia nervosa. *Journal of Family Therapy, 17*, 115–131.

Eveleth, P., & Tanner, J. (1976). *Worldwide variation in human growth*. New York: Cambridge University Press.

Faber, A. J., Edwards, A. E., Bauer, K. S., & Wetchler, J. L. (2003). Family structure: Its effects on adolescent attachment and identity formation. *American Journal of Family Therapy, 31*, 243–255.

Falicov, C. J. (1998). *Latino families in therapy: A guide to multicultural practice*. New York: Guilford Press.

Farrell, A. D., & White, K. S. (1998). Peer influences and drug use among urban adolescents: Family structure and parent-adolescent relationship as protective factors. *Journal of Consulting and Clinical Psychology, 66*(2), 248–258.

Feldman, S., & Elliott, G. (Eds.). (1990). *At the threshold: The developing adolescent*. Cambridge, MA: Harvard University Press.

Fisch, R., Weakland, J. H., & Segal, L. (1982). *The tactics of change: Doing therapy briefly*. San Francisco: Jossey-Bass.

Fisher, L. (1986). Systems-based consultation with schools. In L. C. Wynne, S. H. McDaniel, & T. T. Weber (Eds.), *Systems consultation: A new perspective for family therapy*. New York: Guilford Press.

Fishman, H. C. (1988). *Treating troubled adolescents: A family therapy approach*. New York: Basic Books.

Fishman, H. C. (1993). *Intensive structural therapy: Treating families in their social context.* New York: Basic Books.

Fordham, S., & Ogbu, J. U. (1986). Black students' school success: Coping with the "burden of acting white." *Urban Review, 18,* 176–206.

Forehand, R., Wierson, M., Thomas, A. M., Armistead, L., Kempton, T., & Neighbors, B. (1991). The role of family stressors and parent relationships on adolescent functioning. *Journal of the American Academy of Child and Adolescent Psychiatry, 30,* 316–322.

Frabutt, J. M., Walker, A. M., & MacKinnon-Lewis, C. (2002). Racial socialization messages and the quality of mother/child interactions in African American families. *Journal of Early Adolescence, 22*(2), 200–217.

Freeman, H., & Brown, B. B. (2001). Primary attachment to parents and peers during adolescence: Differences by attachment style. *Journal of Youth and Adolescence, 30*(6), 653–674.

French, S. E., Seidman, E., Allen, L., & Aber, J. L. (2006). The development of ethnic identity during adolescence. *Developmental Psychology, 42*(1), 1–10.

Freud, A. (1958). Adolescence. *Psychoanalytic Study of the Child, 13,* 255–278.

Fromm-Reichmann, F. (1948). Notes on the development of treatment of schizophrenics by psychoanalytic psychotherapy. *Psychotherapy, 11,* 263–274.

Fuligni, A., & Eccles, J. (1993). Perceived parent–child relationships and early adolescents' orientation toward peers. *Developmental Psychology, 29,* 622–632.

Galambos, N. L., Barker, D. T., & Almeida, D. M. (2003). Parents do matter: Trajectories of change in externalizing and internalizing problems in early adolescence. *Child Development, 74*(2), 578–594.

Gallatin, J. (1975). *Adolescence and individuality.* New York: Harper & Row.

Garland, A. F., & Zigler, F. (1993). Adolescent suicide prevention: Current research and social policy implications. *American Psychologist, 48,* 169–182.

Garofalo, R., Wolf, R., Wissow, L., Woods, E., & Goodman, E. (1999). Sexual orientation and risk of suicide attempts among a representative sample of youth. *Archives of Pediatric and Adolescent Medicine, 153*(5), 487–493.

Gilbert, S., & Thompson, J. K. (1996). Feminist explanations of the development of eating disorders: Common themes, research findings, and methodological issues. *Clinical Psychology: Science and Practice, 3,* 183–202.

Gilligan, C. (1982). *In a different voice.* Cambridge, MA: Harvard University Press.

Gilligan, C., Lyons, N. P., & Hanmer, T. J. (Eds.). (1990). *Making connec-*

tions: The relational worlds of adolescent girls at Emma Willard School. Cambridge, MA: Harvard University Press.

Ginsburg, G. S., & Bronstein, P. (1993). Family factors related to children's intrinsic/extrinsic motivational orientations and academic performance. *Child Development, 64,* 1461–1474.

Ginsburg, G. S., & Schlossberg, M. C. (2002). Family-based treatment of childhood anxiety disorders. *International Review of Psychiatry, 14,* 143–154.

Gittelman, R., Mannuzza, S., Shenker, R., & Bonagura, N. (1985). Hyperactive boys almost grown up: I. Psychiatric status. *Archives of General Psychiatry, 42,* 937–947.

Goldner, V. (1985). Feminism and family therapy. *Family Process, 24,* 31–47.

Goldner, V. (1988). Generation and gender: Normative and covert hierarchies. *Family Process, 27,* 17–33.

Goosby, B. (2007). Poverty duration, maternal psychological resources, and adolescent socioemotional outcomes. *Journal of Family Issues, 28*(8), 1113–1134.

Gottesman, I. I. (1991). *Schizophrenia genesis: The origins of madness.* New York: Freeman.

Gottfried, A. E., Fleming, J. S., & Gottfried, A. W. (1998). Role of cognitively stimulating home environment in children's academic intrinsic motivation: A longitudinal study. *Child Development, 69*(5), 1448–1460.

Graber, J. A., Brooks-Gunn, J., & Warren, M. P. (2006). Pubertal effects on adjustment in girls: Moving from demonstrating effects to identifying pathways. *Journal of Youth and Adolescence, 35*(3), 413–423.

Green, R. (2000). "Lesbians, gay men, and their parents": A critique of LaSala and the prevailing clinical "wisdom." *Family Process, 39*(2), 257–266.

Grossman, A. H., & D'Augelli, A. R. (2006). Transgender youth: Invisible and vulnerable. *Journal of Homosexuality, 51*(1), 111–128.

Gutman, L. M., McLoyd, V. C., & Tokoyawa, T. (2005). Financial strain, neighborhood stress, parenting behaviors, and adolescent adjustment in urban African American families. *Journal of Research on Adolescence, 15*(4), 425–449.

Haldeman, D. C. (1994). The practice and ethics of sexual orientation conversion therapy. *Journal of Consulting and Clinical Psychology, 62,* 221–227.

Hale, W. W., Engels, R., & Meeus, W. (2006). Adolescent's perceptions of parenting behaviours and its relationship to adolescent Generalized Anxiety Disorder symptoms. *Journal of Adolescence, 29,* 407–417.

Haley, J. (1987). *Problem-solving therapy* (2nd ed.). San Francisco: Jossey-Bass.

Haley, J. (1997). *Leaving home: The therapy of disturbed young people* (2nd ed.). New York: McGraw-Hill.

Hall, G. S. (1904). *Adolescence.* New York: Appleton.

Halmi, K. A. (1995). Changing rates of eating disorders: What does it mean? *American Journal of Psychiatry, 152,* 1256–1257.

Harrop, C. E., Trower, P., & Mitchell, I. M. (1996). Does the biology go around the symptoms?: A Copernican shift in schizophrenia paradigms. *Clinical Psychology Review, 16,* 641–654.

Harter, S. (1990). Self and identity development. In S. Feldman & G. Elliott (Eds.), *At the threshold: The developing adolescent.* Cambridge, MA: Harvard University Press.

Harter, S. (1999). *The construction of the self: A developmental perspective.* New York: Guilford Press.

Heinze, H. J., Toro, P. A., & Urberg, K. A. (2004). Antisocial behavior and affiliation with deviant peers. *Journal of Clinical Child and Adolescent Psychology, 33*(2), 336–346.

Henggeler, S. W., Clingempeel, W. G., Brondino, M. J., & Pickrel, S. G. (2002). Four-year follow-up of multisystemic therapy with substance-abusing and substance-dependent juvenile offenders. *Journal of the American Academy of Child and Adolescent Psychiatry, 41,* 868–874.

Herek, G. M. (2000). The psychology of sexual prejudice. *Current Directions in Psychological Science, 9,* 19–22.

Hershberger, S. L. (2001). Biological factors in the development of sexual orientation. In A. R. D'Augelli & C. J. Patterson (Eds.), *Lesbian, gay, and bisexual identities in youth: Psychological perspectives.* New York: Oxford University Press.

Hill, J., Fonagy, P., Safier, E., & Sargent, J. (2003). The ecology of attachment in the family. *Family Process, 42*(2), 205–221.

Hill, J., & Lynch, M. (1983). The intensification of gender-related role expectations during early adolescence. In J. Brooks-Gunn & A. Petersen (Eds.), *Girls at puberty.* New York: Plenum.

Hirschi, T. (1969). *Causes of delinquency.* Berkeley: University of California Press.

Hoffman, L. (1981). *Foundations of family therapy: A conceptual framework for systems change.* New York: Basic Books.

Hollis, C. (1996). Depression, family environment, and adolescent suicidal behavior. *Journal of the American Academy of Child and Adolescent Psychiatry, 35*(5), 622–630.

Hooley, J. M. (2007). Expressed emotion and relapse of psychopathology. *Annual Review of Clinical Psychology, 3,* 329–352.

Imber-Black, E. (1991). A family-larger system perspective. In A. S. Gurman & D. P. Kniskern (Eds.), *Handbook of family therapy* (Vol. 2). New York: Brunner/Mazel.

Inclan, J. (2001). Steps toward a culture and migration dialogue: Developing a framework for therapy with immigrant families. In S. H. McDaniel, D. Lusterman, & C. L. Philpot (Eds.), *Casebook for integrating family therapy: An ecosystemic approach*. Washington, DC: American Psychological Association.

Inhelder, B., & Piaget, J. (1958). *The growth of logical thinking from childhood to adolescence*. New York: Basic Books.

Jack, D. C. (1991). *Silencing the self: Women and depression*. New York: HarperCollins.

Jack, D. C. (1999). Silencing the self: Inner dialogues and outer realities. In T. Joiner & J. C. Coyne (Eds.), *The interactional nature of depression: Advances in interpersonal approaches*. Washington, DC: American Psychological Association.

Jarrett, R. L. (1995). Growing up poor: The family experiences of socially mobile youth in low-income African American neighborhoods. *Journal of Adolescent Research, 10*(1), 111–135.

Jessor, R., & Jessor, S. L. (1977). *Problem behavior and psychological development: A longitudinal study of youth*. San Diego: Academic Press.

Johnson, S. M. (2004). *The practice of emotionally focused couple therapy: Creating connection*. (2nd ed.). New York: Brunner-Routledge.

Johnston, L. D., O'Malley, P. M., Bachman, J. G., & Schulenberg, J. E. (2008). *Monitoring the future: National results on adolescent drug use: Overview of key findings, 2007*. Ann Arbor, MI: Institute for Social Research.

Jordan, J. V., Kaplan, A. G., Miller, J. B., Stiver, I. P., & Surrey, J. L. (Eds.). (1991). *Women's growth in connection: Writings from the Stone Center*. New York: Guilford Press.

Josselson, R. (1987). *Finding herself: Pathways to identity development in women*. San Francisco: Jossey-Bass.

Kandel, D. (1978). Homophily, selection, and socialization in adolescent friendships. *American Journal of Sociology, 84*, 427–436.

Kandel, D. B., & Davies, M. (1982). Epidemiology of depressive mood in adolescents. *Archives of General Psychiatry, 39*, 1205–1212.

Kaplan, A. G. (1991). The "self-in-relation": Implications for depression in women. In J. V. Jordan, A. G. Kaplan, J. B. Miller, I. P. Stiver, & J. L. Surrey, (Eds.), *Women's growth in connection: Writings from the Stone Center*. New York: Guilford Press.

Kaplan, A. G., Klein, R., & Gleason, N. (1991). Women's self development in late adolescence. In J. V. Jordan, A. G. Kaplan, J. B. Miller, I. P. Stiver, & J. L. Surrey, (Eds.), *Women's growth in connection: Writings from the Stone Center*. New York: Guilford Press.

Keel, P. K., Klump, K. L., Leon, G. R., & Fulkerson, J. A. (1998). Disordered eating in adolescent males from a school-based sample. *International Journal of Eating Disorders, 23*, 125–132.

Kegan, R. (1982). *The evolving self*. Cambridge, MA: Harvard University Press.

Keim, J. P. (2005). Oppositional behavior in children. In C. E. Bailey (Ed.). *Children in therapy: Using the family as a resource*. New York: Norton.

Kellow, J., & Jones, B. (2008). The effects of stereotypes on the achievement gap: Reexamining the academic performance of African American high school students. *Journal of Black Psychology, 34*(1), 94–120.

Kendall, P. C. (Ed.). (1991). *Child and adolescent therapy: Cognitive-behavioral procedures*. New York: Guilford Press.

Kendall, P. C., Hudson, J. L., Gosch, E., Flannery-Schroeder, E., & Suvey, C. (2008). Cognitive-behavioral therapy for anxiety disordered youth: A randomized clinical trial evaluating child and family modalities. *Journal of Consulting and Clinical Psychology, 76*(2), 282–297.

Kennard, B., Silva, S., Vitiello, B., Curry, J., Kratochvil, C., Simkons, A., et al. (2006). Remission and residual symptoms after short-term treatment in the Treatment of Adolescents with Depression Study (TADS). *Journal of the American Academy of Child and Adolescent Psychiatry, 45*(12), 1404–1411.

Kerr, M., & Stattin, H. (2000). What parents know, how they know it, and several forms of adolescent adjustment: Further support for a reinterpretation of monitoring. *Developmental Psychology, 36*(3), 366–380.

Kinnish, K. K., Strassberg, D. S., & Turner, C. W. (2005). Sex differences in the flexibility of sexual orientation: A multidimensional retrospective assessment. *Archives of Sexual Behavior, 34*(2), 173–183.

Klein, J. B., Jacobs, R. H., & Reinecke, M. A. (2007). Cognitive-behavioral therapy for adolescent depression: A meta-analytic investigation of changes in effect–size estimates. *Journal of the American Academy of Child and Adolescent Psychiatry, 46*(11), 1403–1413.

Kohlberg, L. (1963). The development of children's orientations toward a moral order. *Vita Humana, 6*, 11–33.

Kopeikin, H. S., Marshall, V., & Goldstein, M. J. (1983). Stages and impact of crisis-oriented family therapy in the aftercare of acute schizophrenia. In W. R. McFarlane (Ed.), *Family therapy in schizophrenia*. New York: Guilford Press.

Krautter, T. H., & Lock, J. (2004). Treatment of adolescent anorexia nervosa using manualized family-based treatment. *Clinical Case Studies, 3*(2), 107–123.

Krieder, D., & Motto, J. (1974). Parent–child role reversal and suicidal states in adolescence. *Adolescence, 9*, 365–370.

Kroger, J. (2003). Identity development during adolescence. In G. R. Adams & M. D. Berzonsky (Eds.), *Blackwell handbook of adolescence*. Malden, MA: Blackwell.

Krohne, H. W., & Hock, M. (1991). Relationships between restrictive mother–child interactions and anxiety of the child. *Anxiety Research*, 4(2), 109–124.

Laible, D. J., Carlo, G., & Raffaelli, M. (2000). The differential relations of parent and peer attachment to adolescent adjustment. *Journal of Youth and Adolescence*, 29(1), 45–59.

Laird, R. D., Pettit, G. S., Bates, J. E., & Dodge, K. A. (2003). Parents' monitoring-relevant knowledge and adolescents' delinquent behavior: Evidence of correlated developmental changes and reciprocal influences. *Child Development*, 74(3), 752–768.

Larson, R., & Richards, M. (1994). *Divergent realities: The emotional lives of mothers, fathers, and adolescents.* New York: Basic Books.

LaSala, M. C. (2000). Lesbians, gay men, and their parents: Family therapy for the coming-out crisis. *Family Process*, 39(1), 67–81.

Lau, S. (1989). Sex role orientation and domains of self-esteem. *Sex Roles*, 21, 415–422.

Laumann, E. O., Gagnon, J. H., Michael, R. T., & Michaels, S. (1994). *The social organization of sexuality.* Chicago: University of Chicago Press.

Leff, J., & Vaughn, C. (1981). The role of maintenance therapy and relatives' expressed emotion in relapse of schizophrenia: A two-year follow up. *British Journal of Psychiatry*, 139, 102–104.

le Grange, D., Crosby, R. D., Rathouz, P. J., & Leventhal, B. L. (2007). A randomized controlled comparison of family-based treatment and supportive psychotherapy for adolescent bulimia nervosa. *Archives of General Psychiatry*, 64(9), 1049–1056.

le Grange, D., Eisler, I., Dare, C., & Hodes, M. (1992). Family criticism and self-starvation: A study of expressed emotion. *Journal of Family Therapy*, 14(2), 177–192.

le Grange, D., & Lock, J. (2007). *Treating bulimia in adolescents: A family-based approach.* New York: Guilford Press.

Leon, G. R., Fulkerson, J. A., Perry, C. L., & Early-Zald, M. B. (1995). Prospective analysis of personality and behavioral vulnerabilities and gender influences in the later development of disordered eating. *Journal of Abnormal Psychology*, 104, 140–149.

Lerner, R., & Steinberg, L. (Eds.). (2004). *Handbook of adolescent psychology.* New York: Wiley.

Lev, A. I. (2004). *Transgender emergence: Therapeutic guidelines for working with gender-variant people and their families.* Binghamton, NY: Haworth Press.

Leventhal, T., & Brooks-Gunn, J. (2000). The neighborhoods they live in: The effects of neighborhood residence on child and adolescent outcomes. *Psychological Bulletin*, 126(2), 309–337.

Lewinsohn, P. M., Clarke, G. N., Hops, H., & Andrews, J. A. (1990). Cognitive-behavioral treatment for depressed adolescents. *Behavior Therapy*, 21(4), 385–401.

Lewinsohn, P. M., Rohde, P., & Seeley, J. R. (1996). Adolescent suicidal ideation and attempts: Prevalence, risk factors, and clinical implications. *Clinical Psychology: Science and Practice, 3*, 25–46.

Li, S. T., Nussbaum, K. M., & Richards, M. H. (2007). Risk and protective factors for urban African-American youth. *American Journal of Community Psychology, 39*, 21–35.

Li, X., Stanton, B., & Feigelman, S. (2000). Impact of perceived parental monitoring on adolescent risk behavior over 4 years. *Journal of Adolescent Health, 27*, 49–56.

Liddle, H. A. (1999). Theory development in a family-based therapy for adolescent drug abuse. *Journal of Clinical Child Psychology, 28*, 521–532.

Liddle, H. A., Dakof, G. A., Parker, K., Diamond, G. S., Barrett, K., & Tejeda, M. (2001). Multidimensional Family Therapy for adolescent drug abuse: Results of a randomized clinical trial. *American Journal of Drug and Alcohol Abuse, 27*, 651–688.

Lidz, T., Cornelison, A., Fleck, S., & Terry, D. (1957). Intrafamilial environment of schizophrenic patients: II. Marital schism and marital skew. *American Journal of Psychiatry, 114*, 241–248.

Lindblad-Goldberg, M., & Dukes, J. L. (1985). Social support in Black, low-income, single-parent families: Normative and dysfunctional patterns. *American Journal of Orthopsychiatry, 55*(1), 42–58.

Lipka, O., & Siegel, L. S. (2006). Learning disabilities. In D. A. Wolfe & E. J. Mash (Eds.), *Behavioral and emotional disorders in adolescents*. New York: Guilford Press.

Lock, J., Agras, W., Bryson, S., & Kraemer, H. (2005). A comparison of short- and long-term family therapy for adolescent anorexia nervosa. *Journal of the American Academy of Child and Adolescent Psychiatry, 44*(7), 632–639.

Lock, J., Couturier, J., & Agras, S. (2006). Comparison of long-term outcomes in adolescents with anorexia nervosa treated with family therapy. *Journal of the American Academy of Child and Adolescent Psychiatry, 45*(6), 666–672.

Lock, J., le Grange, D., Agras, W. S., & Dare, C. (2001). *Treatment manual for anorexia nervosa: A family-based approach*. New York: Guilford Press.

Luepnitz, D. A. (1988). *The family interpreted: Feminist theory in clinical practice*. New York: Basic Books.

Lusterman, D. (1985). An ecosystemic approach to family–school problems. *American Journal of Family Therapy, 13*, 22–30.

Maccoby, E., & Martin, J. (1983). Socialization in the context of the family: Parent–child interaction. In E. M. Hetherington (Ed.), *Handbook of child psychology: Vol. 4. Socialization, personality, and social development*. New York: Wiley.

Mackey, S. K. (1996). Nurturance: A neglected dimension in family therapy with adolescents. *Journal of Marital and Family Therapy, 22,* 489–508.

Madanes, C. (1981). *Strategic family therapy.* San Francisco: Jossey-Bass.

Madanes, C. (1984). *Behind the one-way mirror: Advances in the practice of strategic therapy.* San Francisco: Jossey-Bass.

Madon, S., Jussim, L., & Eccles, J. (1997). In search of the powerful self-fulfilling prophecy. *Journal of Personality and Social Psychology, 72*(4), 791–809.

Madsen, W. C. (2007). *Collaborative therapy with multi-stressed families* (2nd ed.). New York: Guilford Press.

Magnusson, D., Strattin, H., & Allen, V. L. (1985). Biological maturation and social development: A longitudinal study of some adjustment processes from midadolescence to adulthood. *Journal of Youth and Adolescence, 14,* 267–283.

Manassis, K., Avery, D., Butalia, S., & Mendlowitz, S. (2004). Cognitive-behavioral therapy with childhood anxiety disorders: Functioning in adolescence. *Depression and Anxiety, 19*(4), 209–216.

Mannuzza, S., & Gittelman, R. (1984). The adolescent outcome of hyperactive girls. *Psychiatry Research, 13,* 19–29.

Mannuzza, S., Klein, R. G., Bonagura, N., & Malloy, P. (1991). Hyperactive boys almost grown up: V. Replication of psychiatric status. *Archives of General Psychiatry, 48,* 77–83.

March, J., Silva, S., Curry, J., Wells, K., Fairbank, J., Burns, B., et al. (2004). Fluoxetine, cognitive-behavioral therapy, and their combination for adolescents with depression: Treatment for Adolescents with Depression Study (TADS) randomized controlled trial. *Journal of the American Medical Association, 292*(7), 807–820.

Marcia, J. (1966). Development and validation of ego identity status. *Journal of Personality and Social Psychology, 3,* 551–558.

Marcia, J. (1976). Identity six years after: A follow-up study. *Journal of Youth and Adolescence, 5,* 145–150.

Marcus, R. F., & Betzer, P. D. S. (1996). Attachment and antisocial behavior in early adolescence. *Journal of Early Adolescence, 16*(2), 229–248.

Markowitz, L. M. (1992). Making house calls. *Family Therapy Networker, 16,* 26–37.

Markstrom-Adams, C. (1989). Androgyny and its relation to adolescent psychological well-being: A review of the literature. *Sex Roles, 21,* 469–473.

Marshall, S. (1995). Ethnic socialization of African American children: Implications for parenting, identity development, and academic achievement. *Journal of Youth and Adolescence, 24*(4), 377–396.

Marshall, W. (1978). Puberty. In F. Falkner & J. Tanner (Eds.), *Human growth* (Vol. 2). New York: Plenum Press.

Massad, C. (1981). Sex role identity and adjustment during adolescence. *Child Development, 52,* 1290–1298.

McFarlane, A. C. (1987). Posttraumatic phenomena in a longitudinal study of children following a natural disaster. *Journal of the American Academy of Child and Adolescent Psychiatry, 26*(5), 764–769.

McFarlane, W. R., Dixon, L., Lukens, E., & Lucksted, A. (2003). Family psychoeducation and schizophrenia: A review of the literature. *Journal of Marital and Family Therapy, 29*(2), 223–245.

McGoldrick, M., Giordano, J., & Garcia-Preto, N. (2005). *Ethnicity and family therapy* (3rd ed.). New York: Guilford Press.

McLean, C. (1996). Boys and education in Australia. In C. McLean, M. Carey, & C. White (Eds.), *Men's ways of being.* Boulder, CO: Westview.

McLoyd, V. C. (1998). Socioeconomic disadvantage and child development. *American Psychologist, 53*(2), 185–204.

McLoyd, V. C., Jayaratne, T. E., Ceballo, R., & Borquez, J. (1994). Unemployment and work interruption among African American single mothers: Effects on parenting and adolescent socioemotional functioning. *Child Development, 65*(2), 562–589.

Meilman, P. W. (1979). Cross-sectional age changes in ego identity status during adolescence. *Developmental Psychology, 15,* 230–231.

Micucci, J. A. (1995). Adolescents who assault their parents: A family systems approach to treatment. *Psychotherapy, 32,* 154–161.

Micucci, J. A. (2006). Helping families with defiant adolescents. *Contemporary Family Therapy, 28*(4), 459–474.

Miklowitz, D. J. (2007). The role of the family in the course and treatment of bipolar disorder. *Current Directions in Psychological Science, 16*(4), 192–196.

Miklowitz, D. J. (2008). *Bipolar disorder: A family-focused treatment approach* (2nd ed.). New York: Guilford Press.

Miklowitz, D. J., Biuckians, A., & Richards, J. A. (2006). Early-onset bipolar disorder: A family treatment perspective. *Development and Psychopathology, 18*(4), 1247–1265.

Miller, J. B. (1991). The construction of anger in women and men. In J. V. Jordan, A. G. Kaplan, J. B. Miller, I. P. Stiver, & J. L. Surrey (Eds.), *Women's growth in connection: Writings from the Stone Center.* New York: Guilford Press.

Minuchin, P., Colapinto, J., & Minuchin, S. (2007). *Working with families of the poor* (2nd ed.). New York: Guilford Press.

Minuchin, S. (1974). *Families and family therapy.* Cambridge, MA: Harvard University Press.

Minuchin, S. (1984). *Family kaleidoscope.* Cambridge, MA: Harvard University Press.

Minuchin, S., & Fishman, H. C. (1981). *Family therapy techniques.* Cambridge, MA: Harvard University Press.

Minuchin, S., Montalvo, B., Guerney, B. G., Rosman, B. L., & Schumer, F. (1967). *Families of the slums.* New York: Basic Books.

Minuchin, S., & Nichols, M. P. (1993). *Family healing: Strategies for hope and understanding*. New York: Free Press.

Minuchin, S., Nichols, M. P., & Lee, W. (2007). *Assessing families and couples: From symptom to system*. Boston: Pearson Education.

Minuchin, S., Rosman, B. L., & Baker, L. (1978). *Psychosomatic families: Anorexia nervosa in context*. Cambridge, MA: Harvard University Press.

Mistry, R. S., Vandewater, E. A., Huston, A. C., & McLoyd, V. C. (2002). Economic well-being and children's social adjustment: The role of family process in an ethnically diverse low-income sample. *Child Development, 73*(3), 935–951.

Monroe, S. M., Rohde, P., Seeley, J. R., & Lewinsohn, P. M. (1999). Life events and depression in adolescence: Relationship loss as a prospective risk factor for first onset of Major Depressive Disorder. *Journal of Abnormal Psychology, 108*(4), 606–614.

Moore, K., Peterson, J., & Furstenberg, F., Jr. (1986). Parental attitudes and the occurrence of early sexual activity. *Journal of Marriage and the Family, 48*, 777–782.

Mueller, C., Field, T., Yando, R., & Harding, J. (1995). Undereating and overeating concerns among adolescents. *Journal of Child Psychology and Psychiatry and Allied Disciplines, 36*, 1019–1025.

Mufson, L., Dorta, K. P., Moreau, D., & Weissman, M. M. (2004). *Interpersonal psychotherapy with depressed adolescents* (2nd ed.). New York: Guilford Press.

Myers, H. F., & Taylor, S. (1998). Family contributions to risk and resilience in African American children. *Journal of Comparative Family Studies, 29*, 215–229.

Neumark-Sztainer, D., Wall, M. M., Story, M., & Perry, C. L. (2003). Correlates of unhealthy weight-control behaviors among adolescents: Implications for prevention programs. *Health Psychology, 22*(1), 88–98.

Newcomer, S., & Udry, J. (1984). Mothers' influence on the sexual behavior of their teenage children. *Journal of Marriage and the Family, 46*, 477–485.

Nichols, M. P. (2004). *Stop arguing with your kids: How to win the battle of wills by making your children feel heard*. New York: Guilford Pres.

Nickerson, A. B., & Nagle, R. J. (2005). Parent and peer attachment in late childhood and early adolescence. *Journal of Early Adolescence, 25*(2), 223–249.

Nolen-Hoeksema, S. (1987). Sex differences in unipolar depression. *Psychological Bulletin, 101*, 259–282.

Oetting, E. R., & Beauvais, F. (1987). Peer cluster theory, socialization characteristics, and adolescent drug use: A path analysis. *Journal of Counseling Psychology, 34*, 205–213.

Offer, D., Ostrov, E., & Howard, K. I. (1981). The mental health professional's concept of the normal adolescent. *Archives of General Psychiatry, 38,* 149–152.

Offer, D., & Schonert-Reichl, K. A. (1992). Debunking the myths of adolescence: Findings from recent research. *Journal of the American Academy of Child and Adolescent Psychiatry, 31,* 1003–1014.

Olfson, M., Marcus, S. C., & Shaffer, D. (2006). Antidepressant drug therapy and suicide in severely depressed children and adults. *Archives of General Psychiatry, 63*(8), 865–872.

Osherson, S., & Krugman, S. (1990). Men, shame and psychotherapy. *Psychotherapy, 27,* 327–339.

Papp, P. (1983). *The process of change.* New York: Guilford Press.

Paschall, M. J., Ennett, S. T., & Flewelling, R. L. (1996). Relationships among family characteristics and violent behavior by black and white male adolescents. *Journal of Youth and Adolescence, 25*(2), 177–197.

Perosa, L. M., Perosa, S. L., & Tam, H. P. (2002). Intergenerational systems theory and identity development in young adult women. *Journal of Adolescent Research, 17,* 235–259.

Petersen, A. C., Compas, B. E., Brooks-Gunn, J., Stemmler, M., Ey, S., & Grant, K. E. (1993). Depression in adolescence. *American Psychologist, 48,* 155–168.

Petersen, A. C., Sarigiani, P. A., & Kennedy, R. F. (1991). Adolescent depression: Why more girls? *Journal of Youth and Adolescence, 20,* 247–271.

Pfeffer, C. R. (1981). The family system of suicidal children. *American Journal of Psychotherapy, 35,* 330–341.

Phinney, J. S. (1989). Stages of ethnic identity development in minority group adolescents. *Journal of Early Adolescence, 9,* 34–39.

Phinney, J. S. (1990). Ethnic identity in adolescents and adults: Review of research. *Psychological Bulletin, 108*(3), 499–514.

Phinney, J. S., & Devich-Navarro, M. (1997). Variations in bicultural identification among African American and Mexican American adolescents. *Journal of Research on Adolescence, 7*(1), 3–32.

Pipher, M. (1994). *Reviving Ophelia: Saving the selves of adolescent girls.* New York: Putnam.

Pleck, J. H. (1981). *The myth of masculinity.* Cambridge, MA: MIT Press.

Pleck, J. H. (1995). The gender role strain paradigm: An update. In R. F. Levant & W. S. Pollack (Eds.), *A new psychology of men.* New York: Basic Books.

Pollack, W. (1998). *Real boys: Rescuing our sons from the myths of boyhood.* New York: Henry Holt and Company.

Power, T. J., & Bartholomew, K. L. (1985). Getting uncaught in the middle: A case study in family–school system consultation. *School Psychology Review, 14,* 222–229.

Quadrel, M. J., Fischhoff, B., & Davis, W. (1993). Adolescent (in)vulnerability. *American Psychologist, 48,* 102–116.

Quintana, S. M. (2007). Racial and ethnic identity: Developmental perspectives and research. *Journal of Counseling Psychology, 54*(3), 259–270.

Rapee, R. M. (1997). Potential role of childrearing practices in the development of anxiety and depression. *Clinical Psychology Review, 17*(1), 47–67.

Reinecke, M. A., & Curry, J. F. (2008). Adolescents. In M. A. Whisman (Ed.), *Adapting cognitive therapy for depression: Managing complexity and comorbidity.* New York: Guilford Press.

Rende, R., Slomkowski, C., Lloyd-Richardson, E., Stroud, L., & Niaura, R. (2006). Estimating genetic and environmental influences on depressive symptoms in adolescence: Differing effects on higher and lower levels of symptoms. *Journal of Clinical Child and Adolescent Psychology, 35*(2), 237–243.

Rheingold, A. A., Herbert, J. D., & Franklin, M. E. (2003). Cognitive bias in adolescents with social anxiety disorder. *Cognitive Therapy and Research, 27*(6), 639–655.

Ricciardelli, L. A., & McCabe, M. P. (2004). A biopsychosocial model of disordered eating and the pursuit of muscularity in adolescent boys. *Psychological Bulletin, 130*(2), 179–205.

Rice, F., Harold, G. T., Shelton, K. H., & Thapar, A. (2006). Family conflict interacts with genetic liability in predicting childhood and adolescent depression. *Journal of the American Academy of Child and Adolescent Psychiatry, 45*(7), 841–848.

Rice, K. G., & Mulkeen, P. (1995). Relationships with parents and peers: A longitudinal study of adolescent intimacy. *Journal of Adolescent Research, 10*(3), 338–357.

Richards, M. H., Miller, B. V., O'Donnell, P. C., Wasserman, M. S., & Colder, C. (2004). Parental monitoring mediates the effects of age and sex on problem behaviors among African American urban young adolescents. *Journal of Youth and Adolescence, 33*(3), 221–233.

Richman, J. (1979). The family therapy of attempted suicide. *Family Process, 18,* 131–142.

Robbins, M. S., Szapocznik, J., Dillon, F. R., Turner, C. W., Mitrani, V. B., & Feaster, D. J. (2008). The efficacy of structural ecosystems therapy with drug-abusing/dependent African American and Hispanic American adolescents. *Journal of Family Psychology, 22*(1), 51–61.

Robertson, J. F., & Simons, R. L. (1989). Family factors, self-esteem, and adolescent depression. *Journal of Marriage and the Family, 51*(1), 125–138.

Robin, A. L., Siegel, P. T., Koepke, T., Moye, A. W., & Tice, S. (1994). Family therapy versus individual therapy for adolescent females with anorexia nervosa. *Journal of Developmental and Behavioral Pediatrics, 15,* 111–116.

Rodgers, K. (1999). Parenting processes related to sexual risk-taking behaviors of adolescent males and females. *Journal of Marriage and the Family*, *61*, 99–109.

Rohner, R. P., & Pettengill, S. M. (1985). Perceived parental acceptance–rejection and parental control among Korean adolescents. *Child Development*, *56*, 524–528.

Rojano, R. (2004). The practice of community family therapy. *Family Process*, *43*(1), 59–77.

Rosenblum, G. D., & Lewis, M. (2003). Emotional development in adolescence. In G. R. Adams & M. D. Berzonsky (Eds.), *Blackwell handbook of adolescence*. Malden, MA: Blackwell.

Rosenstein, D. S., & Horowitz, H. A. (1996). Adolescent attachment and psychopathology. *Journal of Consulting and Clinical Psychology*, *64*(2), 244–253.

Rosenthal, R., & Jacobson, L. (1968). *Pygmalion in the classroom: Teacher expectations and pupils' intellectual development*. New York: Holt, Rinehart & Winston.

Rueter, M. A., Scaramella, L., Wallace, L. E., & Conger, R. D. (1999). First onset of depressive or anxiety disorders predicted by the longitudinal course of internalizing symptoms and parent–adolescent disagreements. *Archives of General Psychiatry*, *56*, 726–732.

Russell, G. F. M., Szmulker, G. I., Dare, C., & Eisler, I. (1987). An evaluation of family therapy in anorexia nervosa and bulimia nervosa. *Archives of General Psychiatry*, *44*, 1047–1056.

Sargent, J. (1987a). Integrating family and individual therapy for anorexia nervosa. In J. E. Harkaway (Ed.), *Eating disorders*. Rockville, MD: Aspen.

Sargent, J. (1987b). *Talking to you* [Videotape].

Savin-Williams, R. C. (1998a). *"And then I became gay": Young men's stories*. New York: Routledge.

Savin-Williams, R. C. (1998b). Lesbian, gay, and bisexual youths' relationships with their parents. In C. J. Patterson & A. R. D'Augelli (Eds.), *Lesbian, gay, and bisexual identities in families: Psychological perspectives*. New York: Oxford University Press.

Savin-Williams, R. C. (2001). Suicide attempts among sexual-minority youths: Population and measurement issues. *Journal of Consulting and Clinical Psychology*, *69*(6), 983–991.

Savin-Williams, R. C. (2005). *The new gay teenager*. Cambridge, MA: Harvard University Press.

Savin-Williams, R. C., & Berndt, T. (1990). Friendship and peer relations. In S. Feldman & G. Elliott (Eds.), *At the threshold: The developing adolescent*. Cambridge, MA: Harvard University Press.

Savin-Williams, R. C., & Diamond, L. M. (2000). Sexual identity trajectories among sexual-minority youths: Gender comparisons. *Archives of Sexual Behavior*, *29*(6), 607–627.

Savin-Williams, R. C., & Dube, E. M. (1998). Parental reactions to their child's disclosure of a gay/lesbian identity. *Family Relations, 47,* 7–13.

Savin-Williams, R. C., & Ream, G. L. (2003). Suicide attempts among sexual-minority male youth. *Journal of Child and Adolescent Psychology, 32*(4), 509–522.

Scaramella, L. V., Conger, R. D., Spoth, R., & Simons, R. L. (2002). Evaluation of a social-contextual model of delinquency: A cross-study replication. *Child Development, 73*(1), 175–195.

Schwartz, R. C. (1987). Our multiple selves. *Family Therapy Networker, 11,* 25–31.

Schwartz, R. C. (1995). *Internal family systems therapy.* New York: Guilford Press.

Seccombe, K. (2000). Families in poverty in the 1990s: Trends, causes, consequences, and lessons learned. *Journal of Marriage and the Family, 62,* 1094–1113.

Seelig, W. R., Goldman-Hall, B. J., & Jerrell, J. M. (1992). In-home treatment of families of severely disturbed adolescents in crisis. *Family Process, 31,* 135–149.

Segal, Z., Williams, M., & Teasdale, J. (2002). *Mindfulness-based cognitive therapy for depression.* New York: Guilford Press.

Selman, R. (1980). *The growth of interpersonal understanding: Developmental and clinical analyses.* New York: Academic Press.

Selman, R. L., Brion-Meisels, S., & Wilkins, G. G. (1996). The meaning of relationship in residential treatment: A developmental perspective. In H. Rosen & K. T. Kuehlwein (Eds.), *Constructing realities: Meaning making perspectives for psychotherapists.* San Francisco: Jossey-Bass.

Selvini-Palazzoli, M. (1986). Towards a general model of psychotic games. *Journal of Marital and Family Therapy, 12,* 339–349.

Selvini-Palazzoli, M., Boscolo, L., Cecchin, G., & Prata, G. (1978). *Paradox and counterparadox.* New York: Aronson.

Selvini-Palazzoli, M., & Viaro, M. (1988). The anorectic process in the family: A six stage model as a guide for individual therapy. *Family Process, 27,* 129–148.

Sexton, T. L., & Alexander, J. F. (2002). Functional family therapy: An empirically supported, family-based intervention model for at-risk adolescents and their families. In F. W. Kaslow & T. Patterson (Eds.), *Comprehensive handbook of psychotherapy, Volume II: Cognitive-behavioral approaches.* New York: Wiley.

Sheeber, L., Hops, H., Alpert, A., Davis, B., & Andrews, J. (1997). Family support and conflict: Prospective relations to adolescent depression. *Journal of Abnormal Child Psychology, 25*(4), 333–344.

Sheeber, L., Hops, H., Andrews, J., Alpert, T., & Davis, B. (1998). Interactional processes in families with depressed and non-depressed adolescents: Reinforcement of depressive behavior. *Behaviour Research and Therapy, 36*, 417–427.

Sheeber, L., Hops, H., & Davis, B. (2001). Family processes in adolescent depression. *Clinical Child and Family Psychology Review, 4*(1), 19–35.

Sheeber, L., & Sorensen, E. (1998). Family relationships of depressed adolescents: A multimethod assessment. *Journal of Clinical Child Psychology, 27*(3), 268–277.

Sherman, R., & Fredman, N. (1986). *Handbook of structured techniques in marriage and family therapy.* New York: Brunner/Mazel.

Silbereisen, R., Petersen, A., Albrecht, H., & Kracke, B. (1989). Maturational timing and the development of problem behavior: Longitudinal studies in adolescence. *Journal of Early Adolescence, 9*, 247–268

Silverstein, O., & Rashbaum, B. (1994). *The courage to raise good men.* New York: Penguin.

Simmons, R., Burgeson, R., Carlton-Ford, S., & Blyth, D. A. (1987). The impact of cumulative change in early adolescence. *Child Development, 58*, 1220–1234.

Simmons, R., & Rosenberg, F. (1975). Sex, sex roles, and self image. *Journal of Youth and Adolescence, 4*, 229–258.

Simon, G. E. (2006). How can we know whether antidepressants increase suicidal risk? *American Journal of Psychiatry, 163*(11), 1861–1863.

Singer, M. T., Wynne, L. C., & Toohey, M. L. (1978). Communication disorders and the families of schizophrenics. In L. C. Wynne, R. L. Cromwell, & S. Matthysse (Eds.), *The nature of schizophrenia.* New York: Wiley.

Smetana, J. (1989). Adolescents' and parents' reasoning about actual family conflict. *Child Development, 59*, 1052–1067.

Smetana, J. G., & Turiel, E. (2003). Moral development during adolescence. In G. R. Adams & M. D. Berzonsky (Eds.), *Blackwell handbook of adolescence.* Malden, MA: Blackwell.

Smith, C., & Krohn, M. D. (1995). Delinquency and family life among male adolescents: The role of ethnicity. *Journal of Youth and Adolescence, 24*(1), 69–93.

Smolak, L., Levine, M., & Gralen, S. (1993). The impact of puberty and dating on eating problems among middle school girls. *Journal of Youth and Adolescence, 22*, 355–368.

Snyder, H. N., & Sickmund, M. (2006). *Juvenile offenders and victims: 2006 national report.* Pittsburgh, PA: National Center for Juvenile Justice.

Snyder, J., Dishion, T. J., & Patterson, G. R. (1986). Determinants and consequences of associating with deviant peers during preadolescence and adolescence. *Journal of Early Adolescence, 6*, 20–34.

Spencer, S. J., Steele, C. M., & Quinn, D. M. (1999). Stereotype threat and women's math performance. *Journal of Experimental Social Psychology*, *35*(1), 4–28.

Steele, C. M. (1997). A threat in the air: How stereotypes shape intellectual identity and performance. *American Psychologist*, *52*(6), 613–629.

Stein, J. H., & Reiser, L. W. (1994). A study of white middle class adolescent boys' responses to "semenarche" (the first ejaculation). *Journal of Youth and Adolescence*, *23*, 373–384.

Steinberg, L. (1987). The impact of puberty on family relations: Effects of pubertal status and pubertal timing. *Developmental Psychology*, *23*, 451–460.

Steinberg, L. (1996). *Adolescence* (4th ed.). New York: McGraw-Hill.

Steinberg, L. (2001). We know some things: Parent–adolescent relationships in retrospect and prospect. *Journal of Research on Adolescence*, *11*(1), 1–19.

Steinberg, L., Lamborn, S., Darling, N., Mounts, N., & Dornbusch, S. (1994). Over-time changes in adjustment and competence among adolescents from authoritative, authoritarian, indulgent, and neglectful families. *Child Development*, *65*, 754–770.

Steinberg, L., Lamborn, S., Dornbusch, S. M., & Darling, N. (1992). Impact of parenting practices on adolescent achievement: Authoritative parenting, school achievement, and encouragement to succeed. *Child Development*, *63*, 1266–1281.

Steinberg, L., & Silverberg, S. (1986). The vicissitudes of autonomy in early adolescence. *Child Development*, *57*, 841–851.

Steinberg, L., & Steinberg, W. (1994). *Crossing paths: How your child's adolescence triggers your own crisis*. New York: Simon & Schuster.

Steiner-Adair, C. (1990). The body politic: Normal female adolescent development and the development of eating disorders. In C. Gilligan, N. P. Lyons, & T. J. Hanmer (Eds.), *Making connections: The relational worlds of adolescent girls at Emma Willard School*. Cambridge, MA: Harvard University Press.

Stern, S., Whitaker, C. A., Hagemann, N. J., Anderson, R. B., & Bargman, G. J. (1981). Anorexia nervosa: The hospital's role in family treatment. *Family Process*, *20*, 395–408.

Stierlin, H. (1973). A family perspective on adolescent runaways. *Archives of General Psychiatry*, *29*, 56–62.

Stierlin, H., Levi, L. D., & Savard, R. L. (1971). Parental perceptions of separating children. *Family Process*, *10*, 411–427.

Surrey, J. L. (1991). Eating patterns as a reflection of women's development. In J. V. Jordan, A. G. Kaplan, J. B. Miller, I. P. Stiver, & J. L. Surrey (Eds.), *Women's growth in connection: Writings from the Stone Center*. New York: Guilford Press.

Swarr, A. E., & Richards, M. H. (1996). Longitudinal effects of adolescent girls' pubertal development, perceptions of pubertal timing, and parental relations on eating problems. *Developmental Psychology, 32,* 636–646.

Tannenbaum, L., & Forehand, R. (1994). Maternal depressive mood: The role of the father in preventing adolescent problem behaviors. *Behaviour Research and Therapy, 32,* 321–325.

Tanner, J. (1972). Sequence, tempo, and individual variation in growth and development of boys and girls aged twelve to sixteen. In J. Kagan & R. Coles (Eds.), *Twelve to sixteen: Early adolescence.* New York: Norton.

Tavantzis, T. N., Tavantzis, M., Brown, L. G., & Rohrbaugh, M. (1985). Home-based structural family therapy for delinquents at risk of placement. In M. P. Mirkin & S. L. Koman (Eds.), *Handbook of adolescents and family therapy.* New York: Gardner.

Taylor, R. D., Casten, R., Flickinger, S. M., Roberts, D., & Fulmore, C. D. (1994). Explaining the school performance of African American adolescents. *Journal of Research on Adolescence, 4*(1), 21–44.

Taylor, R. D., & Roberts, D. (1995). Kinship support and maternal and adolescent well-being in economically disadvantaged African-American families. *Child Development, 66*(6), 1585–1597.

Taylor, R. D., Seaton, E., & Dominguez, A. (2008). Kinship support, family relations, and psychological adjustment among low-income African American mothers and adolescents. *Journal of Research on Adolescence, 18*(1), 1–22.

Treboux, D., & Busch-Rossnagel, N. (1990). Social network influences on adolescent sexual attitudes and behaviors. *Journal of Adolescent Research, 5,* 175–189.

Vitaro, F., Brendgen, M., & Tremblay, R. E. (2000). Influence of deviant friends on delinquency: Searching for moderator variables. *Journal of Abnormal Child Psychology, 28*(4), 313–325.

Wadsworth, M., Raviv, T., Compas, B., & Connor-Smith, J. (2005). Parent and adolescent responses to poverty-related stress: Tests of mediated and moderated coping models. *Journal of Child and Family Studies, 14*(2), 283–298.

Waldrop, A. E., Hanson, R. F., Resnick, H. S., Kilpatrick, D. G., Naugle, A. E., & Saunders, B. E. (2007). Risk factors for suicidal behavior among a national sample of adolescents: Implications for prevention. *Journal of Traumatic Stress, 20*(5), 869–879.

Waller, J. V., Kaufman, M. R., & Deutsch, F. (1940). Anorexia nervosa: A psychosomatic entity. *Psychosomatic Medicine, 2,* 3–16.

Walsh, F. (2006). *Strengthening family resilience* (2nd ed.). New York: Guilford Press.

Weeks, G. R., & L'Abate, L. (1982). *Paradoxical psychotherapy: Theory and practice with individuals, couples, and families.* New York: Brunner/Mazel.

Wender, E. H. (1995). Attention-deficit hyperactivity disorders in adolescence. *Journal of Developmental and Behavioral Pediatrics, 16,* 192–195.

Whitaker, C. A. (1975). The symptomatic adolescent: An AWOL family member. In M. Sugar (Ed.), *The adolescent in group and family therapy.* New York: Brunner/Mazel.

White, M. (1983). Anorexia nervosa: A transgenerational system perspective. *Family Process, 22,* 255–273.

White, M. (1986). Negative explanation, restraint, and double description: A template for family therapy. *Family Process, 25,* 169–184.

White, M. (1987). Anorexia nervosa: A cybernetic perspective. In J. E. Harkaway (Ed.), *Eating disorders.* Rockville, MD: Aspen.

White, M. (1993). Deconstruction and therapy. In S. Gilligan & R. Price (Eds.), *Therapeutic conversations.* New York: Norton.

White, M., & Epston, D. (1990). *Narrative means to therapeutic ends.* New York: Norton.

Wilks, J. (1986). The relative importance of parents and friends in adolescent decision making. *Journal of Youth and Adolescence, 15*(4), 323–334.

Wilson, G. T., Grilo, C. M., & Vitousek, K. M. (2007). Psychological treatment of eating disorders. *American Psychologist, 62*(3), 199–216.

Winnicott, D. W. (1965). *The maturational process and the facilitating environment.* London: Hogarth Press.

Wolfradt, U., Hempel, S., & Miles, J. N. (2003). Perceived parenting styles, depersonalisation, anxiety and coping behaviour in adolescents. *Personality and Individual Differences, 34,* 521–532.

Wood, D., Flower, P., & Black, D. (1998). Should parents take charge of their child's eating disorder? Some preliminary findings and suggestions for future research. *International Journal of Psychiatry in Clinical Practice, 2*(4), 295–301.

Wood, M. D., Read, J. P., Mitchell, R. E., & Brand, N. H. (2004). Do parents still matter? Parent and peer influences on alcohol involvement among recent high school graduates. *Psychology of Addictive Behaviors, 18*(1), 19–30.

Wynne, L., Ryckoff, I., Day, J., & Hirsch, S. (1958). Pseudomutuality in the family relations of schizophrenics. *Psychiatry, 21,* 205–220.

Yasui, M., & Dishion, T. J. (2007). The ethnic context of child and adolescent problem behavior: Implications for child and family interventions. *Clinical Child and Family Psychology, 10*(2), 137–179.

Young, H., & Ferguson, L. (1979). Developmental changes through adolescence in the spontaneous nomination of reference groups as a function of decision context. *Journal of Youth and Adolescence, 8,* 239–252.

Young, S. (2000). ADHD children grown up: An empirical review. *Counselling Psychology Quarterly, 13*(2), 191–200.

Ziffer, R. L. (1985). The utilization of psychological testing in the context of family therapy. In R. L. Ziffer (Ed.), *Adjunctive techniques in family therapy*. New York: Grune & Stratton.

Zimmerman, P., & Becker-Stoll, F. (2002). Stability of attachment representations during adolescence: The influence of ego-identity status. *Journal of Adolescence, 25*(1), 107–124.

Index

Page numbers followed by an *f*, *n*, or *t* indicate figures, notes, or tables.

Abandonment, 69–70
  fear of, 189, 191–192, 197, 209, 215, 216
  fear of, case, 192–198
Abdication, parental, 265
Abdominal pain, 149–150
Abortion, 218
Abuse, physical, 276
Acceptance, 6, 8–9, 247, 328. *See also* ARCH
  conditional, 115, 138
Acculturation, 50–51, 312
Achievement, identity status, 47–51, 47*f*
  See also Identity
"Acting white," 274
"Acting out," *See* Defiance
ADHD, 219, 222, 271, 279, 281, 282, 293, 299
  subtypes of, 271–272
Adolescent problem behavior
  arrest rates, 220
  gender differences, 220
  prevalence, 220–221
  See also Defiance,
Adolescent development
  asynchronicity, 14–15
  autonomy and, 40–43
  brain development, 17–18
  cognitive changes, 19–23
  early years, 14, 16–29, 30*t*, 56–57
  gender-related expectations, 25–29
  hormones and, 17
  identity development, 45–51
  individual differences, 15

intimacy, 51–55
later years, 14, 45–56, 57*t*, 58, 296
leaving home, 55–56, 295–305
middle years, 14, 29–45, 46*t*, 57–58
moral reasoning, 38–40
peer relations, 23–25, 43–45, 54–55
pubertal changes, 16–19
sexuality, 29–38
Adolescence, early, 14, 16–29, 30*t*, 56–57
Adolescence, late, 14, 45–56, 57t, 58, 296
Adolescence, middle, 14, 29–45, 46*t*, 57–58
Adolescents
  as minority, 327
  engaging reluctant, 240–241
  individual therapy with, 246–248, 253–254, 323–328
Advocate, therapist as, 286
African American, 51, 220, 273, 274
Agoraphobia, 208
Alcohol, 218, 221, 225, 226*t*, 253
Alliance, therapeutic, 80–82, 142
Anderson, Carol, 257
Androgyny, 25
Anger, 95, 192, 196
  at parents, 237, 238, 247–248, 249–250, 251, 260, 276
  boys and, 29
  depression and, 162
  girls and, 27
  parental, 159, 169–170, 245, 248
  therapist, at parents, 168
Anorexia, 83, 97, 105, 108–145. *See also* Eating disorder

"Anti–Anorexia League," 115
Anxiety, 71, 137, 185–216, 293
  abandonment and, 191–198
  case examples, 190–191, 192–216
  cognitive behavioral therapy and,
    189–190
  cognitive factors and, 189–191
  disorders, 60
  family dynamics and, 186–189
  parental, 235, 236
Aponte, Harry, 270, 286, 309, 310
ARCH, 8, 247, 328
Arrest rates, 220
Asian families, parenting style, 43
Assessment
  defiant behavior, 226t
  depression, 150–151
  leaving home, 299–302
  school problems, 271–279
  suicide, 151
Assumptions, hidden, 96
Asynchronicity, 14–15
Attachment, 10, 24, 27, 37, 41, 116, 179,
  192
  defiant behavior and, 223–224, 232,
    234, 247, 249
  family dynamics, 53
  parents, 51–54, 126
  patterns, 52
  peers, 53
  strengthening, 249
  symptoms and, 53
  theory, 3, 10, 52–53
"Attack/defend cycle," 93
Attention-deficit/hyperactivity disorder, See
  ADHD
Authoritarian parenting, See Parenting,
  authoritarian
Authoritative parenting, See Parenting,
  authoritative
Autonomy, 6, 9, 13, 14, 21, 40–43, 46t,
  52, 58, 66, 92, 110, 111, 113, 116,
  121, 133, 158, 160, 225, 228, 234,
  236, 247, 284, 299, 310

B

Bateson, Gregory, 256
Beliefs, about problem, 245–246
Biased perceptions, See Complementary
  biased perceptions
Biology, 5, 6, 16, 17–18, 60
  psychosis and, 256–257
Bipolar disorder, 60, 151, 222, 257, 258,
  260–261

Bisexual adolescents, See GLBT
  adolescents
Blos, Peter, 12, 52
Boszormenyi–Nagy, Ivan, 4, 298
Bowen, Murray, 256
Bowlby, John, 3, 7, 52–53
"Boy Code," 27–29
Boys, adolescent
  aggression in, 251
  androgyny in, 25
  anger in, 29
  anxiety in, 188–189
  arrest rates, 220
  coping with stress, 148
  depression in, 147
  deviant peers and, 53
  early-maturing, 18
  eating disorders and, 109–110
  independence, emphasis on, 10, 28, 296
  intimacy expression, 48, 54–55, 57t
  moral development in, 38
  pubertal development, 16
  same–sex attractions, 31–38
  self-esteem in, 26
  shame in, 29
  socialization pressures on, 27–29,
    274–275
  suicide in, 148
  testosterone in, 17
  working with, 28–29
Bruch, Hilde, 110–111
Bulimia, 105, 155. See also Eating disorder

C

Carter, Betty, 66, 175, 295
Catalytic community partnerships, 318
Causality, circular, 91
CBT, See Cognitive-behavioral therapy
Centrifugal families, 299
Centripetal families, 299
Change, 78, 92
  eliciting, 93–94
Child protection worker, 306–308, 315,
  316, 318, 319, 320, 321
Child Protection, Department of, 306, 316,
  321
Circular causality, See Causality, circular
Coaching strategy, 280–283, 281f, 294
  adolescent, 132, 280–281
  parents, 56, 281–283
  pitfalls of, 283
Coalition, 98, 101, 105, 122, 142, 149,
  260, 288, 290, 291, 293, 314, 316,
  324

Cocaine, 221
Cognitive-behavioral therapy, 4, 61, 92, 151–152, 153, 272
  anxiety and, 189–190
Colapinto, Jorge, 275, 315
Colitis, 119
Communication, facilitating, 45, 94–95, 106, 256
Communication deviance, psychosis, 256
Community resources, 317–318
Competence, eliciting, 130–131
Complementarity, 3, 60, 91, 98, 106, 122, 292, 313
  defined, 92
  working with, 92–94
Complementary biased perceptions, 67, 72, 79, 94, 96, 97
  eating disorders and, 121, 122f
Compulsive rituals, 185
  case example, 192–198
Conditional acceptance, 115, 138
Confidentiality, 101–102, 240
Conflict
  adolescent and parents, 17, 90
  family, 95
  interpersonal, 22–23
Conflict avoidance, 7, 35, 68, 283, 291
  bickering and, 142
  eating disorders and, 113, 120, 123, 127–129, 142
Conflict resolution, 22–23, 231
Consequences, choosing appropriate, 244
Constriction, 64, 70–71, 243, 255, 303
Consultation
  benefits and risks, 105–106
  schools with, 292–293
  "Contaminating the suicidal fantasy," 169
Content (vs. process), 76
Contextual therapy, 4
Control, 6, 78, 92, 116, 121, 137, 177, 179, 188, 189, 224, 227, 232, 233–234, 235, 242, 243, 246, 253, 255
Court, 240
Coyne, James, 156, 159
Crisp, Arthur, 110
Criticism, parental, 60, 244, 257
  eating disorders and, 133, 142–143
Crohn's disease, 119
Cultural factors
  development and, 15
  ethnic identity development, 50–51
  leaving home and, 296

low-income families, 312–313
  motivation and, 273
"Culture of thinness," 112
Curfew violations, 229, 234–235
Curiosity, 8–9, 247, 328. See also ARCH Cycle
Cycle
  attack/defend, 93
  pursuit/withdraw, 93
  symptomatic, See Symptomatic cycle

D

Defiance, 217–254, 255, 261
  assessing severity, 225–226
  attachment and, 223–224, 232, 247
  family sessions and, 248–252
  individual sessions and, 246–248
  mild, 228–232
  moderate, 232–237
  parents and, 223–225
  peers and, 222–223, 225
  severe, 238–253
  symptomatic cycle, 224–229, 225, 229–230, 236, 253
  See also Adolescent problem behavior
Delinquency, 220, 252, 298. See also Adolescent problem behavior; Defiance
Depression
  abandonment and, 154–156
  assessment of, 150–151
  biological factors, 151
  cognitive behavioral therapy, 151–152, 153
  family dynamics in, 153–162
  family patterns, 154–162
  gender differences, 147–148
  grief and, 154
  homeostasis and, 159–162
  interactional model, 156, 159
  interpersonal therapy, 152
  maternal, and eating disorders, 143–144
  medications, 152
  mindfulness and, 152
  overprotectiveness and, 156–159
  parental, 143–144, 302
  prevalence, 147
  suicide, 162–172
    case example, 172–183
Detachment, 51
Detouring, 113, 270
Development
  arrested, 64–66
  family, 104–105
  male, 10

Development (*continued*)
  parental, 15
  supporting, 136–139
  symptomatic cycle and, 136
  See also Adolescent development
Developmental trajectory, 15
Diagnosis, dangers of, 4, 175
Diathesis–stress model, 257
Diffusion, identity status, 47–51, 47*f*
Direct intervention strategy, 281*f*,
      286–291, 294
  advantages of, 287
  case example, 288–291
  pitfalls of, 287–288
Disagreeable versus destructive behavior,
      243–244
Disengagement, 69–70, 72, 147, 163, 283,
      291
  depression and, 154–156
Disruptive behavior, *See* Defiance
Divorced parents, 218, 303–304
  working with, 108–141, 190
Double bind, 180
  psychosis and, 256
DSM-IV-TR, 4, 271
Dualistic thinking, 77, 245
"Dysfunctional," 4–5

E

Eating disorder, 18, 88–89, 108–145, 255
  autonomy and, 111
  Bruch, Hilde, on, 110–111
  collaboration, parental, 125–126
  Crisp, Arthur, on, 110
  criticism, parental and, 133, 142–143
  family systems perspectives, 113–115
  family therapy efficacy, 115
  father–daughter relationship, 111–112
  feminist perspectives, 111
  hospitalization, 110
  incidence of, 109
  males, 109–110
  maternal depression and, 143–144
  Maudsley Model, 110, 123
  medical backup, 119
  Milan School on, 113–114
  Minuchin, Salvador, on, 110, 113, 115,
      129
  narrative model, 114–115
  pitfalls, 141–144
  psychodynamic, 110
  redefining the problem, 120, 123
  relapses, handling, 132–136
  sexuality and, 110, 116
      sociocultural perspectives, 112
      supporting individual development,
        136–139
      supporting transformation, 139–141
      target weight, 125–127
      treatment contract, 120, 121–124
      treatment principles, 115–121
      treatment, steps, 119–121
      unresolved conflicts and, 127–131
Eccles, Jacquelynne, 24, 40, 42, 273
Eclecticism, 2
Ecostructural approach, 286
Ecosystem, 270, 275
Egocentricism, adolescent, 20–21, 30*t*
Ejaculation, initial, 16
Elkind, David, 20, 221
Emotionally focused therapy, 3, 95
Emotions
  "softer," 91, 95, 234, 247, 249, 254
  working with, 95–96
Empathy, 10, 90, 142, 184, 197, 202, 247,
      267
"Empirically supported therapy," 153, 189
Empowering parents, 242, 314–315
Enactment, 3, 67, 85–87, 141
  carrying out, 85–87
Engagement, promoting, 79–80
"Enhanced home–school partnership,"
      286–287
Enmeshment, 113, 115, 117, 213
Eno, Mary, 281–282, 286
Epston, David, 97, 115
Erikson, Erik, 45–48, 54
Escalation, 70
Ethnicity, 15, 296. *See also* Cultural factors
"Evolving Self," 43–45
Expectations, parental, 299–300
Expressed emotion, high, 60–61, 257
"Externalizing the problem," 96–97,
      114–115, 123, 142, 143, 197

F

Families of the Slums, 309
Family game, 256
Family life cycle, 104, 295
Family sessions
  defiance, in, 248–252
  whom to include, 81–82
Family systems, ix, x, 2–4, 6, 60–62, 71,
      77, 112–115
Family therapy, x, 3–4, 5, 7, 45, 60–62,
      66, 85, 99, 101, 115, 119–120, 143,
      144, 146, 153, 190, 256, 258, 270,
      275, 297, 309

Father, adolescent relationship with, 28, 111, 175, 251
Feminism, 10, 54, 111–112, 313
Fighting, adolescent, 22, 269, 270, 288, 290
First session, conducting, 80–82
Fishman, Charles, 3, 64, 163, 286–287
Focus, therapeutic, 74–77
Foreclosure, identity status, 47–51, 47f, 300
Formal operations, 19
Formulation of problem, 88
Foster parents, 308
Frame, bidirectional, 240

G

Gang membership, 220
Gay adolescents, See GLBT adolescents
Gender, 15
  depression, role in, 147–149
  identity, 31
  role intensification, 25, 30t, 57
  role pressures, boys, 27–29
  role pressures, girls, 26–27
  role pressures, school achievement, 274–275
Girls, adolescent
  anger in, 26–27, 147
  anxiety in, 188
  appearance concerns, 18, 147
  arrest rates, 218, 221
  coping with stress, 26–27, 148
  depression, 26, 147–148
  early-maturing, 33, 221
  eating disorders and, 18, 109–112
  identity development, 54
  intimacy expression, 54–55, 57t
  gender role pressures, 26–27
  loss of voice, 26, 111, 148
  moral development in, 38
  poor interoceptive awareness, 111
  same-sex attractions, 31–38
  self-esteem, 26
  stereotype threat in, 273
  sexual harrassment of, 274
  working with, 26–27
GLBT adolescents, 31–38, 149–150
  disclosure to others, 34, 36–37
  family issues, 35–36
  identity development, 32–34
  mood disorder, 37
  romantic relationships, 55
  self esteem, 34

  suicide risk, 37
  working with, 36–38
Goal setting
  low-income families, 314–315
  therapy, 74–77, 87–89
Goldstein, Michael, 258
"Good enough" parent, 10
Grounding, 244
Growth spurt, 16
GSA (gay–straight alliance), 38
Guilt, 112, 133, 276, 299
  value of, 234

H

Haley, Jay, 3, 80, 256, 265
  leaving home on, 297
Hall, G. Stanley, 12
Hallucinogens, 217, 221
Harassment, of adolescent, 31, 274, 283
Heterosexism, 36
Hierarchy, parental, 225–226, 228, 231, 241–242
"Holding environment," 114, 169, 172
Holistic perspective, 6
Home-based services, 315
Home visit, 319–320
Homeostasis, 75, 153, 187
  depression and, 159–162
  eating disorders and, 113
Homework problems, 275–277
  case example, 282–283
Homosexuality, ego-dystonic, 32
Honesty, 8–9, 247, 277, 328. See also ARCH
Hormones, 17, 221
Hospitalization
  averting, 265
  eating disorders and, 110
  suicide and, 164
Humor, use in therapy, 93

I

Idealization, of parents, 21
Identity
  crisis, 45, 49–50
  gender, 31
  sexual, 31, 37
Identity development, 45–51, 57t
  aspects of, 48–49
  family and, 48–49
  gender differences, 48
  GLBT adolescents, 32–34
  racial/ethnic, 50–51
  statuses, 47–51, 47f

Illness, parental, 276, 301
Imagery, 197
Imaginary audience, 20–21
Imber-Black, Evan, 270, 316
Imperial stage, 44
Impulse control, 18
    problems with, 222, 271
Impulsive stage, 44
Incorporative stage, 44
Individual differences, 15
Individual sessions, 101–105
    adolescent, 101–105, 246–248,
        253–254, 323–328
    confidentiality issues, 101–102
    early in treatment, 102–103
    eating disorder, 143
    family sessions, versus, 7
    late in treatment, 104–105
    middle phase of treatment, 103–104
Individuation, 295, 298
Induction, 76
Informed consent, 292
Institutional stage, 44
"Internal working models," 52
Interpersonal stage, 44, 222
Interpersonal therapy, 61, 152
Intervention, general principles, 74–80,
    106
Intimacy, 51–55, 57t
    gender differences, 54–55, 57t
    peers, with, 54–55
    parents, with, 51–54
"Invariant prescription," 256
Invulnerability (personal fable), 20–21, 30t
Ipecac, 84, 109, 118
Isolation
    parental, 245, 264
    psychosis and, 255, 258–261
Isomorphism, 270, 289, 291–292

J

Jackson, Don, 256
Johnson, Susan, 3, 95, 249
Joining, 3, 8, 80–82, 101, 102, 157, 311

K

Kegan, Robert, 43–45, 222
Kin network, 317–318
Kohlberg, Lawrence, 38–40, 221

L

"Launching phase," 296–297
"Laziness," 275

Learning disability, 48, 222, 271–272, 279,
    281, 282, 293, 299, 300
Leaving home, problems with, 55–56, 58,
    232, 295–305
    assessing the family, 301–302
    assessing the youth, 299–300
    cultural factors, 296
    framing the problem, 302–303
    interventions, 302–304
    perspectives on, 297–299
Lesbian adolescents, See GLBT adolescents
Liddle, Howard, 249
Lidz, Theodore, 256
Listening, active, 91
Loss of voice, 26, 111, 148
Low-income families,
    Aponte, Harry, on, 309
    characteristics of successful, 310
    power dynamics in, 313–314
    social agencies impact on, 315–316
    working with, 310–318
Lunch session, 141
Lusterman, Don David, 283–285
Lying, 92–93, 247

M

Macrosystem, 270, 280
Madanes, Cloe, 167, 297–298
"Male relational dread," 181
"Mapping the influence of the problem,"
    114
Marcia, James, 47–51, 47f
Marijuana, 217, 218, 221, 225, 250,
    324
Marital problems, parental, 19, 75, 143–
    144, 149, 154, 228, 246, 297, 302
"Marital schism," 256
"Marital skew," 256
Marital therapy, 302
Masculinity, 10, 25, 28, 29, 251, 275
Maudsley Model, 110, 123
McGoldrick, Monica, 66, 295, 296, 313
Mediation strategy, 283–286, 281f, 294
    case example, 284–285
    pitfalls of, 286
Medications, 5, 61, 105, 152, 156, 219,
    258, 272, 299
Menarche, 16
Metacognition, 19
Methylphenidate, 219, 272
Midlife crisis, parental, 15
Milan School, on eating disorders,
    113–114
Military school, 217, 250

Mindfulness, 4, 152
Minuchin, Salvador, 3, 8, 64, 77, 79, 80, 85, 97, 110, 113, 115, 120, 129, 141, 309, 310
MMPI, 139
Models of therapy
 Cognitive-behavioral, 4, 61, 92, 115, 152–153, 189–191, 272
 contextual, 4
 emotionally focused, 3
Milan School, 113
 narrative, 3, 96–97, 114–115, 123, 211, 298, 311
 psychodynamic, 3, 110–111, 114, 255–256
 strategic, 3
 structural family therapy, 3, 115, 309
Monitoring, parental, 143
Mood disorder, *See* Bipolar disorder; Depression
Moodiness, 17
Moral decisions, 38–40, 46*t*
Morality (vs. convention), 40
Moratorium (identity status), 47–51, 46*t*, 47*f*, 300
Motivation
 achievement, role in, 272–273
 cultural factors, 273
 intrinsic, 272
Mourning, in leaving home, 303–304
Multicultural competence, 312–313
"Multifaceted self," 64, 152
Multiple problems, families with, 306–322
 case example, 306–308, 318–321
"Multiple selves," 105
"Multiple voices," 105, 137–139

N

Narrative(s)
 family, 79, 80, 83, 96–97, 311–312
 model, 114, 123
 mutually reinforcing, 66–67
 "problem saturated," 96, 311
 therapy, 3, 96–97
"Narrative of failure," 298
Neglect, parental, 48, 278, 309, 315
Nichols, Michael, 3, 91, 129
Nocturnal emission, 16
Nurturance, 3, 9–10, 13, 41, 245, 249, 253

O

"Other-transforming" strategy, 23
Overprotectiveness, 64, 69, 72, 93
 anxiety and, 188, 190, 199, 200, 204, 215, 216
 eating disorders and, 113, 134
 depression and, 61, 156–159
 leaving home problems and, 296, 300

P

Panic attacks, 300
Papp, Peggy, 113
Paradoxical tasks, 99–100, 113
Parent sessions,
 defiance, 241–246
 eating disorder, 143
Parental monitoring, 31, 223, 310
"Parent–child role reversal," 162
Parentification, 167–168, 192
Parenting
 authoritarian, 40, 41–43, 189, 274, 276, 291–292
 authoritative, 41–43, 274
 indifferent, 41
 indulgent, 41
 reciprocal influence, 42
 role of culture, 42
 styles, 41–43
Parents
 attachment to, 51–54
 conflict with, 17
 defiant behavior and, 223–225
 sessions with, 238, 241–246, 253–254
Patterns
 linking problem to, 88–89
 techniques for changing, 89–100, 106–107
"Peer cluster theory," 24
Peers
 conformity to, 24, 40, 57
 defiant behavior and, 222–223, 225
 deviant, 24, 222–223, 233, 252, 253
 differentiation from, 44, 46*t*
 group composition, 43
 identity development and, 24
 importance of, 23, 30*t*
 intimacy with, 54–55
 moral decisions and, 39
 orientation towards, 40–41, 46*t*
 peers, identification with, 23–24
 pressure, 24
 selection, 24
 sexuality and, 30

Peers (*continued*)
  socialization, 24
  underachievement and, 274–275
"Personal fable," 22–23, 221
Perspective taking, 256
PFLAG, 35
Piaget, Jean, 19, 38, 44
Pipher, Mary, 18, 26, 148, 274
Police, parents calling, 236, 343
Pollack, William, 10, 25, 28–29, 275
"Poor interoceptive awareness," 111
Posttraumatic symptoms, 188
Poverty, 278
  delinquency and, 220
  effects on children, 308–309
  See also Low-income families
Power dynamics, in families, 313–314,
  321
Power struggle, 227, 233, 235, 276, 303
Preganancy, adolescent, 218
Problem behavior, *See* Adolescent problem
  behavior
Problem, history of, 84–85
  process (vs. content), 76
Progressive relaxation, 197
Projection, 181–183, 298
Projective identification, 298
Prosocial behavior, 221
"Pseudomutuality," 252
Psychiatrist, 5, 105, 267
Psychodynamic theory, 3
  eating disorders and, 110–112
  psychosis and, 255–256
Psychoeducational evaluation, 271, 272,
  279, 293
Psychoeducational model, 138–139, 257
Psychological testing, 105, 138–139, 271,
  272, 279, 306
Psychosis, 5, 222, 255–268, 298
  biology and, 256–257
  diathesis–stress model , 257
  family dynamics, 255–256, 267
  high expressed emotion and, 257
  integrated approach, 258
  isolation and, 255, 258–262
  psychoeducational model and, 257–258
  rediscovering voice and, 261–263
  symptomatic cycle and, 259
  treatment team collaboration, 266–267
Puberty, 16–19, 30t, 221
  eating disorder and, 116
  family relationships and, 19
  psychological impact of, 18
  timing, 16

Punctuation, 98
Pursuit–withdraw cycle, 93

R

Rashbaum, Beth, 10, 28, 147, 148, 252,
  275, 296
"Reauthoring," 114
Redefining problem, eating disorder, 120,
  123
Referrals, by school, 278, 292–293
Reframing, 67, 87–88, 143, 169, 285
Relapses, eating disorder, 132–136
Relational aggression, 148
Relationships
  power of, 7–8
  romantic, 54–55, 57t
Resistance, 74, 99, 103, 278, 316
Resources, community, 317–318, 322
Respect, 8–9, 142, 247, 328. *See also*
  ARCH
Rigidity, in eating disorder, 113
Risk taking, 21
"Ritual of leave taking," 304
Rorschach test, 139
Rules and consequences, 238–244

S

Sargent, John, 53, 63, 115, 127, 165
Scapegoating, 291, 292
Schizophrenia, 5, 60, 146, 175, 256, 258.
  See also Psychosis
"Schizophrenogenic mother," 256
School, 320
  conferences, 270, 283, 286, 288–291
  counselor, 270, 278, 281, 282, 285,
    289, 290
  environment, and underachievement,
    273–274
  intervention strategies, 279–291
  problems related to, 269–294
  referrals from, 278, 292–293
  refusal (case), 160–162
  suspension, 269, 284, 306
  therapist as consultant, 292–293
Schwartz, Richard, 105, 137
Second class citizen, adolescent as, 327
Secrets, family, 101–102
"Secure base," 7
Self-esteem, 26, 34, 56, 60, 168
"Self, evolving," 43–45
Self-fulfilling prophecy, 13, 79, 273
Self, multifaceted, 64, 152
Self-soothing, 197

"Self-transforming" strategy, 23
Selman, Robert, 22–23, 221
Selvini-Palazzoli, Mara, 256
"Separate realities," 21
Sexual behavior, adolescent
  consequences of, 29–30
  prevalence, 29
  peer influence on, 30
  promiscuous, 226
Sexual harrassment, 274
Sexual identity, 31, 36, 37
  fluidity of, 33
Sexually transmitted disease (STD),
  218
Sexual minority, 31
Sexual orientation, 15, 31
Sexuality, adolescent, 29–38, 46t, 236
  eating disorder and, 110, 116
Shame, in boys, 29
Silverstein, Olga, 10, 28, 147, 148, 252,
  275, 296
"Simulated families," x
Single parent, 258, 311, 316
Sleep phase shift, 18
Smoking, 227
Social agencies, and low-income families,
  310, 315–317
Socialization, 274
Socioeconomic status, 15
"Softening," 249
Stealing, 217, 220, 226, 236, 243
Stereotype threat, 273
Stierlin, Heim, 298
Stonewalling, 240
"Storm and stress," 12, 56
Strategic therapy, 3
Strengths, family, 78, 82, 96, 129, 253,
  311, 321
"Stroke and kick," 79
Structural family therapy, 3, 115, 309
Substance abuse, 39, 221, 222
Suicide, 148, 298
  assessment of, 151
  case example, 146, 172–183
  ensuring safety, 163–164
  family factors, 162–163
  GLBT youth, 37
  incidence of, 162
  interventions, 162–172
  motives for, 163
  parentification and, 167–168
  pitfalls and complications, 168–172
  promoting dialogue, 164–167
  watch, 163–164

Supersystem, 316
Surrey, Janet, 111
Suspension, school, 269, 284, 306
Symptomatic cycle, ix, x, 3, 7, 53, 74, 78,
  82, 91, 92, 97, 101, 103, 104
  arrested development and, 64–65, 136
  common patterns, 68–72
  consequences of, 64–68
  constriction and, 64
  defiance and, 224–225, 229–230, 229f,
    236, 253
  described, 62–64
  disrupting, 65f, 89–100
  eating disorder and, 116–119, 118f,
    136, 137, 139
  identifying, 82–87
  illustrations of, 63f, 118f, 224f, 229f,
    259
  multifaceted self and, 64
  mutually reinforcing narratives and,
    6–7, 122
  psychosis and, 258–259
Systems, family, See Family systems
Systems, teaching families about, 91

T

Tasks, as interventions
  assigning, 98–100, 138–139
  paradoxical, when to use, 99–100
TAT (Thematic Apperception Test),
  139
Teaching interventions
  skills, 91–92
  systems principles, 91
Team, treatment, 266
Technique
  assumptions, challenging, 96
  communication, encouraging, 94–95
  competence, eliciting, 130–131,
    311–312
  complementarity, working with, 92–94.
    See also Complementarity
  "contaminating suicidal fantasy," 169
  enactment, 67, 85–87, 141
  engagement, promoting, 79–80
  externalizing the problem, 96–97,
    114–115, 123, 142, 197
  humor, use of, 93
  joining, 8, 80, 102–103, 157, 311
  listening, active, 91
  lunch session, 141
  mindfulness, 4, 152
  multiple voices, listening to, 105,
    137–139

Technique (*continued*)
  punctuation, 98
  reframing, 67, 87–88, 143, 169, 285
  strengths, acknowledging, 82
  "stroke and kick," 79
  tasks, assigning, 98–100
  teaching about systems, 91
  teaching skills, 91
  theory, versus, 2
  tracking, 81, 84, 122
  unbalancing, 97–98
  "wiping the slate clean," 342
"Tell me/don't tell me bind," 69, 70, 117, 119, 128–129, 165, 170, 173, 183
Testing, psychological, *See* Psychological testing
Testosterone, 17
Thematic Apperception Test (TAT), 139
Theories of therapy, *See* Models of therapy
Tracking, 81, 84, 122
Transgendered youth, 31
Transitions, developmental, 231, 253, 295, 299
Trauma, 6, 188
Treatment contract
  developing, 87–89
  eating disorder, 120, 121–124
Triangulation, 19, 84, 105, 133, 156, 266, 268, 294
  consultants and, 105–106
  eating disorder and, 113
  identifying and avoiding, 291–293

U

Unbalancing, 97–98
Underachievement, 269–294
  factors contributing to, 271–279
  family dynamics and, 275–277
  family–school relationship and, 277–297
  motivation and, 272–273
  peer influence on, 274–275
  school environment, 273–274
  See also School, problems related to
Undermining, 83, 121, 141–142, 229, 246, 256, 259, 266, 267, 274, 298
  parents and schools, 277–278
Underorganization, in low-income families, 309
"Undifferentiated ego mass," 256
"Unique outcomes," 79–80, 97, 114

V

Values, 21
Vandalism, 220
Violence, 29, 225–226, 236, 253, 253

W

Weakland, John, 3, 84, 256
Whitaker, Carl, 114, 298
White, Michael, 67, 79, 97, 114
Wiltwyck School for Boys, 309
"Wiping the slate clean," 242
Worries, obsessive, 100
Wynne, Lyman, 256